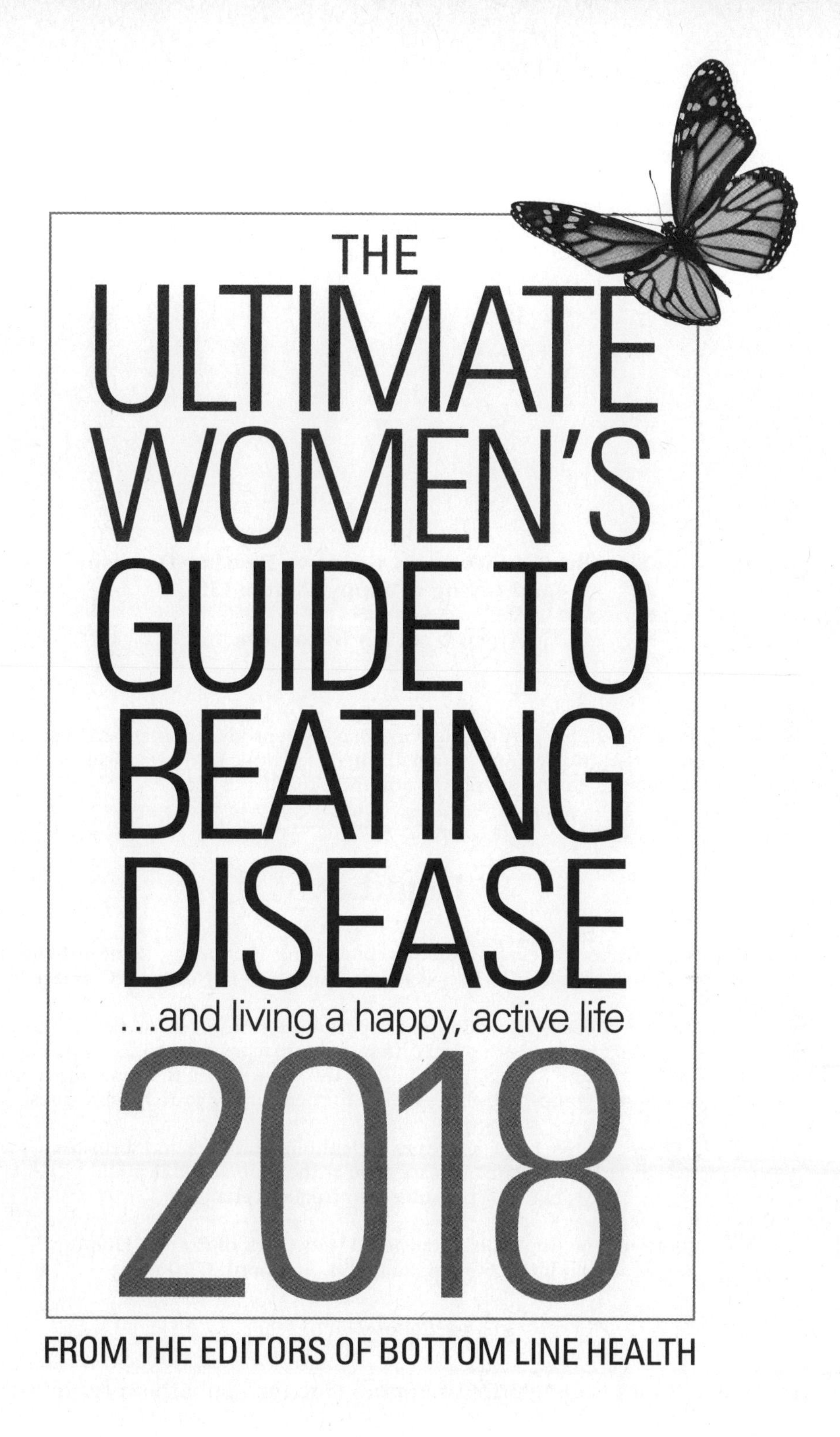

# THE ULTIMATE WOMEN'S GUIDE TO BEATING DISEASE

...and living a happy, active life

# 2018

FROM THE EDITORS OF BOTTOM LINE HEALTH

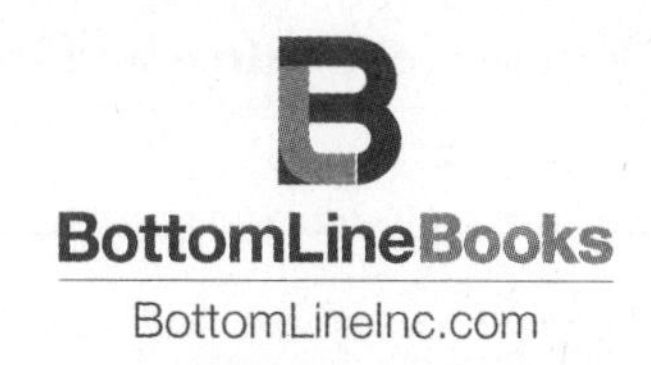

**The Ultimate Women's Guide to Beating Disease and Living a Happy, Active Life**



10 9 8 7 6 5 4 3 2 1



ISBN 0-88723-777-0

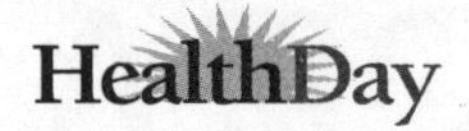


A selection of articles in this book were written by reporters for HealthDay, an award-winning international daily consumer health news service, headquartered in Norwalk, Connecticut.

Bottom Line Books® publishes the advice of expert authorities in many fields. These opinions may at times conflict as there are often different approaches to solving problems. The use of a book is not a substitute for legal, accounting, investment, health or any other professional services. Consult competent professionals for answers to your specific questions.

Offers, prices, rates, addresses, telephone numbers and websites listed in this book are accurate at the time of publication, but they are subject to frequent change.

Bottom Line Books® is a registered trademark of Bottom Line Inc.
3 Landmark Square, Suite 201, Stamford, CT 06901

*www.BottomLineInc.com*

---

Bottom Line Books is an imprint of Bottom Line Inc., publisher of print periodicals, e-letters and books. We are dedicated to bringing you the best information from the most knowledgeable sources in the world. Our goal is to help you gain greater wealth, better health, more wisdom, extra time and increased happiness.

---

Printed in the United States of America

# CONTENTS

## 2 • CANCER BREAKTHROUGHS



## 3 • LUNG HEALTH AND ALLERGIES



## 4 • STROKE RISKS, SYMPTOMS AND HELP WITH RECOVERY

### 11 • EMOTIONAL RESCUE



## APPENDICES

### APPENDIX 1: DIET, NUTRITION AND FITNESS

**APPENDIX 2: OPTIMUM AGING**



**APPENDIX 3: VERY PERSONAL**

# PREFACE

We are proud to bring to you *The Ultimate Women's Guide to Beating Disease and Living a Happy, Active Life 2018*. This essential volume features trustworthy and actionable life-saving information from the best health experts in the world—information that will help women beat the conditions that are most deadly to them.* In the following chapters, you'll find the latest discoveries, best treatments and scientifically proven remedies to keep you living a long, happy and active life.

Whether it's heart care, the latest on stroke, breast cancer prevention and treatment, breakthrough treatments for hot flashes or cutting-edge nutritional advice, the editors of *Bottom Line Health* talk to the experts—from top women's health doctors to research scientists to leading alternative care practitioners—who are creating the true innovations in health care.

In this 2018 edition, we've gone beyond diseases and have included two chapters and an appendix of life-enhancing health information on pain, depression, fitness, diet, quality medical care, sexuality and aging...all of which are essential to living a happy, active life. And it's all backed by breaking studies and top health experts. Also note that respiratory diseases, according to the Centers for Disease Control and Prevention, are now considered one of the top three causes of death in women of all ages (same percentage as stroke).

Over the past four decades, we have built a network of literally thousands of leading physicians in both alternative and conventional medicine. They are affiliated with the premier medical and research institutions throughout the world. We read the important medical journals and follow the latest research that is reported at medical conferences. And we regularly talk to our advisors in major teaching hospitals, private practices and government health agencies for their insider perspective.

*The Ultimate Women's Guide to Beating Disease and Living a Happy, Active Life 2018* is a result of our ongoing research and connection with these experts, and is a distillation of their latest findings and advice. We trust that you will glean new, helpful and affordable information about the health topics that concern you most...and find vital topics of interest to family and friends as well.

As a reader of a Bottom Line book, please be assured that you are receiving well-researched information from a trusted source. But, please use prudence in health matters. Always speak to your physician before taking vitamins, supplements or over-the-counter medication...stopping a medication...changing your diet...or beginning an exercise program. If you experience side effects from any regimen, contact your doctor immediately.

Be well,
The Editors, *Bottom Line Health*
Stamford, Connecticut

*"Leading Causes of Death in Females," Centers for Disease Control and Prevention (*http://www.cdc.gov/women/lcod/2014/index.htm*).

# Chapter 1

# HEART HEALTH FOR WOMEN

## Heart Disease Risk Factors Doctors Miss Most in Women

We've all seen this acted out... a man clutches his chest, showing intense pain and collapses on the floor—heart attack. It's usually the first symptom of heart disease in these movie scenes.

You probably think women are different, right? That's been the "new" story in the last several years—that women have very different symptoms from men, often not experiencing the classic chest pains but more often complaining of nausea or back pain or extreme fatigue.

It turns out that almost everything we think we know about women and heart disease symptoms is wrong. That's the finding of a major recent study of gender differences in heart disease.

When it comes to heart disease, women are indeed very different from men—even chest pain symptoms are subtly different. Plus, doctors often miss important risk factors in women—or order the wrong diagnostic tests.

### A Real-World Look into Women's Hearts

"Every aspect of the evaluation for heart disease seems to differ between men and women, whether looking at risk factor profile, risk scores, symptoms, the tests that doctors selected and the test results," says Pamela Douglas, MD, Ursula Geller Professor for Research in Cardiovascular Disease at Duke University School of Medicine, and leader of the study team.

While most studies have looked at how to evaluate patients who show up in the ER with a suspected heart attack, we know very little about everyday patients who go to their regular doctors with symptoms that may be a sign of heart disease. So Dr. Douglas's team analyzed data from the PROMISE (Prospective Multicenter Imaging Study for Evaluation of Chest Pain) trial, which evaluated about

---

Pamela Douglas, MD, Ursula Geller Professor for Research in Cardiovascular Disease, Duke University School of Medicine. Dr. Douglas is internationally known for her scientific work in noninvasive imaging, exercise physiology, and heart disease in women.

Study titled, "Sex Differences in Demographics, Risk Factors, Presentation, and Noninvasive Testing in Stable Outpatients With Suspected Coronary Artery Disease," by Pamela Douglas, MD, and colleagues, published in *Journal of the American College of Cardiology Imaging.*

10,000 patients with suspected coronary artery disease (CAD)—the most common kind—who were seen in outpatient settings. The average age of women was 62 (for men it was 59).

The differences were so big that Dr. Douglas, along with other experts, believes that there should be unique prevention and diagnostic guidelines just for women. Her team's research is supporting that aim and has already uncovered some key differences that all women should know about to protect their hearts—now. *Here's what they found...*

## Similar Symptoms

Chest pain was the number-one complaint: Nearly 75% of men and women who went to their primary care doctors to be evaluated for heart disease showed up because they had chest pain. However, there were subtle differences in the types of pain. Women were more likely to experience squeezing or crushing chest pain, while men were more likely to experience aching, dull or burning chest pain.

Both men and women were equally unlikely to complain of less classic symptoms—about 16% of both men and women went to the doctor because they were experiencing shortness of breath, for example. There were some differences in more minor symptoms, but these only brought patients to their doctors less than 4% of the time—women complained of back, neck or jaw pain and palpitations, whereas men complained of fatigue or weakness.

***Bottom line:*** When it comes to heart disease symptoms, both men and women should pay attention to chest pain and, to a lesser extent, shortness of breath. Women don't need to worry so much about unusual symptoms like fatigue or nausea.

## Risk Factors: A Lost Prevention Opportunity

When women went to the doctor for suspected heart problems, they had a higher prevalence of risk factors for heart disease than men. They were more likely to have hypertension, high cholesterol, vascular disease and a family history of premature CAD, and about as likely to have diabetes. They were also more likely to have nontraditional risk factors that are not measured on risk scales, such as depression and a sedentary lifestyle.

Here's what it means—women, at least until menopause, are somewhat protected against heart disease. It takes more risk factors for them to get to the point that it starts affecting their heart.

While that's a good thing, it also means there is a big missed opportunity for prevention—treating these risk factors before you turn up at your doctor's office with chest pain! Even if these risk factors show up at, say, your annual physical, some doctors may be letting them slide with women.

***Another trap:*** A low score on a heart disease risk calculator such as the Framingham Heart Risk Score. Because these scores don't include factors such as depression or a sedentary lifestyle, they often can underestimate a woman's real heart disease risk. That is, even if your doctor diagnoses you with depression, it wouldn't raise your official heart risk score—even though it does actually increase your risk.

***Bottom line:*** Primary care physicians shouldn't ignore creeping high blood pressure, cholesterol problems, mood conditions or a couch potato lifestyle in their female patients. Doctors should be more aggressive in treating women for risk factors.

## A Difference in Diagnostic Testing

Compared with men, women were more likely than men to be referred for imaging echocardiography stress tests, which use ultrasound to create an image that shows how well your heart pumps while you exercise. That makes sense since these tests are known to be more accurate than electrocardiograms in women than men, says Dr. Douglas.

But another difference concerned her. Physicians ordered more stress nuclear tests, in which a radioactive dye is injected, over stress echocardiography tests, for women compared with men. Why the concern? For one, there isn't good evidence that nuclear tests are any better than standard non-nuclear echocardiographs. *Second*: Women are more sensitive to the negative health effects of radiation, resulting in a small increase in cancer risk.

***Bottom line:*** If your doctor suggests a nuclear stress test, ask if it's really necessary. (Sometimes there's a good reason, such as comparing new results against previous nuclear test results or because you have breast implants.)

### What We Still Don't Know About Women's Hearts

To really understand how heart disease differs between the genders, much more work like that of Dr. Douglas's team needs to happen.

***One example of what we still don't know:*** Women are less likely to have a result that indicates a problem (a so-called "positive" test result) from one of these diagnostic tests, compared with men. That sounds like good news, but it's really a paradox. It should mean that women's hearts are healthier than men's. But they're not.

The same percentage of women die from cardiovascular disease as men. This would suggest that, somehow, we are missing something here—we're just not sure what.

---

## Women More Likely to Have "Silent" Heart Attacks

Andrea Ohrn, MD, PhD, fellow, University of Tromso, Norway...and Nieca Goldberg, MD, medical director, Women's Heart Program, NYU Langone Medical Center, New York City.

*Journal of the American Heart Association.*

People who are less sensitive to pain may be at increased risk of having a "silent" heart attack, a recent study hints.

Chest pain is one of the "classic" symptoms of a heart attack. But many people have so-called silent heart attacks, where they notice no obvious symptoms.

"Almost everyone knows what a heart attack is. When we hear about it, we think of chest pain and [emergency] medical care," said Andrea Ohrn, MD, PhD, the lead researcher on the recent study.

"But what's less known is, many people experience heart attacks without knowing it—without ever receiving a diagnosis," said Dr. Ohrn, a fellow at the University of Tromso in Norway.

No one knows why that is. But the recent findings suggest that pain tolerance might be a factor.

Using a standard test of pain sensitivity, Dr. Ohrn's team found that people who had a silent heart attack in the past generally had a higher pain tolerance than people who'd sought treatment for heart attack symptoms.

When the researchers dug deeper, the connection appeared to be stronger in women than men.

That's an interesting finding, but it's unclear what to make of it at this point, said Nieca Goldberg, MD, medical director of the Women's Heart Program at NYU Langone Medical Center in New York City.

### Atypical Heart Attack Symptoms

The main takeaway, Dr. Goldberg said, is that people should know the "atypical" symptoms of heart attack.

Those include pain in the upper back or jaw, shortness of breath, nausea and heartburn-like pressure in the upper abdomen.

"We need to be more vigilant in educating people that chest pain is not the only symptom of heart attack," said Dr. Goldberg, who wasn't involved in the study.

### Study Details

The findings, published in the *Journal of the American Heart Association*, came from a long-term health study of people living in Tromso, Norway.

One study visit involved a standard pain-sensitivity test where people plunge a hand into cold water for as long as they can stand it, for up to two minutes.

At the next study visit, participants underwent electrocardiograms—which can detect signs of a past heart attack, even if it was unrecognized at the time.

Of over 4,800 adults who had both tests, it turned out that 8% had previously had a silent heart attack. Just under 5% had a diagnosed heart attack.

When the researchers compared the two groups, they found that people who had a silent attack had, on average, greater pain tolerance.

## Implications

It's possible that people who tolerate cold-induced pain are also less sensitive to pain caused by reduced blood flow to the heart, Dr. Ohrn said.

But, Dr. Goldberg said, it's not clear how often "silent" heart attacks truly caused no pain or other symptoms. Some people may simply have not realized the seriousness of their symptoms, and chose to bear them instead of seeking help.

## Silent Heart Attacks More Likely in Women

There were differences between men and women in the study.

Overall, more men had suffered a heart attack—19% versus 7% of women.

But silent attacks accounted for three-quarters of all heart attacks among women, compared with 58% among men.

According to Dr. Ohrn's team, that's in line with past studies: Women are more likely than men to have atypical heart attack symptoms, and their heart attacks are more likely to go undiagnosed.

It's not clear how pain sensitivity fits into that picture.

In this study, women generally had less pain tolerance than men. But the connection between greater pain tolerance and silent heart attack was stronger among women than in men.

It's possible, Dr. Ohrn said, that women with diagnosed heart attacks have particularly severe symptoms. "It may be that it 'takes more' symptoms to have your heart attack recognized if you are a woman," she speculated.

The bottom line, according to Dr. Ohrn, is that it's important for doctors to be on the lookout for less-obvious heart attack symptoms, especially in women. And for women to be aware of the symptoms, too.

"Absence of chest pain should not lower doctors' alertness toward heart disease," she said.

Sometimes the red flags pop up in the longer term, Dr. Ohrn noted. Breathing problems and swelling in the legs, for instance, can be signs of heart muscle damage from a previous, undiagnosed heart attack, she said.

Silent attacks, Dr. Ohrn said, are just as serious as ones that cause obvious chest pain—carrying similar risks of death or repeat heart attack over the long term.

And that, Dr. Goldberg said, underscores the importance of prevention. A healthy diet, regular exercise and controlling risk factors like high blood pressure and high cholesterol are all critical, she said.

The American Heart Association has more info on hard-to-recognize heart attack symptoms at GoRedForWomen.org. Search "hard to recognize heart attack symptoms."

# This Triples Heart Attack Risk...

Avoid strenuous exercise when you are upset. People who are angry or upset and work out to help themselves handle the emotions triple their risk of having a heart attack within an hour. Both exercise and emotional stress put a strain on the heart, and the combination creates an even greater strain.

***Self-defense:*** If you find that it helps to work out when you are stressed or upset, be careful not to go beyond your normal routine—the intensity of exercise at times of emotional upset raises cardiovascular risk.

Study led by researchers at Population Health Research Institute, McMaster University, Hamilton, Ontario, published in *Circulation.*

## Women Fare Better Than Men After a Heart Valve Replacement

Roxana Mehran, professor of medicine in cardiology, Mount Sinai School of Medicine, New York City.
Molly Szerlip, MD, cardiologist, The Heart Hospital Baylor Plano, Texas.
*Journal of the American College of Cardiology,* news release.

Women have a higher survival rate than men after a specific type of heart valve replacement procedure, a recent study finds.

The procedure is called a transcatheter aortic valve replacement (TAVR). Researchers looked at information from more than 23,000 heart patients. They all had TAVR between 2011 and 2014. The study included nearly an equal number of women and men.

Even though women had more complications after the procedure, their chances of survival over the next year were higher than for men. The reasons for this aren't clear, the study authors said.

The study was published in the *Journal of the American College of Cardiology.*

### About the Procedures

TAVR is a minimally invasive method used on high-risk patients with aortic valve disease.

***Patients with this condition can undergo one of three treatments:*** TAVR; surgical aortic valve replacement (SAVR); or medical therapy, the researchers said. To decide which treatment a patient should receive, doctors use scoring methods to determine the risk of complications or death within 30 days.

### Implications

But these scoring methods were generally designed to predict risk associated with SAVR, not TAVR, the researchers explained.

"These findings are significant because it may mean heart teams are overestimating the risks of TAVR in some women, and that also may mean that valve replacement is underutilized," said study senior author Roxana Mehran, MD. She is a professor of medicine in cardiology at Mount Sinai School of Medicine in New York City.

"In other words, some women who could benefit from TAVR may not be getting it," she said in a journal news release.

Because the study only looked at survival rates after one year, Dr. Mehran said that "further study is needed on the medium- to long-term causes of death in men and women who have had TAVR."

### Expert Commentary

The results of the study should be interpreted with caution, according to Molly Szerlip, MD, a cardiologist at The Heart Hospital Baylor Plano in Texas. She wrote an editorial accompanying the study.

"The findings of this study are only applicable to the population that was studied and should not necessarily be extrapolated to lower-risk populations or to patients who receive newer-generation valves," Dr. Szerlip said.

The American Heart Association has more information about heart valve replacement at heart.org. Search "heart valve replacement."

# Taller, Bigger Women May Face Irregular Heartbeat Risk

Annika Rosengren, MD, professor, internal medicine, University of Gothenburg, Sweden.
Allan Stewart, MD, director, aortic surgery, Mount Sinai Health System, New York City.
Neil Bernstein, MD, cardiac electrophysiologist, Lenox Hill Hospital, New York City.
European Society of Cardiology meeting, Malaga, Spain.

Big or tall women are nearly three times as likely to develop the dangerous irregular heart rhythm known as atrial fibrillation as smaller women, a preliminary study says.

The larger a woman's body size as a young adult, the more likely she is to develop the heart disorder later in life, according to the researchers.

"There was a stepwise elevation in risk with increasing body size," said study author Annika Rosengren, MD.

"The group with the highest body surface area had nearly three times the risk as those with the lowest body surface area," added Dr. Rosengren, a professor of internal medicine at the University of Gothenburg in Sweden.

## About Atrial Fibrillation

Atrial fibrillation is an irregular heartbeat that develops in the atria—the two upper chambers of the heart. The quivering heartbeat increases risk of stroke, heart failure and other heart rhythm problems, according to the American Heart Association.

It's the most common heart rhythm disorder, and everyone has a one in five chance of developing atrial fibrillation during their lifetime, the researchers said in background information. The problem occurs most often in people older than 60.

"The implications may be substantial, because the world population is growing taller as well as heavier," Dr. Rosengren said. "We might be looking at substantially more AF in the future."

A previous study found that husky or tall young men were more likely to develop atrial fibrillation as they aged, particularly if they gained weight, Dr. Rosengren said.

## Study Details

To see if this also occurs in women, Dr. Rosengren and her colleagues reviewed data on 1.5 million Swedish women.

Using a national birth registry, the researchers gathered information on women with a first pregnancy (average age 28). The registry contained data on height and weight, which the researchers used to determine each woman's body surface size. The registry also had information on other heart risk factors such as diabetes, high blood pressure and smoking.

The investigators tracked the women for 16 years on average. During that time, more than 7,000 women were hospitalized with atrial fibrillation, at an average age of 49.

Compared to the smallest women, the largest women had a 2.6-times increased risk of atrial fibrillation, after adjusting for other risk factors, the researchers found. They also found that the risk increased with women's initial body size.

Dr. Rosengren said having a big body means having a big heart with larger-than-usual atria, which raises the risk of atrial fibrillation.

The findings were presented at a meeting of the European Society of Cardiology in Malaga, Spain.

## Expert Commentary

Allan Stewart, MD, is director of aortic surgery for Mount Sinai Health System in New York City. He said heart muscle tissue serves a dual function. Each cell contributes to the regular heart muscle contractions that pump blood through the body. But the cells also pass along an electrical impulse that controls the rhythm of the heartbeat, he explained.

Big atria challenge this heart function. "You have the same number of cells, but when they're stretched and they increase in size, it interrupts the electrical pathway of the heart," Dr. Stewart said. "You go from a normal rhythm to atrial fibrillation."

Just being big in and of itself likely adds to the problem, said Dr. Stewart, who wasn't involved in the study.

"You're more likely to have more pressure against your heart and more pressure against your lungs, and these can cause the atrium to distend," he said.

Still, larger females shouldn't worry. Even in big women, the absolute risk of developing atrial fibrillation remained low in this study, less than 0.5%, noted Neil Bernstein, MD. He's a cardiac electrophysiologist with Lenox Hill Hospital in New York City.

"The more interesting fact will be the data as this group ages, since there is a well-known increase in the incidence of atrial fibrillation with age," said Dr. Bernstein, who had no role in the study.

## Expert Advice

Based on these findings, people who are naturally big or tall need to eat right, exercise and take other lifestyle steps to protect their heart health, Dr. Stewart and Dr. Bernstein said.

It also would pay for doctors to keep a closer eye on the heart health of tall or husky men and women as they grow older, Dr. Stewart added.

For more information on atrial fibrillation, visit the website of the American Heart Association, heart.org, and search "atrial fibrillation."

# What Else Mammograms Can Spot

Mammograms may predict heart disease, too. According to a recent study, digital mammography was about 70% accurate in predicting the presence of calcium in coronary arteries, an early sign of heart disease. Researchers report that mammograms were often more accurate in predicting heart disease than standard predictors, such as high blood pressure and elevated cholesterol. If your mammogram shows calcifications in the breast arteries, be sure to follow up with your primary care doctor.

Harvey Hecht, MD, professor of medicine and cardiology, Icahn School of Medicine at Mount Sinai, New York City.

# Early Onset Hot Flashes May Signal Higher Heart Risks

Rebecca Thurston, PhD, director, Women's Biobehavioral Health Laboratory, University of Pittsburgh School of Medicine.

Jill Rabin, MD, co-chief, division of ambulatory care, Women's Health Programs-PCAP Services, Northwell Health, New Hyde Park, New York.

Rachel Bond, MD, associate director, Women's Heart Health, Lenox Hill Hospital, New York City.

North American Menopause Society, news release.

Hot flashes may be more than a troublesome nuisance for some women during menopause—they may be a signal for increased risk of heart disease, recent research suggests.

## The Study

Researchers tracked the health of 272 nonsmoking women, aged 40 to 60. Among women between 40 and 53 years of age, frequent hot flashes were linked to a reduced ability of blood vessels to dilate, the study found.

This association was independent of other heart disease risk factors, noted the team led by Rebecca Thurston, PhD, of the University of Pittsburgh School of Medicine.

The link seemed restricted to the younger women in the study—there was no such relationship among women aged 54 to 60, the study authors said.

The findings were published in the journal *Menopause*.

## Implications

One obstetrician/gynecologist called the findings potentially "groundbreaking."

At least in those women who undergo menopause early, hot flashes "are not simply a bother, but herald potential microvascular [small-vessel] disease, and may be a risk factor and predictor of subsequent cardiovascular disease," said Jill Rabin, MD.

She's co-chief of ambulatory care in Women's Health Programs at Northwell Health in New Hyde Park, New York.

"The reason the study is so important is that heart disease in women in particular can be very difficult to diagnose until its latter stages. All too often, the diagnosis is made far too late, if at all and at the expense of a woman's life," Dr. Rabin added.

"Overall, this is a very interesting and important study," she said.

"Future research in this area is warranted and eagerly awaited."

According to Dr. Thurston's team, heart disease is the leading cause of death for American women, and the recent findings may help health-care providers assess heart disease risk in menopausal patients.

The researchers noted that 70% of women report having hot flashes during menopause, and about one-third say their hot flashes are frequent and/or severe.

## Expert Commentary

Rachel Bond, MD, helps direct Women's Heart Health at Lenox Hill Hospital in New York City. Reviewing the recent findings, she said that even though hot flashes seemed linked to heart risk in younger menopausal women, "we still do not know the causative effect or mechanism" linking the two.

Perhaps in the future, "by gaining a better understanding of the role hot flashes play on vascular health, we could potentially help identify women who may be at risk much sooner," Dr. Bond said.

"In my own practice in the women's heart health program, early hot flashes may be a red flag for me as a physician to be more aggressive at either screening for or preventing other risk factors and cardiovascular disease," she said.

# Depression Can Fuel Heart Disease in Middle-Aged Women

Xuezhi Jiang, MD, obstetrician-gynecologist, Reading Hospital, Reading, Pennsylvania, and assistant professor, obstetrics and gynecology, Sidney Kimmel Medical College of Thomas Jefferson University, Philadelphia.

Simon A. Rego, PsyD, chief psychologist, and associate clinical professor, psychiatry and behavioral sciences, Montefiore Medical Center/Albert Einstein College of Medicine, New York City.

North American Menopause Society annual meeting, Orlando, Florida.

Women in midlife with a history of depression appear at markedly greater risk of suffering from heart disease, new research suggests.

The finding seems to reinforce the well-known link between depression and heart troubles, but it doesn't prove a cause-and-effect relationship.

Tracking about 1,100 women over 10 years, researchers found that depression was the only significant risk factor for coronary artery disease in women younger than 65 who had no history of heart ailments at the beginning of the study.

In women over age 65, however, age was identified as the only significant predictor for heart disease, the investigators found.

Heart disease is the leading cause of death for both women and men in the United States, responsible for one in four deaths each year, according to the U.S. Centers for Disease Control and Prevention.

"Once we added depression...with the other well-known risk factors for coronary artery disease, depression was the only one to stand out" in women under 65, said study author Xuezhi Jiang, MD, an obstetrician-gynecologist at Reading Hospital in Reading, Pennsylvania. "This is kind of surprising."

### Study Details

Dr. Jiang and his team tracked 1,084 women who received routine mammogram screenings at a radiology facility starting in 2004. Their average age was 55. Each completed a depression questionnaire with three questions inquiring about feeling sad or depressed; helpless; or downhearted and blue.

Other health information was also taken, including participants' heart disease risk factors, such as family history, smoking status, exercise levels, high blood pressure or diabetes. A similar depression questionnaire was mailed to each participant four times over the next 10 years to obtain follow-up information and any change in heart disease status.

Of the 1,030 women who had no history of heart disease at the start of the study, about 18% answered "yes" to at least one depression question. Of those women, 9% experienced one or more instances of cardiac disease over the next 10 years, compared with only 2% who reported "no" to feeling depressed.

The study was presented at the North American Menopause Society's annual meeting in Orlando, Florida.

### Possible Explanation

Depression was the only significant risk factor associated with the development of heart disease in women under age 65. While scientists don't fully understand why depression increases heart disease risk, Dr. Jiang said, depression can increase the production of stress hormones in the body that may play a role in heart problems.

### Expert Commentary

Simon A. Rego, PsyD is chief psychologist at Montefiore Medical Center/Albert Einstein College of Medicine in New York City. He said the recent study highlights the serious impact a mental health condition can have on medical outcomes.

"The take-home message is to increase and broaden our mental health screening procedures in sites that do not traditionally screen for these conditions, in this case, women presenting for routine breast cancer screening," said Dr. Rego. He wasn't involved in the recent research.

Dr. Rego noted that depression can have an impact on healthy behaviors, such as reducing exercise and activity levels, altering eating and sleeping habits, and increasing alcohol and drug use. He said additional research should determine whether such factors may also influence heart disease risks.

## Sex Is Good for Women's Hearts

The sex link to heart health differs for men and women. In a study of more than 2,200 people age 57 and older, men who had sex at least once a week had almost twice the cardiovascular risk of men who were sexually inactive. Women who reported the most satisfying sex had lower risk for high blood pressure and other cardiovascular conditions than other women.

***Why:*** Women may benefit from hormones produced during orgasm, while men might subject themselves to undue stress through exertion or medication for erectile dysfunction.

Hui Liu, PhD, associate professor of sociology, Michigan State University, East Lansing.

## Fitful Sleep May Take Toll on Older Women's Hearts

Rebecca Thurston, PhD, director, Women's Biobehavioral Health Laboratory, and professor, psychiatry, University of Pittsburgh.

Suzanne Steinbaum, DO, cardiologist and director, Women's Heart Health, Lenox Hill Hospital, New York City.

North American Menopause Society annual meeting, Orlando, Florida.

The sleep woes that many women suffer during menopause may be more than a nuisance. Recent research suggests a link between lost sleep and an increase in risk factors for heart disease and stroke.

When loss of sleep was measured both objectively and subjectively, the researchers found it correlated with a higher risk of plaque buildup in blood vessels and a thickening of artery walls.

"Our results indicate that short or poor sleep is associated with some increased risk for cardiovascular events such as heart attack and stroke," said lead researcher Rebecca Thurston, PhD, director of the Women's Biobehavioral Health Laboratory at the University of Pittsburgh.

The increased risk, she said, "is probably somewhere around small to moderate, not large."

Dr. Thurston couldn't explain the link, and added that the study did not prove that sleep troubles cause heart risks to rise.

But, "we measured many things in this study to explain why sleep may be related to cardiovascular disease risk [for example, inflammatory factors, nervous system factors, depression], but they did not explain the association we saw," she said.

Sleep problems are known to be common during menopause, Dr. Thurston said.

"Menopause is also a time of accelerating cardiovascular disease risk," she added. "Whether sleep problems help explain the accelerations in cardiovascular disease risk during the menopause transition, we do not know, but we will be looking into that question in future work."

## The Study

For the study, Dr. Thurston's team assessed 256 women, aged 40 to 60. They wore wrist monitors for three days to objectively assess sleep quality and answered questionnaires about their sleep quality and mood. They also had blood tests and artery ultrasounds done.

None of the women had a history of heart disease, took hormone therapy, worked night shifts or were taking sleep medications.

For each hour of sleep lost, the blood vessel plaque buildup rose. The highest amount of thickening of the artery walls was found in women sleeping only five or six hours a night. Longer sleep, more than seven hours, was not protective, however. Women who reported poorer sleep also had more thickening of the vessels, the study found.

The association lingered even after the researchers took into account other factors such as mood.

Dr. Thurston's findings were presented at the North American Menopause Society's annual meeting, in Orlando, Florida.

## Expert Commentary

The link between poor sleep and heart disease risk has been known for some time, said Suzanne Steinbaum, DO, director of Women's Heart Health at Lenox Hill Hospital in New York City. However, she said the study adds valuable information since it includes both objective and subjective measures of sleep.

"We know that with lack of sleep there is an increased risk of high blood pressure, there is an increased risk of obesity, inflammatory markers go up and stress hormones go up," Dr. Steinbaum said.

With the objective markers in the recent study, Dr. Steinbaum said, it reinforces the idea that "not sleeping is so detrimental to health." Women should expect their doctors to pay attention and offer solutions if they report they aren't sleeping well, she said.

## How to Get a Good Night's Sleep

According to the National Sleep Foundation, healthy sleep habits are vital. The association offers a variety of sleep tips, including going to bed and waking up at the same time daily, even on weekends. A relaxing bedtime ritual away from bright lights (listening to music, for instance) could help, too. Avoiding naps, especially in the afternoon, can help you sleep better at night. Getting regular exercise can also be beneficial, according to the foundation.

To learn more about how much sleep you really need, visit the National Sleep Foundation website, SleepFoundation.org, and search "How much sleep do we really need?"

# What Your Skin Says About Your Heart Health

Jeffrey P. Callen, MD, a professor of medicine and chief of the division of dermatology at the University of Louisville School of Medicine in Kentucky. He is the coeditor of *Dermatological Signs of Systemic Disease*, the author or coauthor of more than 400 scientific papers and the recipient of the 2017 Master Dermatologist Award from the American Academy of Dermatology.

A red, itchy rash...little yellow bumps... extremely dry skin. The list of skin problems can go on and on. But did you know that a skin issue isn't always just about your skin? It might be alerting you to an internal problem, such as heart disease, that your doctor needs to know about and treat.

Plus, some skin conditions may mean that you have an increased risk for other health problems (for example, psoriasis has been shown to increase risk for cardiovascular disease), and you will want to take measures to reduce these risks.

## Signs of Cardiovascular Disease (CVD)

CVD is characterized by narrowed or blocked blood vessels that can cause heart attack or stroke. In many cases, chest pain, heart attack or stroke is the first recognizable sign of CVD. *But several skin changes may indicate that you're at increased risk for CVD...*

- **Yellow plaques on the eyelids.** These waxy growths (known as xanthelasma) are found mostly on the upper eyelids. They may be a sign of elevated cholesterol levels, a risk factor for CVD. In some cases, use of cholesterol-lowering drugs will resolve these growths.

- **Swollen and itchy legs and feet.** Excess accumulation of fluid in patients with congestive heart failure can result in leg swelling (edema). If left untreated, stasis dermatitis, a condition characterized by itchy, red skin, may occur. Treatments that improve heart function, along with compression stockings and topical corticosteroids, help to alleviate symptoms and prevent recurrence.

## A Risky Skin Condition

If you have psoriasis, you and your doctor need to be aware of the possible health risks that are linked to the condition...

This inflammatory autoimmune disease attacks skin cells, producing scales of silvery, thick skin and raised red patches that can be painful as well as itchy. The inflammation associated with psoriasis can increase risk for high blood pressure, heart attack, stroke, peripheral artery disease (poor circulation in the legs) and diabetes.

***What to do:*** Standard treatments for psoriasis include medications, such as steroids, light therapy and stress management. While there's some evidence that treatments may lower CVD risk, it is best to work with your doctor to assess your CVD risk factors. You can then lower your risk by losing weight, exercising regularly, not smoking and, when necessary, using medication to control CVD risk factors such as high blood pressure and elevated cholesterol.

# Fat Near the Heart Is a Hazard for Postmenopausal Women

Samar El Khoudary, PhD, MPH, assistant professor, epidemiology, University of Pittsburgh, Graduate School of Public Health.

Suzanne Steinbaum, DO, director, women's heart health, Lenox Hill Hospital, New York City.

*Journal of the American Heart Association*, online.

When a certain type of fat collects around the heart, it may be a sign of developing heart disease in postmenopausal women, a recent study suggests.

As estrogen levels fall during menopause, deposits of "paracardial" fat increase, the researchers found. This may indicate more calcium buildup in the heart's arteries, an early sign of heart disease.

## About Paracardial Fat

Paracardial fat sits in pockets around the heart. These pockets lie between the heart and another type of fat that covers the heart called epicardial fat, the study authors explained.

Epicardial fat provides energy to the heart, but paracardial fat has no known beneficial function, the researchers said.

"We are showing for the first time that paracardial fat is associated with greater risk of calcification [calcium build-up] in postmenopausal women, more than in premenopausal women," said lead researcher Samar El Khoudary, PhD, MPH. She's an assistant professor of epidemiology at the University of Pittsburgh Graduate School of Public Health.

"Premenopausal women also have this type of fat, but it increases significantly as estrogen levels drop during menopause," she explained.

## The Study

Dr. El Khoudary's team found that a 60% increase in paracardial fat was associated with a 160% greater risk of calcium buildup in the heart's blood vessels in postmenopausal women versus pre- or early menopausal women.

Postmenopausal women are at risk for even more calcification in their coronary artery as their levels of paracardial fat rise, Dr. El Khoudary said.

However, while the study found an association between increased paracardial fat and greater calcium buildup in postmenopausal women, it could not prove a cause-and-effect relationship.

For the study, Dr. El Khoudary and her colleagues collected data, including CT heart scans and blood samples, on 478 US women who took part in the Study of Women's Health Across the Nation.

The women were in varying stages of menopause. Their average age was 51. None of the women was on hormone replacement therapy.

The report was published in the *Journal of the American Heart Association*.

## Possible Explanations

In an earlier study, Dr. El Khoudary's team found that an increase in paracardial fat after menopause results from a drop in the hormone *estradiol*, a form of estrogen. Increased levels of epicardial fat were linked to other risk factors, such as obesity, Dr. El Khoudary said.

"We know that the menopausal transition puts women at greater risk of heart disease," she said.

"For example, their cholesterol increases and they start to have more fat around their waist. We are showing that postmenopausal women have more fat around the heart, which could be more damaging to the heart than fat around the waist, because it produces inflammatory factors that could affect the heart," Dr. El Khoudary said.

## What You Can Do

It's possible to reduce paracardial fat through diet and, in obese women, by weight-loss surgery, she said.

Hormone replacement therapy—which increases estrogen levels—might also reduce paracardial fat deposits, but that's not known, Dr. El Khoudary said. To find out, she is planning to study the effects of hormone replacement on the heart.

Suzanne Steinbaum, DO, is director of Women's Heart Health at Lenox Hill Hospital in New York City.

She said the drop in estrogen and the increase of fat around the heart are part of the natural process of menopause.

"Knowing this, we have to understand the huge impact of our lifestyle in preventing what could be a double whammy," she said. "As soon as you start feeling changes in your hormones, this is when you need to get your risk factors for heart disease under control."

This includes controlling blood pressure, cholesterol and weight. In addition, a healthy diet and exercise can help cut the risk of heart disease, Dr. Steinbaum said.

"Menopause is the time it becomes most important to reduce all the risk factors that lead to heart disease," she said.

For now, Dr. El Khoudary suggested, a healthy diet and lots of physical activity are the best prescriptions for reducing the risks of heart disease.

For more on women and heart disease, visit the website of the US National Heart, Lung, and Blood Institute, NHLBI.nih.gov. Search "How Does Heart Disease Affect Women?"

---

# A Test We All Need for Hidden Heart Disease

Rebecca Shannonhouse, editor, *Bottom Line Health*. American Heart Association, news release.

---

Doctors routinely check for cardiovascular risk factors during annual checkups—things like high blood pressure, elevated cholesterol and diabetes. But unless you have known or suspected heart disease, it's unlikely that you've ever had a cardiorespiratory fitness (CRF) test.

In fact, CRF is the only major heart disease risk factor that isn't evaluated during routine visits. But that may be changing.

***What's new:*** The American Heart Association recently released a report that strongly advises doctors to include a fitness assessment as part of regular exams. Because CRF is potentially a stronger predictor of future heart health than other risk factors, you need to know where you stand.

If you haven't gotten much exercise lately, you have the most to gain. Research has shown that for every one-point increase in aerobic fitness (as measured in METs, a unit used in fitness tests), there's a 10% to 25% improvement in survival.

Your doctor might recommend a cardiopulmonary exercise test, during which you'll be wired to the gills while riding an exercise bike or using a treadmill. It's the best test for CRF, but it can be expensive if your insurance doesn't cover it.

***Do-it-yourself option:*** A one-mile walk test. You map out a course of one mile...walk as fast as you can...check your heart rate when you're done...then enter your heart rate, age, weight and how long it took you to complete the walk into an online calculator, such as ExRx.net/Calculators/Rockport.html. It will give a rating such as "good" or "fair," which you can discuss with your doctor.

---

# How TV Can Kill You

Research letter titled "Watching Television and Risk of Mortality from Pulmonary Embolism Among Japanese Men and Women" by investigators at the Osaka University Graduate School of Medicine, Japan, published in *Circulation*.

---

You may think binge-watching the latest Netflix series is a guilty but harmless pleasure. Think again. It could kill you. Really.

Oh, one or two episodes of *House of Cards* —or *The Bachelor*—won't do you in. But too many hours of binge watching can greatly increase your risk for an often-fatal condition.

## The Five Hour Threshold

Researchers at Osaka University in Japan were studying lifestyle factors related to blood clots. When a blood clot happens in the leg, it's called deep vein thrombosis—but if one breaks free and travels to your lungs, it can cause a pulmonary embolism, which often is fatal.

Researchers already knew that being sedentary for a long period of time—such as a long airplane flight—can increase the odds of getting blood clots. So they decided to look at television watching. They analyzed records of more than 86,000 men and women between the ages of 40 and 79 in 45 regions of Japan.

***Bingo:*** Those who watched between two-and-a-half and five hours of TV a night, on average, were 70% more likely than those who watched less than that to have a fatal pulmonary embolism...and those who watched more than five hours were 250% more likely than those who watched less than two-and-a-half hours of TV.

## Enjoying TV...in Moderation

Granted, the absolute number of deaths was still pretty small. There were 59 total deaths from pulmonary embolism over the 20 years of the study, 40 of them from the 2.5-hours-to-five hours and more-than-five-hours groups combined. Plus, these kinds of observational studies can't actually prove cause and effect.

On the other hand, we already know that watching too much TV is remarkably bad for health—people who watch more than six hours a night on average are likely to die nearly five years earlier than TV abstainers, for example.

We've got nothing against relaxing in front of the TV. But if you find yourself zoning out for more than two or three hours every night, finding more active pursuits can be a very healthy change—it might even make you happier. At the very least, get up and walk around frequently—and try a few quick exercises.

# More Sun, Longer Life

Study titled "Avoidance of sun exposure as a risk factor for major causes of death: a competing risk analysis of the Melanoma in Southern Sweden cohort" by researchers at Karolinska University Hospital, Lund University, both in Sweden, published in *Journal of Internal Medicine.*

Michael F. Holick, PhD, MD, professor of medicine, physiology and biophysics, Boston University School of Medicine, and author of *The Vitamin D Solution.*

Let the sunshine in. It's good for the heart, according to a recent study.

It's no excuse to start sunbathing for hours without sunscreen, to be sure, but the recent research suggests that avoiding the sun might shorten your life.

## A Healthier Heart

Back in the early 1990s, nearly 30,000 Swedish women filled out a questionnaire about how often they spent time in the sun in the summer or went to sunny climates for holiday in the winter. Over the next 20 years, researchers reported a few years ago, those who had the most sun exposure, compared with those with the least, were half as likely to die from all causes.

In the latest study, the researchers determined that the reason the sun seekers were less likely to die earlier was a decreased incidence of cardiovascular disease, which can cause death from heart attacks and stroke.

The sun seekers did have a greater prevalence of cancers, both skin cancers and internal cancers. But that's most likely because they lived longer. Age is one of the strongest risk factors for cancer. Interestingly, those who had nonmelanoma skin cancers, such as squamous or basal cell cancer, which are rarely fatal, tended to have been exposed to the most sun—and had the lowest rates of overall mortality.

How much longer did sun seekers live? Depending on other risk factors, such as smoking, sun seekers lived between six months and two years longer than sun avoiders, on average.

This is an observational study, so it doesn't prove cause-and-effect relationships, but noted it does fit in with other research—in both men and women.

## How Sun Protects the Heart

Vitamin D, which the body produces in response to sun exposure, is of course a likely protective factor. In the famous Framingham Heart Study, men and women with blood levels of vitamin D below 15 ng/mL were 50% more likely to have a heart attack than those with higher levels. For reference, the Endocrine Society recommends blood levels at or above 30 ng/mL.

### Easy Ways to Move for Better Heart Health

**Take five.** If you're going to be sitting for hours—which is bad for your heart—set an alarm on your phone, watch or computer to chime hourly. When you hear the alarm, get up and walk around for five minutes. According to an Indiana University study, walking just five minutes for every hour you sit is enough to help your heart.

*Bottom Line Personal.*

**Fidgeting is good for you.** Sitting for long periods reduces blood flow to the legs and may increase risk for cardiovascular disease. But a small amount of leg fidgeting—such as tapping your foot—increases blood flow to the lower limbs and prevents decline in arterial function.

Study by researchers at University of Missouri, Columbia, published in *American Journal of Physiology: Heart and Circulatory Physiology.*

Vitamin D is heart-healthy in many ways—it helps regulate blood pressure (by tamping down production of the pressure-raising protein renin), improves the functioning of blood vessels (by reducing production of "foam" cells that can lead to atherosclerosis) and helps strengthen the heart muscle itself.

But the sun also stimulates the skin to produce nitric oxide, which is then released into the bloodstream. Nitric oxide allows our blood vessels to relax, and that can reduce blood pressure. Sun exposure also promotes production and release of feel-good beta endorphins—one reason that sunny days may be mood boosters—which reduces stress, protecting the heart.

### Just Enough Sun...Plus Vitamin D Supplements

Before you head out unprotected into the sunshine, remember that Swedes (the subjects of the latest research) are much more likely to suffer a sun drought than most Americans. Stockholm, for example, gets only about 1,800 hours of sunshine a year—compared with 3,200 hours in, for example, Grand Junction, Colorado.

Most Americans can get enough vitamin D in the summer by receiving sensible sun exposure.

To ensure adequate vitamin D all year round, a supplement is recommended—for children, 600 IU to 1,000 IU daily...for most adults 2,000 IU daily...and for obese adults 4,000 IU to 6,000 IU daily. That's because anyone living north of Atlanta can't make enough vitamin D from sun alone between October and April. For the record, vitamin D-2 is just as effective as vitamin D-3, so it doesn't matter which form of the supplement you take.

## Should You Take Aspirin? There's an App for That

Article titled "Aspirin for primary prevention of atherosclerotic cardiovascular disease. Advances in diagnosis and treatment" written by Samia Mora, MD, MHS, Harvard Medical School, and JoAnn E. Manson, MD, DrPH, Harvard T.H. Chan School of Public Health, both in Boston, published in *JAMA Internal Medicine.*

Figuring out whether to take a daily low-dose aspirin is tricky. By reducing the tendency of blood to clot, aspirin can help prevent a heart attack or a stroke...but it can also put you at risk for intestinal, even cerebral, bleeding. Do the benefits outweigh the risks—for you?

Even doctors don't always get it right—in some medical practices, nearly two-thirds of patients on aspirin therapy shouldn't be taking it.

Now a new, free smartphone app makes figuring that out easier, faster and safer.

### Doc in a Pocket

Aspirin Guide (currently available for iPhone and iPad only), an app designed by researchers at Brigham and Women's Hospital and Harvard Medical School, is designed for health-care professionals, but it's patient-friendly, too. All you need to know is some basic medical information, such as your systolic blood pressure (the upper number), and your high-density (HDL) and total cholesterol numbers.

The app uses evidence-based algorithms to calculate your 10-year risk for heart attack, stroke and your risk of bleeding based on your answers to certain questions. It then gives two numbers, one for your likelihood of harm and one for your likelihood of benefit.

## The Best Candidate for App Advice

What kind of patient can most benefit from Aspirin Guide? Probably not someone who has already had a heart attack or an ischemic stroke (the kind caused by a blood clot). That's because a low-dose daily aspirin is a well-established therapy, so it's likely that your doctor has already advised you to take it.

But if you are trying to prevent a first heart attack or stroke, the individualized information from the new app is a great starting point for a health-care conversation. What if your benefit is high but your risk of harm is also high? That's a great question to ask your doctor.

# How to Survive a Heart Attack

Gregory S. Thomas, MD, MPH, medical director for the MemorialCare Heart & Vascular Institute at Long Beach Memorial Medical Center in California and clinical professor at the University of California, Irvine.

Every year, about 750,000 Americans have a heart attack. Even though advances in emergency care and cardiology have greatly improved one's odds of survival, roughly one of every six of these individuals dies.

What determines whether a heart attack sufferer lives or dies? Certainly, the person's age and overall health play an important role. But there's another factor that gets far less attention than it should.

***Lifesaving strategy:*** When a person on the scene knows how to recognize that someone is having a heart attack and then respond to the emergency appropriately, it can have a profound effect on whether the victim lives or dies.

***Sobering research:*** When a heart attack occurs, the average sufferer (particularly women) waits two hours or more before calling 911 and going to the hospital. This delay often occurs because victims can't believe that they are really having a heart attack...or they don't want to feel embarrassed at the hospital if it turns out that it's not a heart attack and they've "wasted" everyone's time.

But each minute of delay during a heart attack destroys more heart muscle, putting the victim at greater risk for disability and death.

## Recognize and Respond

My advice for quickly and accurately identifying heart attack symptoms...*

- **Chest discomfort.** Chest pain is widely believed to be the classic heart attack symptom, but severe chest discomfort usually is a more accurate way to describe it. Pain typically is sharp, but the sensation that usually occurs with a heart attack is not sharp but rather a severe pressure, squeezing or tightness—as if a massive weight had been placed on the chest.

***Also:*** Many women report having no chest discomfort during any part of the heart attack.

***How to respond:*** If a person is having severe chest discomfort, don't assume that it can't be a heart attack because he/she isn't complaining of chest pain. Call 911 immediately. It is important to tell the dispatcher that

*There are some exceptions to the heart attack symptoms described in this article. If you have any question, play it safe and call 911.

you believe the person is having a heart attack because saying this increases the likelihood that an ambulance specializing in heart care will be sent.

• **Referred pain.** The nerves that supply the heart also serve many other areas of the body between the jaw and the navel—places that can produce referred pain during a heart attack.

***Case history:*** A woman who had tooth pain while exercising was referred to me. Her exercise stress test showed that her tooth pain was referred pain. In actuality, the pain was due to angina, a sign that her arteries were significantly blocked, putting her at high risk for a heart attack. Other areas of referred pain during heart attack can include one or both arms or shoulders...the upper back or abdomen...the neck and lower part of the face, including the jaw.

• **Other common symptoms.** A heart attack can produce many other symptoms, including sudden shortness of breath... nausea and vomiting...a cold sweat, or feeling cold and clammy...fatigue...and/or light-headedness.

***Important:*** All of these symptoms (except for feeling cold and clammy) tend to be more common in women than in men.

***How to respond:*** If a man has chest discomfort and at least one other symptom...or if a woman has chest, back or jaw pain and at least one other symptom, it's very likely the individual is having a heart attack. Or if a person's discomfort or pain is particularly severe—even without another symptom—a heart attack is also likely. In either instance, call 911.

***Another red flag:*** Sometimes, a victim has a feeling of "impending doom" and asks a loved one or friend to take him to the hospital. If someone says to you, "I think I should go to the hospital," call 911. Never drive a victim to the hospital—lifesaving treatments start when the paramedics show up. The only exception is if you are within a few minutes of emergency care.

## Know Who's at Greatest Risk

Knowing one's risk for a heart attack also helps prevent delays in treatment.

While some heart attack victims don't have any of the risk factors described below, people generally are at increased risk due to smoking, age (generally, over age 50 for men and over age 60 for women) and being at least moderately overweight. Diabetes or a chronic inflammatory disease, such as rheumatoid arthritis or lupus, can cause heart disease 10 or 20 years earlier than the norm, increasing risk for heart attack.

***Important:*** Diabetes damages nerves, so a diabetic having a heart attack is less likely to have nerve-generated chest discomfort or referred pain—and more likely to have sudden shortness of breath.

## More Lifesaving Actions

In addition to calling 911, do the following to aid a heart attack victim...

• **Position the person correctly.** Contrary to popular opinion, the best position for a conscious heart attack victim is not lying down—this fills the heart with a bit more blood, straining it. The best position is sitting up, which puts the least amount of stress on the heart. An exception is if the person is light-headed, which might indicate low blood pressure. In that case, lay the person down and call 911 immediately.

• **Give aspirin.** Give the person uncoated aspirin—either four 81-mg baby aspirin or one full-strength aspirin (325 mg). The pills should be chewed—this releases clot-busting medicine within 15 minutes into the bloodstream versus up to 30 minutes or more when aspirin is swallowed whole. If someone is already taking a daily blood thinner, aspirin may not be needed. If the person has been prescribed nitroglycerin, it should be taken as directed.

• **Reassure.** A heart attack is frightening—and fear floods the body with adrenaline, speeding up and further stressing the heart. Reassure the person that help is on the way and that he will get through this.

***If the victim is unconscious:*** If the individual doesn't appear to be breathing and you cannot feel a pulse or are unable to check for one, start CPR if you know how to do it. If you don't, simply press down on the victim's chest at least two inches deep (where the ribs meet at the base of the breastbone) and pump as fast as you can (100 times per minute). Like CPR, this technique pushes air into the lungs—the best action you can take until paramedics arrive.

## Don't Drive to the Hospital

If you have heart attack symptoms, don't use a car to get to the hospital. Call 911 for an ambulance because it will have equipment that can restart your heart if it stops—cardiac arrest is rare but is fatal without prompt treatment. And many dispatchers receiving 911 calls about heart attack symptoms send paramedics who are trained to give patients electrocardiograms (ECGs). The ECG results are then sent to the emergency department of the hospital to help speed treatment on arrival.

*Harvard Health Letter.* Health.Harvard.edu

# 4 out of 5 People Prescribed Statins May Not Need Them

Study titled "Accuracy of the Atherosclerotic Cardiovascular Risk Equation in a Large Contemporary, Multiethnic Population" by researchers at Kaiser Permanente Northern California, University of California, San Francisco, et al. published in *Journal of the American College of Cardiology.*

Ever since new guidelines to identify who needs a statin were introduced in 2013, there have been skeptics. One major suspicion was that the cardiovascular risk calculator used to determine statin eligibility widely overestimated heart disease risk.

That could result in many people—potentially millions—taking these drugs when they shouldn't. But those concerns were theoretical, based on competing estimates of risk.

Now we have evidence from the first major study that actually looked at what happens with real patients.

The skeptics were right.

## Real People's Hearts Are So Much Healthier Than We Thought

In this study, researchers put the risk calculator to the test by applying it to the population it was designed for—that is, men and women, ages 40 to 75, who did not already have diagnosed diabetes or cardiovascular disease, with an LDL cholesterol under 190 mg/dL. (If your LDL is above 190, current guidelines recommend a statin even if your risk is low.) Using a large database from Kaiser Permanente Northern California, they identified more than 300,000 men and women who in 2008 fit the profile of the ideal user of the calculator.

According to the cardiovascular risk calculator, the number of these patients who, over the next five years, would have a heart attack or an ischemic stroke (the most common kind) or die from heart disease should have been 10,150 people.

In reality, it was 2,061.

That's good news of course. But it means that cardiovascular disease was overestimated across the board—at every level of risk. It was found among both men and women and also among major ethnic groups including non-Hispanic white, non-Hispanic black, Asian-Pacific Islander and Hispanic people.

Not everyone in the study would have been a candidate for a statin—but about 30% were. And, based on this study, it appears that four out of five of them who would be candidates for statins based on the standard risk calculator don't need them.

How could the tests be so wrong? One possibility—the data from which the testing tool was created is based on studies from the

1990s, when more people smoked and developed cardiovascular disease at younger ages.

## Better Ways to Find Out If You Need a Statin

Here are a few approaches that may be more reliable...

• **Use a better risk calculator.** According to the Centers for Disease Control and Prevention, the Framingham score is an accurate predictor of cardiovascular risk when measured against actual patient outcomes.

• **If your doctor suggests a statin, you may want to discuss getting a coronary artery calcium scan.** It detects actual calcium deposits in your coronary arteries, which can predict heart disease before symptoms develop. There is some exposure to radiation involved.

• **Have you had a digital mammogram?** You can skip the calcium scan. Instead, ask your radiologist about calcium that may have been seen in the arteries of your breasts, which correlates well with the coronary artery calcium score.

# When Statins Don't Mix with Other Heart Drugs

Barbara S. Wiggins, PharmD, a clinical pharmacy specialist in cardiology at the Medical University of South Carolina and adjunct professor at South Carolina College of Pharmacy, both in Charleston. She is the lead author of *Pharmacist's Guide to Lipid Management, 2nd Edition.* She also chaired the committee that created the American Heart Association's 2016 Scientific Statement on statin-related drug-drug interactions.

If you're taking a statin drug to help reduce your risk for heart attack or stroke, you wouldn't expect it to interact with another heart medication that your doctor may have prescribed...but it can.

***What most people don't realize:*** The statin drugs that are taken by about one-quarter of American adults age 40 and older can interact with many medications that are needed to treat related cardiovascular conditions.

Even though combining a statin with other heart medicines usually offers more benefit than harm, it's important that these medications be closely monitored by one's doctor. Keep a list of your current medications and doses so that your doctor (and pharmacist) can evaluate them for potential drug-drug interactions (DDIs).

***Latest development:*** The American Heart Association recently released a statement about these possible drug interactions, along with guidelines on how to avoid them. *What you need to know...*

## What Are the Risks?

Millions of Americans take two or more drugs to reduce the risk for heart attack, stroke and other cardiovascular conditions. Multiple medications often are necessary to optimize treatment in patients who have more than one medical condition and are at risk for cardiovascular disease. Along with statins (used for lowering cholesterol), these drugs include fibrates (for lowering triglycerides)...blood thinners (for reducing clots)...calcium channel blockers (for high blood pressure and other conditions)...and many others.

When statins are combined with one or more of these other heart medications, a DDI can occur.

***Important:*** If you're taking a statin, be sure to tell your doctor (and pharmacist) whenever any medication is added or taken away from your regimen or a drug dose changes.

## Possible Interactions

Statin-related DDIs can range from mild muscle aches or weakness to a severe form of muscle damage known as rhabdomyolysis, which is rare but can be life-threatening. If you notice muscle pain and/or weakness, known as myopathy, tell your doctor right away.

Discuss with your doctor how to minimize side effects if you take the following combinations—even if you aren't currently experiencing side effects. You may not always tolerate these combinations.

• **Statin plus a fibrate.** Patients with high triglycerides or complex lipid disorders—such as metabolic syndrome, obesity and/or diabetes—sometimes are treated with both a statin and a fibrate drug. The fibrates include *gemfibrozil* (Lopid) and *fenofibrate* (Tricor). Gemfibrozil is particularly risky when combined with some statins.

***The risk:*** Blood levels of *lovastatin* (Mevacor) and *simvastatin* (Zocor) can double or triple when combined with gemfibrozil. Gemfibrozil plus *pravastatin* (Pravachol) can increase blood-statin concentrations by more than 200%. When blood levels of a statin you're taking reach such high levels, it can increase risk for rhabdomyolysis.

***Option:*** Choose the fibrate fenofibrate. According to the FDA's Adverse Event Reporting System, reports of rhabdomyolysis are 15 times lower with this drug than with gemfibrozil. However, fenofibrate is much more expensive, and not all patients will tolerate this drug.

***Another option:*** Switch to the statin *fluvastatin* (Lescol). Unlike the three statins mentioned above, fluvastatin doesn't interact with gemfibrozil. For patients who must take one of the higher-intensity statins, such as *atorvastatin* (Lipitor), *rosuvastatin* (Crestor) or *pitavastatin* (Livalo), along with gemfibrozil, a lower statin dose can minimize the risk for side effects.

***Note:*** Because the degree of risk versus benefit is different for all drugs, just lowering the dose is not always an option.

• **Statin plus *warfarin*.** Patients who are candidates for statins may also require a blood thinner. Warfarin (Coumadin) is often prescribed for patients with a high risk for stroke, heart attack or blood clots (including those leading to a pulmonary embolism). It's also used in people who have had a previous stroke or damage to a heart valve.

***The risk:*** Statins may increase the effects of warfarin. When doses of warfarin are too high, it can lead to bleeding.

***Warning signs:*** Bleeding gums when brushing your teeth...bloody urine or dark stools due to internal bleeding...or sudden, unexplained fatigue (possibly due to anemia). Some reports have found that warfarin plus simvastatin can cause up to a 30% change in a patient's International Normalized Ratio (INR), a standard measure of how quickly blood clots.

***Option:*** Patients who show a marked change in INR might be advised to take pitavastatin or atorvastatin. They appear less likely to affect the INR than other statin drugs.

***Note:*** When you first combine warfarin with a statin, or when you change a statin dose, you should have frequent blood tests to check your INR so the warfarin dose can be adjusted if needed—for example, two or three tests in the first week of treatment. Once the drug effects have stabilized and you have good clotting control, testing can be scaled back to once or twice a month.

Or in some cases, patients may be able to switch to *rivaroxaban* (Xarelto) or another one of the newer blood thinners instead of warfarin.

• **Statin plus a calcium channel blocker.** Many patients with high cholesterol also have high blood pressure, stable angina or some heart irregularities (arrhythmias)—all of which may be treated with a calcium channel blocker.

***The risk:*** One drug in this class, *amlodipine* (Norvasc), may increase risk for muscle damage when combined with simvastatin or lovastatin. Other calcium channel blockers, such as *diltiazem* (Cardizem) and *verapamil* (Verelan), increase blood levels of simvastatin, atorvastatin and lovastatin.

***Options:*** The degree of interaction is lower when amlodipine is combined with atorvastatin or pravastatin. Some patients may report occasional fatigue or muscle pain, but the dose of one drug could be lowered to avoid side effects.

The combinations of diltiazem with lovastatin or simvastatin, or verapamil with the same statins, can cause "moderate" increases in statin levels. However, lowering the statin dose might be all that's needed to prevent side effects, such as muscle pain and fatigue.

• **Statin plus antiarrhythmic drugs.** Patients with heartbeat irregularities (arrhythmias) often need to combine a statin with an antiarrhythmic drug.

***The risks:*** Blood levels of *digoxin* (Lanoxin), a common drug in this class, may increase when it's combined with atorvastatin, leading to digoxin toxicity (nausea, vomiting, diarrhea, blurred vision, headaches and other symptoms). Patients who require this combination will need frequent tests (including blood tests) to detect toxicity before any troublesome symptoms kick in.

*Dronedarone* (Multaq), another antiarrhythmic agent, may increase blood levels of simvastatin, possibly leading to statin side effects.

Patients taking the antiarrhythmic drug *amiodarone* (Cordarone) may experience statin side effects when also using lovastatin or simvastatin.

***Options:*** It's generally safe to use a heart-rhythm drug with one of the following statins—rosuvastatin, atorvastatin, pitavastatin, fluvastatin or pravastatin.

In patients taking lovastatin or simvastatin with an antiarrhythmic that increases the statin's blood level, a lower statin dose may be used and/or blood tests may be given to check for muscle damage.

# 9 Little Ways to Keep Your Blood Pressure Low All Day Long

Samuel J. Mann, MD, professor of clinical medicine, New York Presbyterian Hospital/Weill-Cornell Medical College, New York City. He is a nationally recognized hypertension specialist and author of *Hypertension and You; Old Drugs, New Drugs, and the Right Drugs for Your High Blood Pressure.*

Whether your blood pressure is normal, borderline or high, you probably think of it as a Big Number. If it's less than 120/80, it's normal. If it's between that and 139/89, you've got borderline high blood pressure. If it's 140/90 or higher, that's high blood pressure.

But your blood pressure isn't just one reading—it fluctuates all day and night long. Everything from emotions to meals to alcohol to physical activity to aromas can make it go up—or down—throughout the day.

Blood pressure generally drops to its lowest levels when you're sleeping—by about 10% to 15%. Getting that nighttime "dip" is linked with the prevention of hypertension…and better control if you do develop it. That's why getting a good night's sleep is so important. The dip happens during the deepest "slow wave" phase of sleep. (Protecting that "dip" is also why people who take blood pressure medications should, unless otherwise instructed, take them at night.)

As you wake up, your blood pressure starts to rise and keeps rising throughout the day and then gradually falls in the late afternoon and evening. Since blood pressure is generally highest in the afternoon, that's a key time to avoid pressure-boosting stresses and to take pressure-lowering steps. *Here are suggestions from Samuel Mann, MD, professor of clinical medicine at New York Presbyterian Hospital/Weill-Cornell Medical College to do just that…*

## Stop…

• **Eating big meals.** A large meal can trigger the release of norepinephrine, one of the stress hormones that can raise blood pressure. Eat smaller, more frequent meals, especially in the afternoon and early evening when blood pressure is already on the rise.

• **Exposing yourself to BPA.** Bisphenol A (BPA), a hormone-disrupting synthetic chemical, is everywhere, including in many plastics, food-can linings and cash register receipts. Exposure may raise blood pressure—quickly. In one study, simply drinking a beverage from a can with BPA in the lining pushed up blood pressure by 5 points systolic (the upper number) over the next two hours.

***Bottom line:*** Avoid canned foods and beverages (unless specifically labeled BPA-free), look for BPA-free plastic bottles or glass bottles, and skip receipts if you don't need them.

• **Pouring that extra drink.** Moderate consumption of alcohol actually lowers systolic blood pressure by 2 to 4 points. But if you have more than one drink a day for women, two drinks for men, it can raise blood pressure. Binge drinking—four or more drinks for women, five or more for men, within two hours—is even worse. It not only raises blood pressure in the short term, but it's associated with an increased risk of developing chronic high blood pressure.

• **Drinking lots of coffee—if you're a slow metabolizer.** The jury is out on whether coffee—or caffeine in general—raises blood pressure significantly, but some studies show that drinking a lot of it (about 24 ounces a day) can raise it. One study published in *Journal of Hypertension* found that coffee raised adrenalin levels and blood pressure—but only in people whose bodies were slow to metabolize caffeine.

***Self-test to see if you are a slow metabolizer:*** Check your blood pressure for a baseline reading. Then drink some coffee, and check your blood pressure again an hour later. If systolic goes up 5 to 10 points you should cut back on caffeine.

## Start...

• **Taking mini exercise breaks.** Blood pressure actually rises slightly while exercising, but studies consistently show that it goes down soon after exercising, and the results last for as much as eight hours.

***If a long morning run or gym session isn't in the cards, there's good news:*** Spreading your exercise out over the day has blood pressure benefits. One study in *Medicine & Science in Sports & Exercise* of men with borderline high blood pressure (aka, prehypertension) showed that taking three 10-minute walks throughout the day was more effective at preventing increases in blood pressure than working out for 30 minutes once a day.

• **If you can't exercise, get up and stretch.** If exercise lowers blood pressure, the reverse—being sedentary—keeps it high. Just standing up can help. Another study in *Medicine & Science in Sports & Exercise* of overweight volunteers with prehypertension found that those who stood up for a total of two-and-a-half hours over an eight-hour day had better blood pressure readings than those who sat continuously for an eight-hour workday.

• **Calm yourself.** When stressors hit—whether you're fighting with your spouse or coping with a demanding boss—it's easy for blood pressure to rise. Anger can make your blood pressure go up. So does fear. Stress hormones raise levels of the enzyme renin, which boosts heart rate and constricts blood vessels. The stress surge will subside on its own...but you can speed the process using relaxation techniques. Just five minutes of deep breathing, for example, has been shown to lower blood pressure. So can short bouts of meditation. This is especially true if you practice meditation—then you can elicit the "relaxation response" in just two or three minutes.

• **Take a midday snooze.** An afternoon nap lowers blood pressure in people with hypertension. According to one study presented at a European Society of Cardiology conference, habitual mid-day snoozers (average nap was one hour) had blood pressure readings that were about 4% lower than people who didn't nap. Nappers had greater nighttime drops in blood pressure, and they needed less hypertension medication.

• **Breathe in the scent of lemon or lavender.** Aromatherapy can quickly lower blood pressure.

***Most effective scents:*** Lemon, lavender, peppermint, chamomile, neroli. In one study published in *Physiology & Behavior*, simply smelling oil of lemon for 15 minutes reduced blood pressure by about 5 points systolic (the upper number) and 3 points diastolic (the bottom number). Try putting two to

## Heart-Healthy Beverages

**Beer may be good for women's hearts.** Women who drank one or two beers per week had 30% lower risk for heart attack over three decades than those who drank beer several times per week/daily or never drank beer.

***Possible reason:*** Beer may reduce triglycerides, blood fats that can raise heart attack risk.

Study of about 1,500 women over more than 30 years by researchers at Sahlgrenska Academy, University of Gothenburg, Sweden, published in *Scandinavian Journal of Primary Health Care.*

**Enjoy your tea time.** Moderate tea drinkers (those who drank at least one cup of black or green tea every day) had less calcium buildup in their coronary arteries and a lower rate of cardiovascular events, such as heart attack, than those who drank less tea or the same amount of other beverages, such as coffee, according to a recent study of 6,500 adults.

***Possible reason:*** Antioxidants in tea may inhibit the formation of coronary artery calcium, a marker for potential heart disease.

Paul Elliott Miller, MD, instructor of medicine, The Johns Hopkins Hospital, Baltimore.

**You can't beat beet juice.** Drinking a 2.4-ounce glass of beet juice daily reduced systolic (top number) blood pressure by five to 10 points in a small, weeklong study of older patients with a common form of heart failure that affects the pumping ability of the left ventricle. A 24% boost in aerobic endurance was also reported. Beet juice tastes sweet and is packed with inorganic nitrate, a nutrient that has been shown to improve vascular health and oxygen metabolism.

Dalane Kitzman, MD, professor of cardiology, Wake Forest Baptist Medical Center, Winston-Salem, North Carolina.

four drops of essential oil on a cotton ball and keeping it in your office or at home...or putting just a drop or two on your pillow at night. You don't have to take a whiff to have the effect...just having it in the room helps.

Doing these little things doesn't get you off the hook to tackle big issues such as losing weight, eating a healthy diet, getting regular exercise and, if you have blood pressure that doesn't respond to these lifestyle changes, taking medication.

But sometimes the best way to accomplish the Big Things is to start with little things.

# Are Calcium Supplements Now Safe for Your Heart?

Connie Weaver, PhD, distinguished professor and head of the department of nutrition science at Purdue University in West Lafayette, Indiana. She is an expert on mineral bioavailability, calcium metabolism and bone health. She is author or editor of four books, including *Nutritional Influences on Bone Health*, and a member of the National Academy of Science's Institute of Medicine.

Until a few years ago, taking a daily calcium supplement was considered a safe, effective way to protect against the bone loss that comes with aging and to reduce the risk for fractures—especially for women, who are more prone to osteoporosis than men.

Then the standard advice came under fire...big time. Not only was serious doubt raised about calcium's usefulness in preventing fractures, but some studies suggested that calcium supplements actually cause harm—increasing the risk for heart disease.

Now a large recent British study—with more than half a million subjects—appears to show that calcium supplements actually are safe for your heart. Should we believe this study? Are calcium pills suddenly safe again? And even if they are, do we really need them to keep our bones strong?

To get answers, we spoke with Connie Weaver, PhD, distinguished professor and head of the department of nutrition science at Purdue University in West Lafayette, Indiana. She is a world-renowned mineral and bone-health expert.

## The Great Calcium/Heart Debate

***A little background:*** Until 2010, the only serious health concern from taking calcium was thought to be a very small increase in the risk for kidney stones. But that year, in a study published in *The BMJ*, New Zealand researchers analyzed several studies of people (mostly women over age 70) who took calcium supplements. They found that calcium supplements were associated with a 30% increase in the risk for heart attack and a smaller increase in the risk for stroke. Even calcium supplements that contain vitamin D, which other studies have suggested protects the heart, were associated with a small increased risk for heart attack and stroke, the same team reported in 2012.

Such statistical links can never be proof of causation, however, and from the start some researchers had their doubts about whether this danger would turn out to be real. The New Zealand researchers speculated that taking calcium supplements gives the body a surge in calcium all at once, which then ends up in our arteries and contributes to the formation of plaque, the substance that leads to atherosclerosis (hardening of the arteries). Yet animal studies conducted at Purdue University (and elsewhere) showed no such mechanism, notes Dr. Weaver. When animals were given high levels of calcium as supplements (or as dairy products), "there was no increased calcification of arteries."

Even the statistical link was an outlier. In a comprehensive review of studies by the U.S. Preventive Services Task Force (USPSTF), a government panel of 16 experts that evaluates health research and makes official health recommendations, none showed any increased cardiovascular risk.

The 2010 and 2012 calcium studies got plenty of press, though, and suddenly people were seriously worried that the calcium they were taking was hurting their hearts...and some stopped taking it.

The recent British study, presented in 2016 at the World Congress of Osteoporosis, Osteoarthritis, and Musculoskeletal Diseases, dealt a strong new blow against the heart-harm hypothesis. More than a half-million participants ages 40 to 69 were followed for seven years. Their use of calcium with or without vitamin D was tracked over the entire period of the study. Then the researchers analyzed their heart-disease–related hospitalizations and deaths, using hospital records.

***Result:*** No link was found between calcium or calcium/vitamin D supplementation and hospital admissions or death related to heart disease.

Bottom line? To Dr. Weaver, this large recent study—combined with the fact that nearly all other studies have found no heart risk and that careful animal studies find no plausible mechanism—makes a compelling case. Her conclusion? "The new research adds to the now large body of evidence that there is no cardiovascular risk of calcium supplementation."

## But Do You Need a Calcium Supplement?

Just because calcium pills are safe for the heart, though, doesn't mean you should take them. According to the USPSTF, there simply isn't enough evidence to recommend a calcium/vitamin D supplement for the prevention of fractures—even in postmenopausal women. It's true that in postmenopausal women, as well as in older men, calcium plus vitamin D supplements halt bone loss and modestly increase bone density, but there's no good evidence that any particular supplementation level will actually prevent fractures.

Still, there's no question that both calcium and vitamin D are important for bone health. For women age 51 and older (and men age 71 and older), the Institute of Medicine's current recommended dietary allowance (RDA) for calcium is 1,200 mg.

To get enough, and to protect your bone health, Dr. Weaver recommends an approach that starts with dietary calcium and vitamin D and looks to supplements only if necessary...

- **Eat plenty of calcium-rich foods,** especially dairy foods such as milk and yogurt (by far the most calcium-dense foods)—but also nondairy calcium-rich foods such as kale, broccoli and turnip greens. Nuts, especially almonds and hazelnuts, also are good sources of calcium, as are canned sardines and canned salmon (be sure to eat the bones).

***Tip:*** If you're a yogurt fan, eat some traditional American-style yogurt, not only Greek-style yogurt—traditional American has twice as much calcium, ounce for ounce.

- **Factor in fortified foods.** Many foods are fortified with calcium, including orange juice, breakfast cereal and soy foods such as tofu and soymilk. Remember to include these amounts when adding up your daily calcium intake.

- **If you're not getting enough dietary calcium,** discuss taking a supplement with your health-care provider. A typical serving of most dairy foods includes about 300 mg of calcium. Nondairy foods contribute, but you would need about three cups of cooked kale to get to that 300 mg. Add in the calcium in fortified foods that you eat daily (check labels), and if you're still below 1,200 mg, consider a supplement for just what you're missing.

- **For vitamin D,** the RDA is 600 IU for people age 70 and younger. For those 71 and older, the RDA is 800 IU. It's very hard to get this amount without taking a supplement.

- **Eat a wide variety of whole foods.** Many nutrients contribute to bone strength and the prevention of osteoporosis, not just calcium and vitamin D but also boron, manganese, silicon, zinc, magnesium and potassium. Eating enough protein is important, as is moderating how much sodium and caffeine you consume and eating plenty of fruits and vegetables. To increase your body's ability to absorb calcium, especially if you are over age 50, *Bottom Line's* medical consultant, naturopathic doctor Andrew Rubman, ND, advises also taking digestive enzyme supplements that include betaine HCL.

---

## Watch Your Numbers

Aggressive blood pressure treatment could save 100,000 lives a year. Current guidelines call for systolic pressure (top number) to be below 140 mmHg. But a recent study says that more lives would be saved with a goal of 120 mmHg or lower in people who are at high risk for heart disease.

***Caution:*** Too-low pressure can cause dizziness that can lead to falls and broken bones.

Analysis of a 2015 National Institutes of Health study led by researchers at Loyola University Medical Center, Maywood, Illinois, presented at a recent meeting of the American Heart Association.

---

## Don't Fall for These Blood Pressure Traps

Holly Kramer, MD, MPH, an associate professor in the department of public health sciences and the department of medicine, Division of Nephrology and Hypertension, at Loyola University Medical Center in Maywood, Illinois. She received the 2016 Garabed Eknoyan Award from the National Kidney Foundation.

---

When it comes to treating serious medical conditions, you would think that high blood pressure (hypertension) would be one of the nation's great success stories. Doctors test for it. Patients know the risks. And there are dozens of medications that treat it.

Yet the results are still disappointing. About one in every three American adults has hypertension…but only about half of them keep it under control.

Why are we still losing the battle against hypertension? Scientists now are discovering some of the traps that prevent people from adequately controlling their blood pressure. *What you need to know…*

***TRAP #1:*** **Not treating soon enough.** Even though normal blood pressure is defined as below 120/80 mmHg, researchers continue to debate optimal blood pressure targets. In reality, most doctors don't consider treatment until readings reach 140/90 mmHg or above—the official definition of hypertension.

But recent research has shown us that is too late. The risks associated with hypertension—stroke, heart attack, kidney disease and vision loss, among others—start to rise at lower levels.

***Important recent finding:*** When researchers compared target blood pressure readings in more than 9,350 adults with hypertension and other cardiovascular risk factors, the results were striking. Those who got intensive treatment to lower their systolic (top number) pressure to below 120 mmHg were 27% less likely to die from any cause over a three-year period than those whose target was below 140 mmHg. In the study, diastolic (bottom number) pressure was not measured because it tends to decline as people get older.

Starting treatment earlier than 140 mmHg to achieve a normal reading could save more than 100,000 American lives a year, the researchers estimated.

***My advice:*** If your systolic blood pressure is 120 mmHg or above (or your diastolic pressure is 90 mmHg or above), tell your doctor that you want to be treated.

***Note:*** If your systolic blood pressure is less than 150 mmHg, you may be able to avoid medication if you adopt healthier habits—not smoking…losing weight, if necessary…getting regular exercise…eating a well-balanced diet, etc. If these steps haven't lowered your blood pressure after six months, you may need medication. If systolic pressure is above 150 mmHg, medications may be needed in addition to lifestyle changes.

***Caution:*** Intensive blood pressure treatment usually involves taking multiple blood pressure–lowering drugs, which increases risk for side effects, such as dizziness and light-headedness. Therefore, blood pressure should be checked frequently (see below) and regular tests should be given for potassium and electrolyte levels. Electrolytes and kidney function should be checked within one month of starting a diuretic or when a dose is increased. After that, levels should be checked every six to 12 months.

***TRAP #2:*** **Not testing at home.** Don't rely only on the blood pressure tests that you get at your doctor's office. They can be too intermittent—and too rushed—to give accurate readings. Your pressure is likely to be artificially high…or artificially low, since people who are seeing a doctor often abstain from some of the things (such as drinking coffee) that raise it.

## Watch Out for Too Little Salt

Too little salt may be riskier than too much. The current recommendation is no more than 2.3 grams (g) of sodium a day—about one teaspoon of salt.

***However:*** In people without high blood pressure, consuming more than 7 g of salt was not associated with a rise in disease or death risk—but consuming less than 3 g was associated with a 26% higher risk for death or cardiovascular events such as heart disease or stroke. In people with high blood pressure, consuming more than 7 g daily was associated with 23% higher risk, but consuming less than 3 g was associated with an even higher risk—34%.

Review of four studies including 133,118 people across 49 countries by researchers at McMaster University, Hamilton, Ontario, Canada, published in *The Lancet.*

***My advice:*** Buy a digital blood pressure monitor, and use it at home. Omron upper-arm blood pressure monitors (available at pharmacies and online for about $40 and up) are about as accurate as office monitors. A *JAMA* study found that 72% of people who tested at home had good blood pressure control versus 57% of volunteers who were tested only by their doctors.

***What to do:*** Every day, check your blood pressure in the morning before eating, exercising or taking medication…and again in the evening. (If your blood pressure is normal, test every few months.)

Before testing, empty your bladder (a full bladder will cause higher readings). Then sit with both feet on the floor, and relax for five minutes. Rest your arm, raised to the level of your heart, on a table, and place the cuff on bare skin.

***Do each reading twice:*** Measure your blood pressure once…wait a few minutes…then repeat—the second reading will be more accurate. Write down the readings, and share them with your doctor during your office visits.

***TRAP #3:* Taking the wrong drug.** About 70% of patients with hypertension require two or more drugs to achieve good control. Many will be given prescriptions for one of the newer drugs, such as an angiotensin-converting enzyme (ACE) inhibitor or an angiotensin receptor blocker (ARB). Some patients (such as those with heart failure) will need one of these drugs. Most people do not—at least not right away.

If you've recently been diagnosed with hypertension, consider a thiazide diuretic, such as chlorthalidone. It's an older drug that is available as a generic. It costs pennies a day, and studies have shown that thiazide diuretics lower blood pressure as effectively as other drugs, with less risk for heart failure and stroke. Thiazide diuretics may be paired with an ARB or ACE inhibitor, since these drugs are synergistic (each drug increases the other's effectiveness).

***The caveats:*** Even though diuretics generally are safe, you'll urinate more often (they're known as "water pills" for a reason). Thiazide diuretics might also lower potassium levels in some patients—if so, your doctor may advise you to take potassium supplements. And diuretics can raise urate levels, triggering gout in some people.

***TRAP #4:* Not timing your medication.** Most people take medications when it's convenient—or at a set time, such as with their morning coffee. But blood pressure medication should be scheduled.

It's natural for blood pressure to vary by about 30 points at different times of the day. It almost always rises in the morning, which is why strokes and heart attacks are more common in the early hours. One study found that patients who took at least one of their blood pressure medications at night were about one-third less likely to have a heart attack or stroke than those who took all of their pills in the morning.

***My advice:*** With your doctor's OK, take at least one of your blood pressure medications (not a diuretic) at bedtime to help protect you from blood pressure increases in the morning. Diuretics should be taken in the morning so that frequent urination won't interrupt sleep.

## High Blood Pressure: A Silver Lining for Ovarian Cancer Patients?

Roswell Park Cancer Institute, news release.

A woman's prognosis after an ovarian cancer diagnosis may be affected by a number of unexpected factors, recent research suggests.

The study found that diabetes is linked to a 12% higher risk of death for women with ovarian cancer. The research also showed that women with a specific type of ovarian cancer actually seemed to benefit from having a high blood pressure (hypertension) diagnosis.

"This is a coincidental and unintended consequence of hypertension and its treatment," said study co-lead author Kirsten Moysich. She's a professor of oncology at Roswell Park Cancer Institute in Buffalo, New York.

"But it's a silver lining to a serious but largely manageable medical condition that has reached epidemic prevalence in the US and many other countries worldwide," Moysich said in an institute news release.

The researchers reviewed data from 15 studies of women. All had invasive epithelial ovarian cancer. The study didn't find an overall association between high blood pressure or heart disease and death risk.

However, high blood pressure was linked to a 46% lower risk of progression for women with endometrioid ovarian cancer. This type of cancer is a subtype of epithelial ovarian cancer. Endometrioid ovarian cancer usually has better outcomes, the researchers said.

It's possible that medications to treat high blood pressure may play a role, the study authors suggested.

The study only found an association—not a cause-and-effect link—between ovarian cancer outcomes and conditions such as diabetes and high blood pressure. The study authors said more research is needed.

"Our findings emphasize the importance of understanding the full clinical profile for women with ovarian cancer in order to predict ovarian cancer outcomes," said co-lead author Albina Minlikeeva, a postdoctoral research affiliate at the institute.

Normally, doctors and researchers look at only clinical factors, such as the stage of a tumor, when predicting cancer prognosis, she said.

More than 22,000 cases of ovarian cancer are diagnosed each year in the United States, and about 14,000 women die from the disease, the researchers said.

The study was published recently in the journal *Cancer Causes & Control.*

## Loss Can Be Heartbreaking

Losing an intimate partner raises risk for atrial fibrillation (Afib)—an irregular heartbeat linked to stroke and heart attack—especially for people under age 60.

***Details:*** In a recent study of nearly one million adults, the newly bereaved were 41% more likely to develop Afib in the first 30 days after a partner's death. Risk was even higher when the death was unexpected.

***Why:*** Severe stress may trigger inflammation and disrupt heart rhythm.

Simon Graff, MD, researcher, department of public health, Aarhus University, Denmark.

## Think Positive!

Researchers have found that heart patients who were encouraged to be optimistic about postsurgical outcomes did better at six months than those who weren't encouraged to expect the best.

*BMC Medicine.*

## What a Tender Temple Could Mean...

Alan M. Rapoport, MD, clinical professor of neurology, David Geffen School of Medicine at UCLA, Los Angeles, and immediate past president of the International Headache Society.

A tender temple should not be ignored. Tenderness of the temple that's accompanied by symptoms such as headache, scalp tenderness, fever, pain in the jaw when chewing, fatigue, weight loss and vision loss can signal a condition known as giant cell arteritis (GCA)—sometimes referred to as temporal arteritis.

Most common in people over age 50, this inflammatory condition typically affects the temporal artery but can affect other medium- and large-sized arteries throughout the body as well, especially those within the brain and eye. The cause of this condition is inflammation in the lining of the arteries, but the reason for the inflammation is not known.

If GCA is untreated, it can lead to devastating, irreversible consequences including stroke, permanent vision loss, damage or rupture of the aorta and even death.

***Important:*** You should see your doctor right away for a thorough evaluation. This exam typically includes a blood test to measure a marker of inflammation (erythrocyte sedimentation rate, or ESR), which may be followed by a biopsy from the temporal artery.

GCA is treated with corticosteroids. If it's treated promptly, most people with GCA recover fully, but relapses are common.

## Post-Heart Attack Danger Is Real

Nearly 25% of people who had a heart attack developed heart failure within four years, in a recent study of nearly 25,000 heart attack survivors. Risk for post–heart attack heart failure was even higher in those who also had atrial fibrillation (abnormal heartbeat)...diabetes...and/or chronic obstructive pulmonary disease (COPD).

***If you've had a heart attack:*** Make sure your doctor monitors you for symptoms of heart failure, such as edema and shortness of breath.

Johannes Gho, MD, PhD, cardiology resident, University Medical Center Utrecht, the Netherlands.

## Better Cardiac Rehab

Heart disease patients who attended weekly group stress-management sessions in addition to exercise-based cardiac rehabilitation were half as likely to have complications, such as stroke, heart attack, recurrent angina or even death, as those in a cardiac-rehab group without stress management. Both groups had better cardiac biomarkers than those who didn't participate in cardiac rehab.

James A. Blumenthal, PhD, professor of psychiatry and behavioral sciences, Duke University School of Medicine, Durham, North Carolina.

## Fish Oil and Heart Attack

Adults who took high doses (4 g per day) of fish oil supplements for six months after a heart attack had better heart function and less scarring of heart muscle than those who didn't take fish oil, according to a recent study of 360 heart attack survivors.

***Possible reason:*** Omega-3 fatty acids in fish oil reduce inflammation that harms the heart.

***Important:*** Check with your doctor before taking fish oil—it can interact with blood thinners and certain other medications.

Raymond Kwong, MD, MPH, director, cardiac magnetic resonance imaging, Brigham and Women's Hospital, Boston.

## Marry for Healthy Heart

Married people recover better from heart surgery than unmarried people.

***Recent finding:*** 28.8% of patients who were divorced or separated and 33.8% of those who were widowed died or developed a new dependency, such as being unable to walk, bathe or dress themselves, within two years of their operation, versus only 20% of patients who were married.

Study of 1,567 people by researchers at Perelman School of Medicine, University of Pennsylvania, Philadelphia, published in *JAMA Surgery.*

# The Best Way to Reverse AFib (It's Not Drugs or Surgery)

Study titled "Long-Term Effect of Goal-Directed Weight Management in an Atrial Fibrillation Cohort" by researchers at University of Adelaide, Australia, et al., published in *Journal of the American College of Cardiology*.

Prashanthan Sanders, MBBS, PhD, director, Centre for Heart Rhythm Disorders, and Knapman-NHF Chair of Cardiology Research, University of Adelaide, and director, Cardiac Electrophysiology and Pacing, Royal Adelaide Hospital, both in Australia.

If you're diagnosed with atrial fibrillation, commonly known as AFib—a chronic condition that creates abnormal heart rhythms, increasing the risk for stroke and heart failure—your doctor may prescribe medications that you need to take for life, and, if that doesn't work, advise a surgical procedure. Not only does each approach have risks, but in many cases you're only controlling the condition, not treating the reasons you have it.

There's a better way.

If you do it the right way, you can virtually reverse this life-threatening condition—while simultaneously dramatically reducing your risk for heart disease and diabetes, finds a recent Australian long-term study. You may wind up needing no medications for this condition at all—and no surgery.

What is this revolutionary new treatment? It's actually pretty old-fashioned—weight loss and managing the associated risk factors such as elevated blood pressure, blood cholesterol and blood sugar. But we're not talking about quick weight-loss schemes here—and losing weight and then regaining a lot of it back can actually backfire, the researchers found.

The good news is that many of the participants in this research lost weight and kept it off for five years. There are lessons here for anyone who needs to lose weight for health.

For someone with AFib, it could be lifesaving.

## The 10% Solution

Obesity is a well-established risk factor for AFib, but the Australian researchers wanted to know the long-term impact of weight loss on heart-rhythm control in obese people with AFib. They were specifically looking at how much weight loss was necessary to see benefits and what the effect of losing and regaining weight (a common occurrence in dieters) would have on AFib.

They studied 355 overweight or obese AFib patients, who were offered weight-loss programs, and followed in a weight-loss registry for five years. To qualify, a 5'10" man would need to weigh more than 188 pounds, although in practice the average weight for someone that height was 235 pounds. Some lost less than 3% of their starting body weight...others lost between 3% and 9%... and some lost at least 10% (an average of 35 pounds). *Results...*

- **The 135 participants who lost at least 10%** were six times more likely to be free from arrhythmia without any need for medication than 220 participants who lost less weight.
- **Losing weight led to normal heart rhythms for many without any need for medication.** That was true for 46% of those who lost at least 10% of their weight...22% of those who lost 3% to 9% of their body weight...and 13% of those who lost less than 3% of their body weight.
- **Two-thirds of the patients who lost at least 10% of their weight were able to maintain the weight loss.**
- **Those who lost more than 10% of their weight had markedly better control of their associated risk factors.**
- **The benefits were drastically reduced in those whose weight fluctuated by more than 5%,** possibly because repeated loss and regain causes physical changes in the heart and can increase the risk for high blood pressure and diabetes. Looking at all the participants, including those still taking medications, researchers found that 85% of the group that lost 10% of their body weight and kept it off were free of AFib—compared with

only 44% among those whose weight fluctuated 5% or more.

Researchers don't know exactly how losing weight improves AFib, but obesity causes a number of conditions that are all risk factors for AFib, such as impaired glucose tolerance, high cholesterol, hypertension and sleep apnea. Weight loss in obese patients reduces these risk factors. In fact, the study found that those who lost weight also had reduced blood pressure, better glucose control, lower cholesterol numbers and reduced inflammation. All in all, they were simply much healthier.

Results often happen quickly. With the loss of five or more pounds, patients start feeling much better. Soon they notice they have less AFib and so they become more motivated.

## The Best Way to Lose Weight

The study also demonstrated that losing weight and keeping it off for years is definitely possible—with the right type of program and support system. The weight-loss program in this study included motivational counseling in a physician-led weight-management program, with regular in-person visits to discuss goals, progress and outcomes—and extra visits if patients requested them. The diet was high protein, low glycemic and calorie-controlled. Most patients just adapted their own eating habits to the guidelines—only 1% to 2% needed meal replacements.

The first lesson was participation—those who followed up more often with the clinic staff were more likely to keep the weight off. *The success of dieters depends on a few key factors...*

- **Individualization.** Look at your own dietary habits, and identify where there is room for improvement. Keep a diary of your food intake and exercise. Specific diets were not the answer. It's more a matter of where you can pare down your diet and how to avoid those foods that are causing trouble. For most people in the Australia diet program, the focus was on eliminating snacking between meals, reducing carbs and sugars, paring meal portions and limiting alcohol.
- **Reasonable goals.** Set achievable, progressive targets to provide a sense of success.
- **Support system.** It's important to have someone to answer to or check in with. While the Australian study relied solely on physicians to help patients identify their problem areas, you can rely on a dietician or nutritionist, says Dr. Sanders. The subjects in the study met with someone once every three months, but those who were having trouble losing weight talked with or e-mailed their doctors weekly.
- **Increased physical activity.** This is important for everyone on a weight-loss program, but anyone with AFib needs to take special precautions. Talk first with your cardiologist and then, if given the green light, set small and achievable goals based on your current level of exercise. For example, if you're walking 10 minutes a day, gradually increase so you're walking 20 minutes on some days and work up to 30 minutes of brisk walking every day. In this study, participants were told to do low-intensity exercise for 20 minutes a day three times a week and then increase that to at least 200 minutes of moderate-intensity activity per week—50 minutes four days a week, for example.
- **Regular medical evaluations—especially for medications.** While waiting for weight loss, make sure you work with your doctor to manage other risk factors that cause AFib, such as high blood pressure, diabetes, sleep apnea. As your weight loss progresses, you may need lower doses—or be able to stop some medications entirely. The treatment for these risk factors needs to be regularly evaluated. Often, with weight loss, patients can be weaned off.

## A New Approach to AFib

Currently, if you have AFib, your doctor will discuss medications and possible surgical approaches—and, if you're lucky, mention lifestyle. The new research suggests that the order should be the opposite—the first line of treatment for someone with AFib is to treat the risk factors, including obesity, that led to it.

For each risk factor that is applicable, work with your doctor to set achievable goals and supervise its management. If, after trying this, you continue to have symptoms, then consider appropriate rhythm-control strategies—such as catheter ablation, in which tiny areas in the heart that are responsible for the abnormal electrical impulses are destroyed.

***The good news:*** Even if you do need treatment, any weight loss you've achieved will likely improve your results. For ablation, for example, patients who lose weight and reduce other risk factors are five times more likely to have their hearts remain in a normal rhythm.

# AFib May Be Linked to Cancer

Women diagnosed with the heart-rhythm abnormality AFib are 48% more likely to be diagnosed with cancer than women without AFib. But this does not mean that AFib causes cancer—more likely, there are underlying risk factors for both conditions, including smoking and obesity.

***Self-defense:*** Lose weight if you are overweight...quit smoking...exercise regularly.

David Conen, MD, MPH, cardiology researcher at Basel University Hospital, Basel, Switzerland, and leader of a 20-year study published in *JAMA Cardiology.*

# Have Your Green Veggies and Coumadin, Too

Timothy S. Harlan, MD, associate professor of medicine at the Tulane University School of Medicine in New Orleans. He is author of *The Dr. Gourmet Diet for Coumadin Users* and *Vegetable Recipes for Coumadin Users.* DrGourmet.com

Could a spinach salad ever be considered dangerous? That may sound impossible. But if you're one of the millions of Americans who takes the popular blood thinner *warfarin* (Coumadin, Jantoven, Marevan, etc.) to help prevent stroke, heart attack or pulmonary embolism, chances are your doctor has told you to limit your intake of spinach and other vitamin K–rich foods.

It's true that vitamin K promotes blood clotting, and consuming too many foods that contain abundant amounts of this nutrient could weaken warfarin's effect.

Taken to the extreme, however, this dietary advice often causes warfarin users to become fearful of eating any of the highly nutritious foods that contain vitamin K.

What many people don't realize is that following this guideline too strictly creates almost as much of a problem as getting too much of this crucial nutrient, which has been shown to promote heart and bone health.

***The solution:*** There is a simple way that you can have your warfarin—and your green veggies, too! *Here's how...*

## The Stay-Safe Formula

If you watch TV, you've no doubt seen plenty of ads for the newer generation of blood thinners, such as *apixaban* (Eliquis), *rivaroxaban* (Xarelto) and *dabigatran* (Pradaxa). These medications work similarly to warfarin by blocking production of blood-clotting proteins in the body, but they use a different mechanism that doesn't require vitamin K vigilance.

Even though these newer blood-thinning drugs are being prescribed more and more, warfarin is still the most widely used medication for stroke and heart attack patients.

But the use of warfarin requires a delicate balancing act that weighs the risk for excessive bleeding against the risk for unwanted clotting. To keep tabs on how long it takes a patient's blood to clot, frequent blood testing is used (initially on a daily basis, then gradually decreased until a target level has been reached) to determine the patient's INR, which stands for "international normalized ratio." For most patients, the target for this standardized measurement ranges from about 2.0 to 3.0.

***Other risks:*** In addition to the dietary considerations, warfarin interacts with a number of medications (such as certain antibiotics, other heart medications, cholesterol drugs and antidepressants) as well as supplements (including St. John's wort and ginkgo biloba).

***Dr. Harlan's stay-safe formula:*** There is no definitive research pointing to optimal levels of vitamin K for warfarin users, but I find that most patients thrive on a plan in which their daily intake of this vitamin is about 75 micrograms (mcg) per day—a level that is lower than the recommended daily allowance for adults (90 mcg per day for women...and 120 mcg per day for men). That intake of vitamin K seems to strike the balance between offering an adequate amount of healthful foods rich in the vitamin while allowing warfarin to do its job.

## A New Way to Eat Vitamin K

It's amazing to see how much the vitamin K content varies depending on the food. Some foods are absolute vitamin K powerhouses—one cup of raw parsley, for example, has a whopping 984 mcg...one cup of cooked spinach contains 888 mcg...and one cup of raw kale, 547 mcg. *Note*: Cooking a vegetable will decrease its volume, but won't change the vitamin K content.

To avoid slipping into a vitamin K danger zone, I advise warfarin users to regularly incorporate vegetables with low-to-moderate amounts of vitamin K into their diet (up to 20 mcg per serving).

***Good choices (serving sizes are one cup unless otherwise indicated):*** Arugula (one-half cup), beets, carrots, celery (one stalk), corn, eggplant, sweet red or green peppers, peas (one-half cup), turnips, tomatoes and zucchini.

Other foods that are naturally low in vitamin K include most fruits, cereals, grains, beans, seeds and tubers (such as white potatoes, sweet potatoes and yams).

***A good rule of thumb:*** Stick to side dishes with 20 mcg to 25 mcg of vitamin K per serving and main courses with 35 mcg to 40 mcg per serving. That should keep you at a safe level.

But what if you reach your daily limit and are still craving some sautéed greens or a big kale salad? Don't despair. You can still enjoy these foods...as long as your intake of vitamin K is consistent.

This means that you can exceed 75 mcg of vitamin K per day—but you must consume the same amount of the vitamin every day. So, you can have a spinach salad, but you need to eat that same size salad (or another dish with an equivalent amount of vitamin K) every single day.

***Important:*** Be sure to first tell your doctor if you plan to increase your intake of vitamin K so that you can be closely monitored and, if needed, your dose of warfarin adjusted. The frequency of monitoring depends on the patient's specific circumstances.

***To find the vitamin K content of various foods:*** Go to Dr. Harlan's website, DrGourmet.com/md/warfarincomprehensive.pdf.

## The "Safe" List

Unless you're a nutritionist, you probably don't know the vitamin K content of most foods off the top of your head. *To help you stay safe when you're close to reaching your limit of the vitamin, here are some healthful foods that contain virtually no vitamin K in a single serving...*

Acorn squash...raw mushrooms ...cooked grits...yellow sweet pepper...cooked salmon, halibut or sole...cooked pork...light-meat turkey (no skin)...lemon, lime or orange...almonds...nonfat sour cream...rosemary, garlic powder or ground allspice, ginger or nutmeg.

## Hot Peppers May Protect Against Heart Disease

Hot peppers may protect against heart disease. People who regularly ate hot red chili peppers were 13% less likely to die during a two-decade period—mainly because the group had fewer deaths from heart attack or stroke. The reason for hot peppers' protective effect is not known, but it may be related to the peppers' content of capsaicin, a compound that can improve coronary blood flow.

Benjamin Littenberg, MD, professor of medicine, University of Vermont College of Medicine, Burlington, and coauthor of a study of data on 16,179 Americans, published in *PLOS ONE*.

## What You Don't Know About Heart Attacks Could Kill You

Suzanne Steinbaum, DO, attending cardiologist and director of Women and Heart Disease, Lenox Hill Hospital, New York City. Trained as a DO and board-certified as an MD, she combines the holistic approach of osteopathy with conventional medicine. Dr. Steinbaum lectures nationally on cardiovascular health and has appeared on numerous TV shows, including *The Doctors, The Early Show, Good Morning America, Dr. Oz* and *20/20*. She also is author of *Dr. Suzanne Steinbaum's Heart Book*. SRSheart.com

Heart disease has historically been thought of as a man's disease, but it turns out that it is the number-one killer of women. We recently spoke with cardiologist Suzanne Steinbaum on what women need to know about heart health.

*What should every woman know about heart disease?*

***Dr. Suzanne Steinbaum:*** Heart disease is the number-one killer of all women, greater than all cancers combined. It is critical for all women to understand that 80% to 90% of the time, heart disease is preventable. So if she knows her family history and pays attention to her risk factors, she can actually prevent heart disease from happening to her.

*What are the differences in heart attack symptoms between men and women?*

***Dr. Steinbaum:*** Men oftentimes get chest pain—it's very classic. In women, we know that two weeks before a heart event, very often there might be sleep disturbances or flulike symptoms or even shortness of breath or chest discomfort. And during a heart attack, one of the most common symptoms is shortness of breath or chest pain. There could be jaw pain, back pain, arm pain, nausea and, again, that flulike symptom. But if a woman finds herself having difficulty doing things that she used to do...especially when combined with these symptoms...then she needs to go see her doctor, because maybe something is wrong with her heart.

*What about women's need to take care of everybody else—does that play a factor in all of this?*

***Dr. Steinbaum:*** Women are under an exorbitant amount of stress today. It is so important that every woman pays attention to her health and her heart, and reaches out not only to doctors for support, but to all levels of emotional and physical care, whether it be from friends, therapists, psychologists, psychiatrists. Sometimes women ignore all symptoms, and in women, depression, which is very, very common, is something that is dismissed. Women need to put themselves first, before they can take care of anyone else.

The bottom line on women and heart disease is that women's risk factors and symptoms are often ignored, so make sure your doctor is keeping an eye on them, and so are you.

# Chapter 2

# CANCER BREAKTHROUGHS

## Good News for Older Women with Early Form of Breast Cancer

Older women treated for a very early form of breast cancer, called ductal carcinoma in situ (DCIS), do not have an overall increased risk of early death compared with their peers, a recent study finds.

"Being diagnosed with DCIS can be extremely distressing, and research indicates that many women overestimate the risks involved and are confused about treatment. This study should provide reassurance that a diagnosis of DCIS does not raise the risk of dying," said Lotte Elshof, MD. She is an epidemiologist at the Netherlands Cancer Institute in Amsterdam.

Dr. Elshof presented the findings at the European Cancer Congress in Amsterdam.

### About DCIS

According to the National Breast Cancer Foundation, DCIS "is a noninvasive cancer where abnormal cells have been found in the lining of the breast milk duct. The atypical cells have not spread outside of the ducts into the surrounding breast tissue. Ductal carcinoma in situ is very early cancer that is highly treatable."

Untreated, DCIS can progress into invasive life-threatening breast cancer. However, it is usually treated with either surgery alone, or a combination of surgery and radiation therapy.

### Study Details

To determine the prognosis of older women diagnosed with DCIS, Dr. Elshof's team tracked 10-year outcomes for 10,000 Dutch women who were diagnosed with the condition between 1989 and 2004.

Women older than 50 who had been treated for DCIS actually had a 10% lower risk of dying from all causes combined, compared with women in the general population, the researchers found.

Specifically, the DCIS patients were less likely to die from other types of cancer and

Lotte Elshof, MD, research physician and epidemiologist, Netherlands Cancer Institute, Amsterdam.

Philip Poortmans, MD, PhD, president-elect, European Cancer Organization, Brussels.

Eleonora Teplinsky, MD, medical oncologist, Northwell Health Cancer Institute, Lake Success, New York.

Stephanie Bernik, MD, chief, surgical oncology, Lenox Hill Hospital, New York City.

European Cancer Congress, news release.

from circulatory, respiratory and digestive diseases, the findings showed.

"It might seem surprising that this group of women actually has a lower mortality rate than the general population. However, the vast majority would have been diagnosed via breast screening, which suggests they may be health-conscious and well enough to participate in screening," Dr. Elshof explained.

The study also looked at the risk of death from breast cancer. The investigators found that women treated for DCIS had a 2.5% risk of breast cancer death after 10 years, and a 4% risk after 15 years.

Both of those rates are higher than in the general population, Dr. Elshof's team noted. However, rates were lower in women whose DCIS had been diagnosed more recently, the study authors added.

And Philip Poortmans, MD, PhD, president-elect of the European Cancer Organization, pointed out that "the increased risk of dying from breast cancer is completely offset by a lower risk of dying from other causes compared to women in the general population."

## Expert Commentary

Two US oncologists who reviewed the new study said it should reassure patients.

"The important take-away message is that women diagnosed with DCIS can be expected to live to a normal age as a whole," said Stephanie Bernik, MD. She is chief of surgical oncology at Lenox Hill Hospital in New York City.

However, she agreed with the authors that there's a good explanation as to why women with DCIS tended to have better life expectancy than other women.

"If a woman is diagnosed with breast cancer, she will find herself with doctors' visits at every turn," Dr. Bernik noted. "This group of women is often encouraged to go to their primary medical doctor for any issue that may arise and screening for other cancers is more likely to occur. This may explain why women diagnosed with DCIS have a better overall survival."

### Three Step-Plan Lowers Breast Cancer Risk

Women can lower their risk for breast cancer by one-third by maintaining a healthy body weight...getting at least 30 minutes of moderate-intensity exercise daily...and avoiding alcohol or limiting it to no more than one drink per day.

Alice Bender, MS, RDN, head of nutrition programs, American Institute for Cancer Research, Washington, DC.

Eleonora Teplinsky, MD, is an oncologist at Northwell Health Cancer Institute in Lake Success, New York. She called the recent study "excellent," and said the next steps should look at "factors that contribute to the progression of DCIS to invasive disease."

The U.S. National Cancer Institute has more on DCIS at Cancer.gov, Search "DCIS."

# Soy Safe, Even Protective, for Breast Cancer Survivors

Fang Fang Zhang, MD, PhD, assistant professor, epidemiology, Friedman School of Nutrition Science and Policy, Tufts University, Boston.

Omer Kucuk, MD, professor, hematology and medical oncology, and director, Integrative Medicine Center, Emory University Winship Cancer Institute, Atlanta.

*Cancer*, online.

The pros and cons of soy for breast cancer patients have been debated for years.

Now, research involving more than 6,200 breast cancer survivors finds that those who ate the most soy had a lower risk of death from all causes during the nearly 10-year follow-up period.

"We didn't find any harmful effects of women diagnosed with breast cancer consuming soy in terms of mortality," said study leader Fang Fang Zhang, MD, PhD. She's an assistant professor of epidemiology at Tufts University's Friedman School of Nutrition Science and Policy in Boston.

"Overall, consuming higher levels of soy is associated with a 21% reduction in the risk of death compared to women who consumed soy at a lower level," she said.

Concerns around soy's "risk/benefit" profile have arisen because the food has estrogen-like compounds called isoflavones. That's important, experts say, because in so-called hormone-receptor positive breast cancers—the most common tumor type—higher estrogen levels may spur cancer cells' growth.

But the recent study should settle the soy controversy once and for all, said Omer Kucuk, MD, a professor of medical oncology and director of the Integrative Medicine Center at Emory University's Winship Cancer Institute, in Atlanta.

He wrote an editorial accompanying the study, which was published in the journal *Cancer*.

Dr. Kucuk said the study's large population is one point in its favor. The recent findings also echo the results of a prior study that found higher soy intake lowered the odds of breast cancer's return.

"When you have decreased recurrence, you have decreased mortality," Dr. Kucuk noted.

"I think now we can say women with breast cancer should not worry about eating edamame, miso soup, tofu and other soy products, and [to] drink soy milk," Dr. Kucuk said.

## Study Details

All of the 6,200 participants in the recent study were enrolled in the Breast Cancer Family Registry, which began in 1995. At the study's start, the women averaged 52 years of age.

During the study, just over 1,200 of the participants died.

Dr. Zhang's team tracked data on all the women's diets, some obtained even before they had received their diagnosis of breast cancer.

The researchers found an association between higher soy intake and better survival after breast cancer diagnosis. However, the study wasn't designed to prove cause-and-effect.

Still, Dr. Zhang's team noted that the benefit was strongest for women who did not have hormone-receptor positive cancers—the type that's sensitive to estrogen. These women had a 50% reduced risk of dying from any cause during the follow-up.

Women who had never taken hormone therapy as breast cancer treatment also appeared to gain a substantial benefit from high soy intake—they had a 32% reduced risk of death during the follow-up period.

## Amount of Soy Eaten

How much soy was needed to see an effect? According to the researchers, women in the "low-soy" group ate less than 0.3 milligrams (mg) of soy isoflavones daily, while those in the highest took in 1.5 mg or more. Most women ate more than 1.5 mg/day, with the average intake being 1.8 mg of soy isoflavones daily.

But even that amount is not a lot of soy, Dr. Zhang said. An intake of 1.8 mg, she noted, is equal to about one-half to one full serving of soy foods, such as soybeans or tofu, per week.

## Possible Reasons for Benefit of Soy

The experts could only speculate as to why soy might be protective against breast cancer death.

"The plant-based estrogen, once it attaches to the surface of the cell, makes estrogen less likely to be able to attach to the same cell," Dr. Zhang pointed out. In essence, the soy isoflavone bumps estrogen out of its preferred spot on the cancer cell, keeping its effects at bay.

Another idea, Dr. Zhang said, is that the soy components may inhibit the growth of nutrient-rich blood vessels that help feed a tumor.

## Expert Advice

Most women—especially those in the United States, where soy consumption is lower—don't need to worry about taking in too much soy, Dr. Kucuk noted. In Asian countries, intakes of 20 to 25 mg of soy isoflavones a day are not unusual, he said.

"If you drink a glass of soy milk, that is about 27 mg of soy isoflavones," he said.

There's more on soy and breast cancer at the Fred Hutchinson Cancer Center, FredHutch.org. Search "soy and cancer survivors."

# Flossing Fights Breast Cancer

Risk of developing breast cancer is 14% higher in postmenopausal women with periodontal disease than in those without the condition, according to recent research. Harmful mouth bacteria may travel into the bloodstream and affect breast tissue.

Jo Freudenheim, PhD, professor of epidemiology and environmental health, University at Buffalo, New York.

## Better Mammograms

Digital breast tomosynthesis (DBT, also known as 3-D mammography), increased cancer detection and resulted in fewer false-positives than traditional two-dimensional mammography in nearly 24,000 women recently studied over a four-year period. DBT provides radiologists with a clearer view of overlapping layers of breast tissue. The test has a bit more radiation than a conventional mammogram and may be covered by insurance.

Emily Conant, MD, chief of breast imaging, Hospital of the University of Pennsylvania, Philadelphia.

# Many Women Who Get Breast Cancer Gene Test Don't Need It

Fangjian Guo, MD, PhD, assistant professor of obstetrics and gynecology, University of Texas Medical Branch at Galveston.

University of Texas Medical Branch at Galveston, news release.

An increasing number of American women who don't have breast or ovarian cancer are being tested for BRCA1 and BRCA2 gene mutations associated with those diseases, a recent study shows.

## About the Breast Cancer Gene Test

Mutations in the BRCA1 and BRCA2 genes significantly increase a woman's risk of breast cancer. These mutations are linked to 5% to 10% of all breast cancer and about 15% of ovarian cancers, the U.S. National Cancer Institute says.

## Study Findings

The recent study found that more than 60% of BRCA tests are done on women without breast or ovarian cancer. In 2004, that number was just 24%.

This increase is likely due to increased marketing of BRCA testing. This may lead women at low risk for BRCA mutations to self-refer for testing, the researchers said.

While the number of low-risk women being tested has increased, BRCA testing is being underused by at-risk women, the study noted.

The study was published in the *American Journal of Preventive Medicine.*

## Implications

"Next-generation sequencing technologies are dramatically reducing costs for genetic testing and sequencing. However, current guidelines and practices are not always identifying women who carry BRCA mutations," said lead investigator Fangjian Guo, MD, PhD, from the University of Texas Medical Branch at Galveston.

BRCA testing strategies that promote equal access and rational use of BRCA testing and also maximize the detection of mutation carriers are needed, Dr. Guo said.

### Recommendation for Testing

If women are considered high-risk because of personal or family history of breast or ovarian cancer, the U.S. Preventive Services Task Force recommends BRCA testing.

The U.S. National Cancer Institute has more on BRCA gene mutations and testing at Cancer.gov. Search "BRCA gene testing."

## IVF Does Not Raise Breast Cancer Risk

IVF (in vitro fertilization) involves raising certain sex hormones to five or 10 times their normal level, and high levels of two of the hormones—estrogen and progesterone—can increase risk for breast cancer.

***Recent finding:*** After more than two decades, there was no increase in breast cancer risk among women who had IVF or other, less intensive treatments to improve fertility.

Study of more than 25,000 Dutch women by researchers at Netherlands Cancer Institute, Amsterdam, published in *JAMA*.

## Many Breast Cancer Survivors Don't Get Life-Extending Therapy

Dezheng Huo, MD, PhD, associate professor of public health sciences, University of Chicago.
University of Chicago Medical Center, news release.

Hormonal therapies such as *tamoxifen*, or a class of drugs called aromatase inhibitors, can reduce the likelihood that women diagnosed with certain breast cancers will experience a recurrence of their disease.

However, a recent study finds these treatments—used in breast cancers that are responsive to hormones such as estrogen—are too seldom utilized or often used incorrectly.

According to the research team, if all US breast cancer survivors who needed them followed recommendations for hormone therapy, that could mean almost 15,000 lives saved over a decade.

Unfortunately, these drugs are "still underused, and in some cases, misused—offered to patients who lack [estrogen] hormone receptors" on their tumor cells, explained study senior author Dezheng Huo, MD, PhD. He's associate professor of public health sciences at the University of Chicago.

### About Hormonal Therapies

As the researchers explained, hormonal therapies are associated with a 29% lower risk of death for women with hormone receptor-positive breast cancer.

The treatment involves drugs such as tamoxifen or aromatase inhibitors that block hormones and prevent cancer from coming back. These drugs work by slowing or stopping the growth of tumors that feed on certain hormones. Patients are encouraged to take these pills daily for at least 10 years.

### Study Details

The study involved nearly one million women with hormone-sensitive breast cancers who were included in a nationwide cancer registry. Of these women, one out of six who should have had post-surgical hormonal treatments never received them.

The study authors estimated that 14,630 women who did not get the recommended hormone therapy went on to die from a recurrence of their cancer between 2004 and 2013. These deaths might have been prevented, Dr. Huo's team suggested.

***There was some good news, however:*** During the study period, adherence to guidelines on the use of the drugs did improve, the investigators found.

Their use "slowly gained popularity over this time," Dr. Huo said. "It improved after 2004, rising from 70% in 2004 to almost 84% in 2011. Then it declined slightly to 82% in 2013, when the study ended."

Still, 18% of women who could have benefited from this treatment were not receiving it by the end of the study, the researchers noted. Also, about 3% of women received the therapies inappropriately, where they might not have been indicated for their particular breast cancer type.

### Side Effects

There are some downsides to hormonal treatments, the researchers noted. The drugs may cause unpleasant side effects, such as nausea or hot flashes, which may help explain why they are underused.

Other risks vary by the type of drug. For example, patients taking tamoxifen are at greater risk for stroke, while those on aromatase inhibitors are more likely to develop osteoporosis, Dr. Huo's group noted.

### Possible Explanation

The researchers also stressed that the long-term survival benefits of hormonal therapy after breast surgery are tough for the average patient to recognize—the benefits aren't immediate and noticeable. That might also influence women's decisions on whether to continue the therapy.

Some women are also more likely than others to adhere to the therapy, the study found. Those groups include women who underwent breast surgery, or those treated at a large hospital. Asian and white women were also more likely than black or Hispanic women to continue their therapy, the research showed.

The findings were published in *JAMA Oncology*.

The U.S. National Cancer Institute has more on hormone therapy for breast cancer at cancer.gov. Search "hormone therapy and breast cancer."

## Melatonin Fights Breast Cancer

Melatonin, a hormone that regulates sleep, reduced both the size and number of breast tumors in lab research. Researchers speculate that a lack of melatonin, common in sleep-deprived individuals, could increase cancer risks.

*Genes & Cancer.*

## Weighty Cancer Risk

Overweight people are known to be at increased risk for cancer of the colon, esophagus, kidney, breast and uterus.

***Now:*** A review of more than 1,000 studies found that eight more cancers are linked to excess weight and obesity—stomach, liver, gallbladder, pancreas, thyroid, ovary, meningioma (brain) and multiple myeloma (blood). The higher a person's body-mass index (BMI), the greater the risk.

***Why:*** Excess fat produces hormones and inflammation linked to cancer growth.

Marie-Béatrice Lauby-Secretan, PhD, scientist, International Agency for Research on Cancer, Lyon, France.

## Smog Linked to Cancers

Long-term exposure to microscopic airborne particulates of dust, dirt, soot, smog or smoke raised risk of dying not only from lung cancer but also malignancies of the liver, pancreas, breast and other organs by 22% or more, according to a recent 10-year study of nearly 67,000 adults age 65 and older. Risk increased with greater concentration of particulates in the air.

***Possible reason:*** Particulates can impair DNA repair, weaken immunity and trigger inflammation.

Thuan Quoc Thach, PhD, scientific officer, School of Public Health, The University of Hong Kong.

## Feed Teens Fiber

Women who ate a high-fiber diet as teenagers had lower risk for breast cancer. Those who ate the largest amount of vegetables, fruits, beans and whole grains in the years when their breasts were still developing had a 24% lower risk for breast cancer before menopause, and their lifetime risk was 16% less than those who recalled eating the smallest amount of fiber.

Survey of more than 44,000 US nurses by researchers at Harvard T.H. Chan School of Public Health, Boston, published in *Pediatrics*.

## Healing Hops?

The flowers that make beer zesty contain natural estrogens.

***Recent finding:*** An enhanced hops extract increased cell detoxification and could help prevent breast cancer.

*Chemical Research in Toxicology.*

## Implants and Mammograms

Getting implants doesn't increase the risk for cancer, but women with breast implants should continue to have mammograms to screen for breast cancer. *Note*: Women with implants will need extra views at the time of their mammograms to move the implants out of the way, since the X-rays cannot go through silicone or saline implants well enough to view the tissue underneath. The good news is that implants often push the breast tissue closer to the skin and can make it easier to detect a lump. The benefits of getting a mammogram outweigh the risk of damaging the implants. Speak with your doctor about having a mammogram before the surgery and within a year after surgery.

Melissa A. Lazar, MD, assistant professor of surgery, Thomas Jefferson University Hospital, Philadelphia.

## Laptop Concern

A lap is a dangerous place for your laptop. Laptops and tablets, like all electronic devices, emit two types of radiation—from the wireless connection and the device itself. Radiation from wireless devices has been linked to increased cancer risk, headaches, lower immunity and sleep problems.

A radiation shield could block radiation to your lap from a laptop, but bounce it to your abdomen, breasts and brain. And there are no standards to ensure that these shields actually work.

***My advice:*** Lower your radiation exposure by placing your laptop on a table and plugging it in with an ethernet cable instead of using a wireless connection. Ethernet cables (available for less than $10 at office-supply stores) are used for connecting to the Internet with a modem and router. You should also turn off the laptop's Wi-Fi settings. Laptops do not belong on laps!

Devra Davis, PhD, MPH, president, Environmental Health Trust, Teton Village, Wyoming.

## Weight Loss Tied to Lower Risk of Uterine Cancer

Juhua Luo, PhD, associate professor of epidemiology and biostatistics, Indiana University Bloomington's School of Public Health.

Jennifer Ligibel, MD, expert in cancer prevention, American Society of Clinical Oncology.

*Journal of Clinical Oncology*, news release.

Weight loss may lower older women's risk of cancer of the endometrium, the lining of the uterus, a recent study suggests.

"Many older adults think it's too late to benefit from weight loss, or think that because they are overweight or obese, the damage has already been done. But our findings show that's not true," said study author Juhua Luo, PhD.

"It's never too late, and even moderate weight loss can make a big difference when it comes to cancer risk," Dr. Luo added. She's an associate professor of epidemiology and biostatistics at Indiana University Bloomington's School of Public Health.

## About Endometrial Cancer

Endometrial cancer is the most common gynecologic cancer and the fourth most common cancer among women in the United States, the researchers said. More than 75% of endometrial cancers occur in women aged 55 and older.

## The Study

The researchers reviewed data from more than 35,000 American women between the ages of 50 and 79. The study included an average of more than 10 years of follow-up.

Though the study didn't prove cause and effect, losing weight was associated with a significantly lower risk of endometrial cancer, and that benefit was greatest in obese women, the researchers said.

Women over 50 who lost 5% or more of their body weight had a 29% lower risk of endometrial cancer, regardless of their age or how much weight they lost, according to the researchers.

Obese women who lost 5% or more of their body weight had a 56% reduction in their risk. Overweight or obese women who achieved a normal body mass index (BMI—an estimate of body fat based on weight and height) had the same risk as women who maintained a normal BMI, the study authors said.

The researchers also found that women who gained more than 10 pounds had a 26% increased risk of endometrial cancer.

The study was published in the *Journal of Clinical Oncology*.

## Implications

"There have been more than a thousand studies linking obesity to an increased risk of endometrial and other cancers, but almost none that look at the relationship between weight loss and cancer risk," said Jennifer Ligibel, MD, an American Society of Clinical Oncology expert in cancer prevention.

"This study tells us that weight loss, even later in life, is linked to a lower risk of endometrial cancer. The findings also support the development of weight loss programs as part of a cancer prevention strategy in overweight and obese adults," she said.

The U.S. National Cancer Institute has more information on endometrial cancer at Cancer.gov. Search "endometrial cancer."

---

# 6 Ways to Beat Back Cancer

Lorenzo Cohen, PhD, the Richard E. Haynes Distinguished Professor in Clinical Cancer Prevention and director of the Integrative Medicine Program at The University of Texas MD Anderson Cancer Center in Houston.

From time to time, we all hear about cancer patients who defy the odds and live longer than anyone predicted—or even, in some cases, have a complete remission. Why does this happen? No one knows for sure. Researchers are trying to understand this puzzle. *Here's what we've learned so far...*

## Spontaneous Remissions

Some cancers simply disappear. We know, for example, that about 5% of patients with advanced kidney cancer will have spontaneous remissions. This doesn't mean that they're cured—the cancer could return at some point. But for some reason, these patients do much better than others.

Genetic factors surely play a role. Researchers have identified a number of "response mutations" in various types of tumors that somehow make them more likely to respond positively to treatments such as chemotherapy or radiation.

## Improve Your Odds

Research is ongoing, but there's evidence suggesting that the six steps below are important in getting the best possible outcome—and can help prevent cancer from developing in the first place...

• **Take control and manage stress.** "Negative" emotions, such as anxiety and depression, are a normal response to a life-changing illness. Yet there's good evidence (both from human and animal studies) that chronic stress can make your body more susceptible to cancer growth—and that reducing stress may make a difference.

***Important research:*** A study published in the journal *Biological Psychiatry* found that breast cancer patients who participated in a 10-week stress-management program had an increase in cancer-controlling gene expression (such as type 1 interferon response genes) for improved immune function and a decrease in genes that control inflammatory molecules that promote cancer growth. An analysis of the 11-year survival data found that the women in the stress-management group lived significantly longer than those in the control group.

***My advice:*** Engage in a stress-management activity every day (for example, meditation, yoga, relaxation techniques, etc.)...strive to bring that state of calm with you throughout the day...and get counseling if you need it.

• **Get a good night's sleep.** Poor sleep and disruptions in the body's biological clock (as occurs with shift work, for example) have been linked to the development of certain malignancies, including breast and prostate cancer. Now research is suggesting that sleep may play a role in cancer survival.

***My advice:*** The sweet spot seems to be about seven hours of sleep a night. Some people need a bit more, but you don't want to get much less. Research has shown that the risk of dying from all causes—not just cancer—is higher in those who get less than six hours of sleep a night.

• **Watch your weight.** People with a higher body mass index (BMI) have greater concentrations of inflammatory molecules...more insulin resistance...and more estrogen and cancer-related growth factors.

And the effects can be significant. Obese patients are not only more likely to be diagnosed with cancer but also to have a cancer recurrence. They tend to have more complications from surgery, chemotherapy or other treatments as well.

***My advice:*** People with a BMI of 27 or higher should make a serious effort to lose weight. They'll get a double benefit because the two main weight-loss strategies—a healthier diet and more exercise—will also improve cancer recovery and survival.

***Important:*** Consult your doctor about the ideal time to lose weight during your treatment—it may not be appropriate at all stages of cancer care.

• **Get more exercise.** It is well known that regular exercise can help prevent many types of cancer. But can it also help cancer patients live longer? The jury is still out.

Thus far, observational studies—those that look at large populations of people—do suggest that it might make a difference. Exercise is believed to decrease circulating levels of cancer-promoting inflammatory markers and increase aspects of immune function that can help to control cancer growth.

***My advice:*** Exercise at least 30 minutes a day at least five or six days a week. Any amount of activity helps—even 10-minute bouts every few hours count. Also avoid sitting for hours at a time.

• **Reduce exposure to toxins.** Cancer-causing chemicals are all around us. Hormone disrupters, such as bisphenol A (BPA) and parabens, are in some plastic bottles and cosmetics and can alter hormonal functioning and increase cancer risk. Carcinogens, such as formaldehyde and benzene, can be in wallpaper, paint, wood floor finishes and other household products.

***My advice:*** Avoid personal-care products that contain parabens, phthalates, triclosan and synthetic fragrance. Use glass and stainless steel containers instead of plastic. Ventilate your home when painting or refinishing floors.

### The Healthy Plate Formula...

To help fight cancer, it's important to make wise food choices throughout the day.

***Here's how:*** Fill half your plate with vegetables (organic, if possible) at every meal, including breakfast. The other half should contain protein, fruits (preferably organic) and whole grains. Try replacing meat with sardines, salmon and other cold-water fish (loaded with omega-3 fatty acids) and beans at least four times a week for a healthy source of animal and plant proteins. Add spices and herbs, which are filled with healthy phytochemicals. It's also smart to eat fewer "white" foods, including white bread, white rice, etc. These and other high-glycemic foods are quickly converted to glucose, which increases levels of insulin and insulin-like growth factor (a cancer promoter).

***Helpful:*** Meet with a dietitian to help guide you in healthy eating. To find a registered dietitian near you, consult the Academy of Nutrition and Dietetics, EatRight.org.

---

## Freeze Therapy: An Alternative to Breast Cancer Surgery?

Deanna Attai, MD, assistant clinical professor, surgery, David Geffen School of Medicine, University of California, Los Angeles, and immediate past president, American Society of Breast Surgeons.

Laura Kruper, MD, director, Women's Center, and chief, Breast Surgery Service, City of Hope Cancer Center, Duarte, California.

*Annals of Surgical Oncology.*

---

A freezing technique known as cryoablation might be a viable alternative to lumpectomy for treating small, early stage breast cancers, researchers report.

In the small study of 86 patients, "cryoablation was shown to successfully [treat] the majority of small breast cancers with few side effects or complications," said study coauthor Deanna Attai, MD. She's an assistant clinical professor of surgery at the University of California, Los Angeles David Geffen School of Medicine.

Using this minimally invasive approach to destroy cancer cells, there should be little to no change in the appearance of the breast, said Dr. Attai, immediate past president of the American Society of Breast Surgeons.

The major risk, Dr. Attai said, is not killing all the cancerous cells.

Another surgeon noted that although further research is still needed, cryoablation appears to be "a potential new tool that we can offer women."

"This is promising data. It's the first step," said Laura Kruper, MD, chief of the breast surgery service at the City of Hope Cancer Center in Duarte, California. However, "it's certainly not going to be for everyone," she added.

For one thing, "the tumor can only be about a centimeter," Dr. Kruper said. That's less than half an inch.

The freezing technique has been used for years to treat cancers of the liver, lung and kidney, as well as noncancerous breast tumors, Dr. Attai and her colleagues said.

### Study Details

For the recent study, the researchers performed the freezing technique on breast cancer patients in 19 centers across the United States. The tumors had to be 2 centimeters (about three-quarters of an inch) or smaller.

Because the study was designed to assess the technique's effectiveness in advance of government approval, the researchers surgically removed the tumors 28 days after the extreme-cold treatment. Then they examined the tissue in a pathology lab.

Overall, freezing was successful for 92% of the cancers. And it worked for all tumors measuring less than 1 centimeter, the study found.

The outpatient procedure is done with local anesthesia. A doctor uses ultrasound imaging to help guide a thin, needle-like probe into the tumors. There, the probe emits liquid nitrogen, which creates an ice ball that freezes the tissue, Dr. Attai said.

Afterward, the body gradually reabsorbs the "dead" tissue, said Dr. Attai, who added that the residual scar is small.

Potential complications of cryoablation include infection, bleeding, cold damage to the skin, pain and scarring, Dr. Attai said. To prevent cold damage, tumors close to the skin surface should not be treated in this way, she said.

Some of the patients in the study told Dr. Attai they would have preferred to skip the surgery that followed cryoablation. However, she said a subset of patients probably would feel more comfortable with traditional surgery.

The study was published in the *Annals of Surgical Oncology.*

## Implications

It could be years before the approach might be recommended for standard practice, Dr. Attai said.

"We know cryoablation will kill small tumors. In order to truly compare with lumpectomy, we need a study where the patients undergo ablation and then are not treated with surgery," Dr. Attai said.

"We need to follow them for at least five years to determine if recurrence rates are higher with ablation alone," she explained.

Also yet to be decided is if radiation therapy would be needed after the cryoablation, Dr. Attai said.

City of Hope also plans to research the technique further, said Dr. Kruper, who wasn't involved in the current study.

"We need more long-term data," she agreed.

For more information on cryoablation, visit the website of the University of Arizona, UACC.arizona.edu, and search "cryoablation."

# Estrogen-Supressing Drug Benefit

Harold J. Burstein, MD, breast oncologist, Dana-Farber Cancer Institute, Boston.

Breast cancer patients benefit from longer use of an estrogen-suppressing drug. Postmenopausal women who took an aromatase inhibitor called *letrozole* for 10 years rather than the standard five years had a 34% lower risk for cancer recurrence within six years, according to a recent study of nearly 2,000 postmenopausal women. Women who stayed on letrozole also had a reduced risk for cancer in the other breast—1%, compared with 3% for those taking the drug for five years.

***Bonus:*** This drug has fewer side effects, such as blood clots and increased risk for stroke, than older hormone suppressants, such as *tamoxifen*, which are typically taken for five years.

***But:*** Longer aromatase-inhibitor therapy can have significant side effects, including ongoing menopausal symptoms and osteoporosis, so it is not for everyone.

# New Method Improves Radiation Therapy

Many radiation treatments given for cancer last for about two minutes, but because chest movement while breathing can increase the risk for damage to surrounding tissue, the therapies are often given over several shorter sessions. *New research*: Women with breast cancer were successfully trained to safely hold their breath for a few minutes, which allowed them to receive their daily dose of radiation in a single breath-hold. This resulted in more accurate targeting of the tumor and spared more healthy tissue.

Mike Parkes, DPhil, senior lecturer in applied physiology, University of Birmingham, UK.

# Know Your Risk for Ovarian Cancer—and the Symptoms

David Fishman, MD, director of the cancer center and gynecologic oncology at New York-Presbyterian/Queens.

NewYork-Presbyterian/Queens, news release.

A major shift is needed in the early detection and treatment of ovarian cancer, according to a doctor who specializes in the disease.

"Ovarian cancer is often diagnosed too late," said David Fishman, MD, director of the cancer center and gynecologic oncology at New York-Presbyterian/Queens.

"It's important for women to know their risk [of] contracting this deadly disease, and its earliest warning signs," he added.

## Risk Factors, Symptoms and Survival Rates

All women are at risk of ovarian cancer, and one in 75 will develop the disease, Dr. Fishman said. More than 250,000 women worldwide are diagnosed with ovarian cancer every year, and 140,000 die from it.

Dr. Fishman stressed that a clean pap test does not mean a woman's ovaries are cancer-free. Pap tests diagnose cervical disease, not ovarian cancer.

Some call ovarian cancer a "silent" killer. Its early symptoms are mild and easy to ignore, according to Dr. Fishman. They include bloating, indigestion and nausea, pain in the abdomen and back, feeling full quickly, frequent urination, weight gain and shortness of breath. Women who have these symptoms for more than a week should consult a doctor, he suggested.

Ovarian cancer is highly treatable if detected early. If the cancer is just in the ovary (stage 1), the average five-year survival rate is 90%. However, the odds of survival are much lower if the cancer is more advanced, Dr. Fishman said.

Women who have had breast cancer or certain other types of cancer are at increased risk. Other ovarian cancer risk factors include certain gene mutations, infertility, early menstruation, obesity and age. Women over age 70 have higher odds of developing the disease, researchers have found.

## Reducing Risk

Several factors can reduce a woman's risk, including following a healthy, low-fat diet; having given birth; using birth control; and having tubal ligation surgery.

Some women at high risk have their ovaries and fallopian tubes removed as a precaution, said Dr. Fishman, who is also vice chairman of obstetrics and gynecology at the hospital.

For example, actress Angelina Jolie disclosed that she had her ovaries and fallopian tubes removed because she had a significantly increased risk of ovarian cancer due to the BRCA1 gene mutation.

The U.S. Office on Women's Health has more information on ovarian cancer at Womenshealth.gov. Search "ovarian cancer."

# Dye "Lights Up" Ovarian Cancers

Surgeons depend on the naked eye (and fingertips) to identify ovarian tumors during surgery.

***New approach:*** A fluorescent dye that binds to receptors that are found on 90% of ovarian cancers.

*Clinical Cancer Research.*

# Ovarian Cancer Deaths Are Down

US ovarian cancer deaths are down 16%. The decline is from 2002 to 2012 (latest data available). *Reasons*: Long-term use of oral contraceptives, which are known to protect against ovarian cancer…and reduced use of menopausal hormone therapy, which can raise cancer risk.

Study by researchers at University of Milan, Italy, published in *Annals of Oncology*.

## Drinking Alcohol Can Cause Seven Types of Cancer

An analysis of studies conducted over the last 10 years determined that drinking increases the risk for cancer of the mouth and throat, esophagus, larynx (voice box), liver, colon, rectum and breast. Heavy drinkers were found to be at the highest risk, but even low-to-moderate drinkers were more likely to get these cancers than nondrinkers.

Analysis conducted by researchers at University of Otago, Dunedin, New Zealand, published in *Addictions*.

# Birth Control Pills Tied to Decline in Ovarian Cancer Deaths

Carlo La Vecchia, MD, professor of epidemiology, University of Milan, Italy.

Paolo Boffetta, MD, chief, division of cancer prevention and control, department of oncological sciences, Mount Sinai School of Medicine, New York City.

*Annals of Oncology*, news release.

Ovarian cancer deaths are down dramatically in many parts of the world, and researchers believe the use of birth control pills may be a main reason why.

## Study Details

The analysis of World Health Organization data found that the ovarian cancer death rate fell 16% in the United States and almost 8% in Canada between 2002 and 2012.

In the European Union, the ovarian cancer death rate fell 10%, though some countries saw far more significant drops. The United Kingdom's ovarian cancer death rate went down by 22%. Denmark and Sweden each saw a drop of 24% in their death rate from ovarian cancer, the researchers said.

Ovarian cancer deaths also decreased about 12% in both Australia and New Zealand. In Japan, the ovarian cancer death rate declined 2%, the study found. Japan has low rates of birth control use, the researchers said.

Ovarian cancer death rates are expected to continue to decline 15% in the United States, and 10% in the European Union and Japan by 2020.

In Latin America, the results were mixed. Argentina, Chile and Uruguay had decreases in ovarian cancer death rates between 2002 and 2012. But, Brazil, Colombia, Cuba, Mexico and Venezuela all had increases, according to the study.

The study was published in the journal *Annals of Oncology*.

## Possible Explanations

The study wasn't designed to prove cause-and-effect. However, a big reason for the decline in ovarian cancer death rates in some parts of the world is likely the use of birth control pills and the long-term protection against ovarian cancer they provide, study leader Carlo La Vecchia, MD, a professor of epidemiology at the University of Milan, Italy, and colleagues, suggested.

Other factors may include reduced use of hormone replacement therapy to manage menopausal symptoms and better diagnosis and treatment of ovarian cancer, the researchers said.

## Expert Commentary

"As our understanding of preventable causes of this major cancer progresses, early detection strategies are developed and novel therapeutic options become available, we enhance our ability to reduce ovarian cancer mortality," Paolo Boffetta, MD, the journal's associate editor, wrote in an accompanying editorial. Dr. Boffetta is also chief of the division of cancer prevention and control of the department of oncological sciences at the

Mount Sinai School of Medicine in New York City.

The American Cancer Society website, Cancer.org, has more on ovarian cancer. Search "ovarian cancer."

# Heart Risks May Boost Women's Colon Cancer Risk, Too

Juhua Luo, PhD, associate professor, epidemiology and biostatistics, Indiana University Bloomington's School of Public Health.

Candyce Kroenke, ScD, research scientist, Kaiser Permanente Northern California, Oakland, California.

Andrew Chan, MD, associate professor of medicine, Harvard Medical School, and attending gastroenterologist, Massachusetts General Hospital, Boston.

Xiaoyun Liang, PhD, department of epidemiology, Beijing Normal University, China.

*Cancer Epidemiology, Biomarkers & Prevention.*

Even normal-weight women may be at greater risk for colon cancer if they have certain traits, such as elevated levels of blood fat, high blood sugar, high blood pressure and low levels of good cholesterol, a recent study suggests.

Among older women of normal weight, those with so-called metabolic risk factors had a 49% increased risk for cancers of the colon, rectum and sigmoid colon (the lower part of the intestine connecting the rectum and colon) compared with healthy counterparts.

Current guidelines recommend colon cancer screening primarily based on a person's age. But identifying at-risk individuals by their metabolic type could help prevent these cancers and catch them at an earlier stage, saving more lives, the study authors concluded.

***The takeaway:*** "Know your own metabolic health, even if your weight is normal," said Juhua Luo, PhD, the study's senior author. She's an associate professor of epidemiology and biostatistics at Indiana University Bloomington's School of Public Health.

Candyce Kroenke, ScD, a research scientist at Kaiser Permanente Northern California and a study coauthor, said the findings "further point to the need for better measures than BMI [body mass index] to assess health risks." Body mass index is a rough estimate of a person's body fat based on height and weight measurements.

The study involved normal-weight postmenopausal women, aged 50 to 79.

It's reasonable to suspect that the findings may apply to men or younger women, too, Dr. Luo said. "But we would need additional study to answer this for sure," she added.

Andrew Chan, MD, is a gastroenterologist and associate professor of medicine at Harvard Medical School in Boston. He agreed that the findings suggest that other factors beyond weight may be independently associated with colon cancer.

"It's really hard to prove cause and effect with this type of study, but it does raise some interesting questions," said Dr. Chan, who wasn't involved in the research.

## About Colon Cancer Risk

Excluding skin cancers, colon cancer is the third most common cancer diagnosed in women and men in the United States, the American Cancer Society says.

The "absolute" risk of developing colon cancer over a specified period of time varies by age, sex and other risk factors. The U.S. Centers for Disease Control and Prevention says a 50-year-old woman has a 2% to 3% chance of having colon cancer over the next 30 years. A 60-year-old male has a 4% chance of developing it over the same three-decade period.

While being overweight or obese is a known risk factor, few studies have examined colon cancer risk among people with unhealthy metabolic factors, especially in normal-weight individuals, the study authors noted.

## About Metabolic Syndrome

***Having "metabolic syndrome" means you have three or more of these traits***: high blood pressure, high triglycerides (a type of blood fat), high blood sugar, low levels of good HDL cholesterol and a large waist measurement.

Thirty percent of normal-weight adults worldwide are believed to be metabolically unhealthy, according to lead study author Xiaoyun Liang, PhD, of Beijing Normal University in China.

### Study Details

The research team's analysis involved more than 5,000 women enrolled in the Women's Health Initiative, a 15-year study led by the U.S. National Institutes of Health.

Women with a body mass index of 18.5 to less than 25 are considered normal weight. Someone who's 5 feet 6 inches tall and weighs 142 pounds would have a BMI of about 23, according to the CDC.

One-third of the women in the study were deemed metabolically unhealthy, meaning they had two or more risk factors of metabolic syndrome. The researchers didn't include waist measurement as one of the factors.

After adjusting for factors that affect cancer risks, women with metabolic syndrome had more than a twofold higher risk of colon and rectal cancers compared with metabolically healthy women, the findings showed.

### Conclusions

Why these women seem at higher risk isn't clear. It's possible that poor metabolic health may promote inflammation in the body that boosts cancer risk, the study authors suggested.

Dr. Chan said it's becoming clear that risk factors for heart disease may overlap with risk factors for many types of cancer.

"So I think that gives people an additional reason for really thinking about trying to maintain a healthy lifestyle," he said.

Learn more about metabolic syndrome from the U.S. National Institutes of Health, NHLBI. nih.gov. Search "metabolic syndrome."

## Better Colonoscopy Prep

It could be time to drop the "no eating" rule the day before having a colonoscopy, according to a recent study.

***Details:*** Participants who were allowed to eat a small amount of low-fiber food (such as mac and cheese, yogurt and ice cream) were less hungry and their bowels were better prepared for the procedure than those restricted to the traditional clear-liquid diet.

***Why:*** Low-fiber foods liquefy and don't stay in the bowel...and eating stimulates bowel movements, which help to clear the colon before colonoscopy.

Jason Samarasena, MD, assistant clinical professor of medicine, University of California, Irvine.

## Beware of Colorectal Cancer Symptoms

About 10% of colorectal cancer cases are diagnosed before age 50 (when screening usually begins). Younger patients also tend to have more advanced disease, perhaps because they're diagnosed only after the cancer causes obvious symptoms.

***Takeaway:*** At any age, consult a doctor if you have symptoms of colorectal cancer, such as frequent pencil-thin stools...persistent diarrhea and/or constipation...or blood in the stool. If you have a family history or other risk factors, ask your doctor if you should be screened before age 50.

Samantha Hendren, MD, MPH, associate professor of surgery, University of Michigan, Ann Arbor.

## Possible Colorectal Cancer Stopper

Twenty-three percent reduction in colorectal cancer risk is linked to regular use of glucosamine and chondroitin supplements. Glucosamine and chondroitin are thought to have anti-inflammatory properties, and this could explain why users of the supplements may have a lower risk for colorectal cancer.

Elizabeth D. Kantor, PhD, MPH, epidemiologist and coleader of a study of colorectal cancer at Harvard T.H. Chan School of Public Health, Boston, published in *International Journal of Cancer.*

# "You've Got a Spot on Your Lung"

Andrew J. Kaufman, MD, an expert in advanced minimally invasive thoracic surgery and thoracic surgical oncology. He is chief of the department of thoracic surgery at Mount Sinai Beth Israel and director of the Thoracic Surgery Airway Program and the Asian Thoracic Surgery Program at Mount Sinai Hospital, both in New York City.

Imagine for a moment that your doctor has told you to get a routine chest X-ray or CT scan because you are having chest pain...are about to have shoulder surgery...or may have cracked a rib.

Then your doctor calls to say that the test unexpectedly detected a "spot" on your lung. Your first thought is, *It might be lung cancer!*...but take a deep breath.

Here are the steps you need to take to preserve your health and your sanity...

***STEP 1:*** **Don't panic.** Most lung spots (dense areas within the lung that appear as white, shadowy areas on imaging tests) are not cancer. In fact, when doctors screen high-risk patients (people over age 55 who have smoked roughly 30 "pack years"—a pack year is defined as smoking one pack of cigarettes a day for a year) specifically for lung cancer, only about 1% to 2% of nodules that are detected on CT scans are cancerous.

When the spot is found incidentally—that is, during an imaging test that wasn't given because cancer was suspected—the risk is even lower.

Many conditions that don't have anything to do with cancer can cause a spot on the lung. These include...

- **Infection from tuberculosis,** pneumonia, bronchitis or other illness involving the lungs.
- **Inflammation from an autoimmune disease**—rheumatoid arthritis, for example, is a common cause of inflammatory lung nodules.
- **Scarring from pulmonary fibrosis or other lung disease.**
- **Environmental irritants,** such as asbestos, coal dust or silicone.
- **Environmental infection,** such as histoplasmosis, caused by fungus spores in bird or bat droppings. People can be exposed while demolishing old buildings, for example, or by spending time in bat-filled caves.

***STEP 2:*** **Talk about your history.** If you've been told that you have a spot on your lung, make an appointment with the doctor who knows you best to review your medical history...take stock of your lung cancer risk... and decide your next steps.

First, your doctor, often in consultation with a radiologist, will want to compare the latest chest X-ray or CT scan with any previous imaging tests of your chest. It is possible that the spot has been there for years but wasn't previously identified. If the spot was present and hasn't grown for many years, the chance that it is malignant is low.

Next, discuss your recent health and personal risk factors for lung cancer with your doctor. Have you had a cough, the flu or a severe cold? Do you have an autoimmune disease? Have you had any risky environmental exposures? These all have the potential to cause lung spots.

If you have a history of another malignancy somewhere in your body, your doctor will want to rule out a metastasis to the lungs.

Of course, smoking history is very significant. Smokers have a higher risk for lung cancer...former smokers have a lower risk than active smokers...and nonsmokers have the lowest risk. For everyone, however, the risk for lung cancer increases with age.

***Important:*** For reasons no one understands, the incidence of lung cancer is rising among never-smokers, especially women. Therefore, people who have never smoked should not assume that they can't have lung cancer. Any lung spot should be evaluated by an expert even if you don't have serious risk factors for lung cancer.

***STEP 3:*** **Get follow-up testing.** If your nodule was found incidentally, you'll need focused follow-up imaging. For most people, the best option is a low-dose CT (LDCT) scan without IV contrast. This test gives a clear view of the nodule with minimal radiation.

The dose of radiation used in an LDCT is about the same as that used in a standard mammogram. The LDCT will let doctors see the size and qualities of the nodule.

For example...*

• **Small nodules**—spots that are less than one-fifth of an inch (5 mm) are very low risk but should be followed with surveillance in most cases. For example, such nodules should usually be monitored for two years at set time intervals to reveal if there is any growth in the nodule. A stable nodule without growth for two years is safely considered benign.

• **Larger nodules**—spots that are about one-third of an inch (8 mm) or greater demand a thorough workup. This may include a positron emission tomography (PET) scan, which involves an injection of radioactive tracers that light up to indicate areas that may be cancerous and would require a biopsy for confirmation, or a needle or surgical biopsy if the person's risk factors are high and the radiographic appearance warrants a tissue diagnosis.

• **Spiky nodules**—or those with an irregular surface—are generally more concerning than smooth nodules.

• **Solid and part-solid nodules**—meaning they have a solid density measurement throughout the entire spot or some solid component—are typically more concerning than nonsolid nodules.

• **More is usually better.** If your doctor says that you have multiple nodules (that is, more than one), the nodules are less likely to be cancer.

Because surveillance is the most practical way to determine whether a spot is dangerous, it's important to get expert recommendations. That's why decisions regarding surveillance are usually made by a multidisciplinary team that includes pulmonary doctors, thoracic surgeons and radiologists.

Even if a nodule is deemed benign, depending on your personal medical history, your doctor may recommend a yearly follow-up scan.

For example, if a person has a close relative with cancer (a first-degree relative such as a parent or sibling) or a history of heavy smoking, he/she will likely need an annual screening to check for new nodules that may develop and possibly become cancerous.

***Important:*** You should not settle for an X-ray as a follow-up. An LDCT provides greater detail.

Among current or former heavy smokers, LDCT has been shown to reduce the risk for lung cancer deaths due to early detection. In the National Lung Screening Trial, more than 53,000 men and women (ages 55 to 74) who were current or former heavy smokers were randomly assigned to receive annual screenings with either LDCT or standard chest X-ray for three consecutive years. The LDCT group had 20% fewer lung cancer deaths than the X-ray group.

***STEP 4:* Get a closer look.** If follow-up scans show that a nodule is getting larger and/or changing in appearance, your physician will need to take a biopsy to determine whether it's malignant.

If the nodule is easy to reach—for example, in the airway—a biopsy may be done with a very thin lighted instrument that is threaded through the mouth or nose and down the throat to snip off a piece of the nodule.

A needle biopsy may be preferred if the nodule is in the peripheral lung or near the chest wall.

A surgical biopsy that involves making an incision to remove a tissue sample may be needed if the approaches described above fail to make an adequate diagnosis or if the likelihood of cancer is considered high.

If lung cancer is diagnosed, then it is crucial to make a prompt appointment with a thoracic surgeon and/or oncologist to begin treatment.

*The sizes and characteristics of nodules that require follow-up (as well as the schedule for such testing) may vary depending on the medical facility where you are receiving care. Many medical centers use the *Fleischner Guidelines for Pulmonary Nodules*, FleischnerSociety.org.

# Lymphoma: New Treatments, New Hope

Elizabeth M. Adler, PhD. Trained in neurobiology, Dr. Adler conducted research and taught at Williams College. Following her own diagnoses with lymphoma and breast cancer, she shifted her focus from science research to science communication and cancer advocacy. She is author of *Living with Lymphoma: A Patient's Guide, 2nd Edition.*

Enormous scientific advances are radically transforming lymphoma treatment. If you're diagnosed with this cancer, your outlook is dramatically better than it would have been 20 years ago.

## Is It Lymphoma?

The most common symptom is swollen lymph nodes—lumps, usually painless, that typically appear in the groin, in the armpit, on the neck or along the chin or collarbone. Other symptoms may include persistent fatigue, unexplained weight loss, fever, soaking night sweats, itching, coughing or trouble breathing and pain or swelling in the abdomen. A diagnosis is usually suggested by a physical exam and a profile of symptoms, followed by a biopsy. If confirmed, blood tests and radiology can hone the diagnosis.

What you need to know about the many new weapons in the fight against lymphoma...

## Treatment Evolution

Lymphoma is a blood cancer that involves cells in the immune system called lymphocytes. There are many different kinds of lymphoma—the main types are Hodgkin's lymphoma and non-Hodgkin's lymphoma. Some grow so slowly—they are called "indolent"—that doctors may recommend a wait-and-see approach. Others are more aggressive.

Chemotherapy is the primary treatment. If a tumor is localized in one or a few lymph nodes, radiation may be used, but the cancer frequently affects more of the body.

In some cases, more advanced disease may require a combination of drugs and radiation. Surgery is rarely used for lymphoma treatment, although surgical biopsies are used in lymphoma diagnosis.

Unfortunately, the standard chemotherapy drugs—including *doxorubicin* (Adriamycin), *vincristine* (Vincasar PFS) and *cyclophosphamide* (Cytoxan)—kill not just cancer cells but also damage other rapidly dividing cells, such as those in the mouth, intestines, hair follicles and elsewhere. Side effects can include hair loss, painful sores in the mouth, increased risk for serious infection (due to a decrease in white blood cells), nausea, fatigue and "chemo brain."

The new drugs don't yet entirely replace these standard agents. But they reflect significant progress in our understanding of the biology behind lymphoma cells' growth and survival.

## The Immunotherapy Revolution

One major advance is a new era in immunotherapy, which uses the immune system's power to quell cancer. It's shown progress against different kinds of cancers and is now an important part of many lymphoma treatment plans.

Some approaches to immunotherapy rely on antibodies, compounds made by white blood cells that are one of the principal weapons of the immune system. Their function is to home in on a specific bacterium, virus or other enemy (such as a tumor cell) and tag it for destruction. In some forms of cancer immunotherapy, patients are given monoclonal antibodies synthetically cloned so that they can seek out a specific protein on the surface of malignant lymphocytes. That is, they turn your immune system against the cancer. Immunotherapy may also use other agents, including drugs, to unleash the immune system against the cancer.

The major immunotherapy drugs approved by the FDA against lymphomas and what they do...

• **Harnessing the immune system.** *Rituximab* (Rituxan), approved in 1997 against non-Hodgkin's lymphoma, is a monoclonal antibody that marks lymphoma cells for the immune system to destroy. This drug has been a major contributor to improved outcomes over the past two decades. It also inhibits tumor growth and promotes a process that signals lymphoma cells to die off.

• **Magnifying the effect.** *Obinutuzumab* (Gazyva) and *ofatumumab* (Arzerra) are two more recently approved monoclonal antibodies. Both work like rituximab but have been tweaked to modify their interactions with the immune system.

• **Opening the immune gates.** *Nivolumab* (Opdivo), another monoclonal antibody, approved in the treatment of Hodgkin's lymphoma in 2016, works to block "immune checkpoints." These are molecules that keep T-cells from attacking normal cells. Lymphoma cells can take over checkpoints for their own nefarious purposes. Monoclonal antibodies and other compounds can be used to neutralize those hijacked checkpoints, unleashing the body's immune system against the cancer.

• **Acting like a Trojan horse.** Monoclonal antibodies can also be engineered to deliver cancer-killing chemicals or radioisotopes. *Brentuximab vedotin* (Adcetris), first approved against lymphoma in 2011, recognizes a protein on the surface of certain cancerous lymphocytes and binds to it. Then it introduces a compound that only becomes toxic inside the lymphoma, causing less toxicity to other cells.

## Other Promising New Drugs

Immunotherapy isn't the only new thing in lymphoma therapy...

• **Honing the attack.** Unlike conventional chemotherapy, which targets rapidly dividing cells, new "targeted chemotherapy" drugs disrupt the molecular pathways that cancer cells must maintain to survive. Two drugs—*ibrutinib* (Imbruvica) and *idelalisib* (Zydelig)—work this way.

• **Helping cancer cells die.** *Venetoclax* (Venclexta), approved in 2016 for a specific type of lymphoma (chronic lymphocytic leukemia), blocks a protein that supports tumor cell survival. Several other drugs that work similarly are now in development.

The search for new ways to treat lymphoma continues. Other innovations include antibiotics to quell infections that promote survival of certain kinds of malignant lymphocytes, and a technique that takes immune cells from the body, genetically alters them to fight cancer, and returns them to circulation.

## Life after Lymphoma

Even when lymphoma is successfully treated, fatigue may persist. Medications such as tricyclic antidepressants, low doses of steroid and even stimulants may help in some cases. Acupuncture and, when needed, treatment for an underactive thyroid, may also help. Many people find that regular exercise is a most effective antidote.

The new drugs are approved only for specific lymphomas, often when they haven't responded to standard treatments, so which newer ones are right for you depends on your specific kind of lymphoma. Even with all these advances, survival carries no guarantee—even after five or 10 years, the disease can sometimes return.

Treatment can increase the risk of other cancers, and can harm the heart and other organs. Discuss with your doctor what follow-up cancer screenings you should have, and reduce your risk for heart disease by not smoking, maintaining a health weight, eating healthfully and being active. Plus, the new immunotherapy can in some cases cause the immune system to attack other organs, leading to serious side effects, some life-threatening.

But none of that changes the fact that the prognosis for many people diagnosed with lymphoma is still better than it's ever been.

# Your Cell Phone Can Cause Cancer

Devra Davis, PhD, MPH, president of Environmental Health Trust, a nonprofit scientific and policy think tank focusing on cell-phone radiation. She is author of *Disconnect: The Truth About Cell Phone Radiation.* EHTrust.org

You may have heard that cell phones have been linked to cancer but wondered if that could really be true. A recent study offers strong evidence that this is the case—cell phones and other wireless devices emit a type of microwave radiation termed radiofrequency radiation (RFR) that can cause brain cancer and other cancers.

Here are the findings and what to do to minimize this risk to your health...

## The Newest Evidence

The government's National Toxicology Program (NTP) conducts scientific studies on toxins to see how they might affect the health of Americans. More than 90 studies show that the radiation emitted by cell phones and other wireless devices can damage DNA, the first step on the road to cancer.

In May 2016, the NTP published preliminary results from a two-year animal study on the health effects of cell-phone radiation—this was the largest study on animals and cell-phone radiation ever published.

One out of every 12 of the animals studied were affected by the radiation. Some of those that were exposed to daily, frequent doses of cell-phone radiation from birth developed glioma, a rare, aggressive type of brain cancer already linked to cell-phone use in people. (Glial cells surround and support neurons.) Other animals had precancerous changes in glial cells. And some developed rare tumors of the nerves around and within the heart called schwannomas. In contrast, a control group of animals not exposed to wireless radiation had no gliomas, no precancerous changes in glial cells and no schwannomas.

There are two crucial takeaways from this recent study...

**1. For decades, many scientists and governments have embraced the following scientific dogma—the only unsafe radiation is "thermal" radiation that heats tissue, such as an X-ray.** "Nonthermal" RFR doesn't heat tissue and therefore is safe. The latest study—during which animals exposed to RFR were monitored to ensure that there was no heating of tissue—contradicts this dogma.

**2. Epidemiological studies that analyze health data from hundreds or thousands of people have linked gliomas and schwannomas to long-term cell-phone use**—and this latest study found the same type of cancers in animals exposed to wireless radiation, strengthening the link.

## Even More Dangers

Gliomas and schwannomas aren't the only dangers. *Research links wireless-device use to a range of other cancers, diseases and conditions...*

- **Meningioma.** A recent study published in *Oncology Reports* showed that heavy users of mobile and cordless phones had up to twice the risk for meningioma, cancer in the protective coverings that surround the brain.
- **Salivary gland (parotid) tumors.** Salivary glands are below the ear and in the jaw—exactly where many people hold cell phones during conversation. A study published in *American Journal of Epidemiology* showed a 58% higher risk for these (usually) noncancerous tumors among cell-phone users.
- **Acoustic neuroma.** Studies show that heavy or longtime users of cell phones have nearly triple the risk of developing acoustic neuromas (also called vestibular schwannomas), noncancerous tumors on the nerve that connects the inner ear to the brain. Symptoms can include gradual hearing loss and tinnitus in the affected ear, along with balance problems, headaches and facial numbness and tingling.
- **Breast cancer.** A study published in *Case Reports in Medicine* describes four young

American women, ages 21 to 39, who had tucked their smartphones into their bras for up to 10 hours a day for several years. Each of them developed breast tumors directly under the antennas of their phones. None of the women had the cancer-causing BRAC1 or BRAC2 gene, a family history of cancer or any other known risk factors.

• **Sleeping problems.** Research shows that people who use cell phones and other wireless devices in the hours before bedtime have more trouble falling asleep and staying asleep. Both wireless radiation and the "blue light" from screens suppress melatonin, a sleep-inducing hormone.

## How to Protect Yourself

Every step you take to reduce radiation is protective because exposure to radiation is cumulative—the higher the exposure, the higher your risk for cancer and other health problems.

The devices you should be concerned about include cell phones, cordless phone handsets and bases, Wi-Fi routers, wireless computers, laptops, iPads and other tablets, smartwatches, wireless fitness bands, iPods that connect to the Internet, wireless speakers, cordless baby monitors, wireless game consoles and any other type of wireless device or equipment such as thermostats, security networks, sound systems and smart meters.

• **Keep it at a distance.** To decrease your exposure to wireless radiation, keep wireless devices as far away from you as possible. *Just a few inches can make a big difference...*

• Never put the phone next to your head. Instead, use the speakerphone function or a wired headset or an earpiece.

• Never place a turned-on device in a pocket or jacket or tucked into clothing. Keep it in a carrier bag, such as a briefcase or purse. Never rest a wireless device on your body. This includes laptops and tablets—keep them off your lap.

• Never fall asleep with your cell phone or wireless tablet in the bed or under your pillow. Many people fall asleep streaming radiation into their bodies.

• Prefer texting to calling. And avoid using your cell phone when the signal is weak—radiation is higher.

• **Turn it off.** Putting your cell phone in "airplane" mode stops radiation. Also, look for the function key on your wireless device that turns off the Wi-Fi. Turn it off when the device isn't in use. There's also a function key to turn off Bluetooth transmissions. If you must use a Wi-Fi router at home, locate it as far away from your body as possible. And turn it off at night.

To stop a gaming console from emitting radiation, you need to turn it off and unplug it.

• **Don't use your cell phone in metal surroundings such as a bus, train, airplane or elevator.** Using the phone creates radiation "hot spots" that increase exposure.

***Exception:*** It is OK to use a cell phone in a car if your phone is hooked into the car's Bluetooth system—this reduces radiation to the user.

• **Trade in the cordless phone.** Cordless phones and wireless routers that use a technology called DECT emit as much radiation as cell phones whether you are using them or not. At home, install telephones that get their signal by being plugged into a jack. Forward your cell phone to your landline whenever you're home.

---

# Just Diagnosed with Cancer?

Mark J. Fesler, MD, an assistant professor of hematology and medical oncology at Saint Louis University Cancer Center and director of the Blood and Marrow Transplant Program at SSM Health Saint Louis University Hospital.

Getting a diagnosis of cancer is one of the scariest, most stressful situations a person can experience. Reeling from the distressing news and overcome with emotion, virtually all new cancer pa-

## Stubborn UTIs May Signal Bladder Cancer

In a recent study of more than 13,000 adults with a bladder malignancy, the cancer diagnosis took longer for those with UTIs—possibly because UTI symptoms, such as blood in the urine and frequent urination, also occur with bladder cancer. People with UTIs that don't improve after a single course of antibiotics should consult a urologist, who may recommend cystoscopy to examine the bladder.

Kyle Richards, MD, assistant professor of urology, University of Wisconsin School of Medicine and Public Health, Madison.

tients find it hard to know exactly what actions should be taken next.

***What works best:*** Following certain steps the first week after a cancer diagnosis greatly reduces stress and sets the course for a treatment plan that involves good decision-making, stronger support systems and perhaps even an improved chance of recovery. The steps below can be adapted to each patient's personal situation, but they will help bring order to what can otherwise be a chaotic and tremendously challenging time...

- **Don't keep your cancer a secret.** Many patients keep their diagnosis to themselves at first. They may be in denial, don't have all the facts yet and/or don't want to worry loved ones. But it's much better to reach out to key family members and close friends right away.

Meet with close family members and friends individually or in a group to share your diagnosis and let them know that you would appreciate their support. You can give them more information at a later time. You could also call your friends and family members to give them the news, but don't communicate this information via text or social media.

The love and moral support as well as practical help with meals and rides that they can give will lessen your burden and anxiety much more than you realize.

- **See an oncologist within the first week after diagnosis.** There's a tremendous amount of anxiety during the time between the cancer diagnosis and the initial visit with an oncologist. I have observed that patients who see their oncologists right away tend to be less anxious.

Oncologists should make it a point to see newly diagnosed patients quickly, certainly within a week of diagnosis and sometimes even sooner. You should try to see at least one oncologist who specializes in your specific cancer subtype, for example, a gynecologic oncologist—if not on the first appointment, then during a second opinion (see next page).

At the appointment, you'll get detailed information about the stage of your cancer... where it's located in your body...what kind of prognosis to expect...what treatment is most appropriate...and how it will affect your life. Having this knowledge often helps to ease anxiety.

To prepare for your appointment...

- **Write down a list of questions.** You no doubt will have questions for the oncologist based on the initial conversation with your doctor. Be sure to write them down so that you don't forget them during the stress of your appointment.

In preparation for your appointment, you may also want to research your condition online, but restrict your browsing to well-respected sites, such as Cancer.gov (National Cancer Institute)...Cancer.org (American Cancer Society)...and Cancer.net (American Society of Clinical Oncology).

***Important:*** Be cautious about drawing conclusions from information on the web. Data on cancer can be complicated, and treatments can change over a short period of time. And prognoses and other stats are usually based on medians or averages. Use the information you glean from the web to add to your list of questions for the oncologist.

- **Bring one to three people with you to the first oncologist visit.** Patients are often so emotionally overwhelmed by the diagnosis that their brains do not process all the important information that's given to them during the appointment. Loved ones and/or friends can help listen, take notes and ask questions. They may also be able to tell the doctor about symptoms they've noticed that the patient isn't even aware of. I advise bringing as many as three loved ones or close friends because they can help the patient in different ways and will ask different questions. With your doctor's permission, you could also record the appointment (a recorder app on your smartphone is easy to use).

• **Consider a second opinion.** Ideally, you should get a second opinion before treatment begins, and it should be from a doctor not affiliated with the first. You should not feel uncomfortable telling your doctor about your plans for a second opinion—in the case of cancer, it's a very common practice and is even required by some insurance providers. Your doctor may facilitate the process of getting a second opinion with an unaffiliated doctor.

Having information you already received corroborated by a second opinion can be reassuring. And if the second opinion conflicts with the first, it's better to know that sooner than later. Insurance will usually cover the cost of a second opinion, but check with your insurance company or your insurance case manager, if you have one.

• **Address your stress.** After a cancer diagnosis, you may suffer from anxiety and/or lack of sleep. To take care of yourself, cut back on nonessential tasks so that you can focus on activities that will help relieve stress, such as getting more exercise and eating well. Talk to your doctor about the best exercise and diet for your specific situation.

Be sure to tell your doctor about any anxiety or depression you're feeling. He/she may refer you to a mental health provider, such as a therapist, psychologist or psychiatrist, and/or may prescribe a short-term medication, such as *alprazolam* (Xanax), to relieve anxiety and help you get some rest.

***Also:*** Support groups can be beneficial. A good resource is Cancer.net (click on "Coping with Cancer," then on "Finding Support and Information" and finally on "Support Groups"). But some patients feel that support groups make them overly consumed by their diagnosis and choose not to join one. That's OK—the patient should decide the form of support that is best for him.

• **Learn about clinical trials.** Even though most people assume that clinical trials enroll only patients who are in very advanced stages of their illnesses, that's not true. There are clinical trials designed for different types and stages of cancer, but they may have very specific requirements. That's why you should ask your doctor early on about clinical trials that may be right for your case.

• **Ask about support services.** Keeping up with all the details of your illness can be overwhelming. A social worker can help with health insurance, financial aid, etc., free of charge. The medical center where your doctor practices may have social workers on staff or be able to refer you to one.

# New Drug for Advanced Bladder Cancer

The FDA approved the immunotherapy drug *atezolizumab* (Tecentriq) for patients with metastatic urothelial carcinoma—the most common form of the bladder cancer. The drug is approved only for urothelial cancer that arises in the urinary tract. It is the first new treatment for this type of bladder cancer in more than 20 years. For that reason, the FDA approved it after only a Phase II clinical trial. Pricing, availability and insurance coverage are not yet known.

Jonathan Rosenberg, MD, a medical oncologist at Memorial Sloan Kettering Cancer Center, New York City, and leader of a study published in *The Lancet.*

# Get the Very Best Cancer Care

Barrie R. Cassileth, PhD, the former Laurance S. Rockefeller Chair and chief of the integrative medicine department at Memorial Sloan Kettering Cancer Center in New York City. She is also author of *Survivorship: Living Well During and After Cancer.*

A cancer diagnosis is always fraught with fear and anxiety—not to mention nagging questions about the best possible treatments.

***Bridging the gap:*** While surgery, chemotherapy and radiation have long been the mainstay treatments for cancer, major cancer centers throughout the US now offer a variety of additional "complementary" therapies that help patients cope with a wide range of cancer-related problems.

***Latest development:*** Recent studies continue to be added to the growing body of evidence supporting the use of such nondrug and nonsurgical therapies, which are used along with conventional cancer treatment.

## Look for Proven Benefits

Only a small number of complementary therapies have been thoroughly tested with randomized, placebo-controlled clinical trials—the gold standard of scientific research. Some of these approaches have now been proven to work.

Common cancer symptoms that can be relieved with complementary approaches—some services may be covered by insurance, so check with your health insurer...

- **Less nausea.** Nausea and/or vomiting are among the most common symptoms cancer patients have—and among the most feared. Antinausea medications help, but they're not a perfect solution. That's why they're sometimes used in tandem with acupuncture, a complementary therapy that has been shown to be particularly effective.

***Scientific evidence:*** When acupuncture was tested in a group of breast cancer patients being treated with a form of chemotherapy that's notorious for causing nausea, those who were given acupuncture for five days had one-third fewer episodes of nausea than those who were treated only with medications that were used for nausea, such as *lorazepam* and *diphenhydramine.* Self-acupressure, in which patients merely press on certain points, such as the PC6 point on the wrist (without using needles), can also help.

***To find the PC6 point:*** Turn your hand so your palm is facing up and locate the area, which is between the tendons three finger widths from the base of the wrist. Massage the area for four to five seconds...or longer, as needed.

- **Pain relief.** Both gentle massage and acupuncture can reduce the pain that's caused by cancer (such as bone cancer) and cancer treatments (such as radiation)—and sometimes allow patients to take lower doses of medication, which can help reduce troubling side effects, including constipation.

***Scientific evidence:*** A study that looked at nearly 1,300 cancer patients found that massage improved their pain scores by 40%... and the improvements lasted for hours and sometimes days after the massage.

Imaging studies show that acupuncture also helps by deactivating brain areas that are involved in pain perception. In one study, patients with chronic cancer pain were treated with either auricular acupuncture (needles placed in the ear) or with sham treatments. After two months, patients in the acupuncture group reported reductions in pain intensity of 36% versus 2% in the placebo group.

- **Less fatigue.** Only about 10% of cancer patients are physically active during treatment. But the vast majority can safely exercise before, during and after treatments...and exercise is among the best ways to reduce treatment-related fatigue.

***Scientific evidence:*** When researchers at the University of Connecticut analyzed 44 studies focusing on patients with cancer-related fatigue, they found that those who exercised had more energy than those who were sedentary.

Any form of exercise seems to help. Yoga that focuses on gentle postures and breathing is good because it's easy on the body and has been shown to reduce anxiety and other stress-related symptoms.

***Bonus:*** Cancer patients who exercise tend to live longer than those who don't stay active. A study of more than 900 breast cancer patients found that those who engaged in brisk walking for two and a half hours a week—the same level of exercise that's recommended for the general population—were 67% less likely to die during the nine-year study period than those who were sedentary.

- **Fewer hot flashes.** Both men and women who have hormone-dependent cancers (such as breast and prostate cancers) often experience hot flashes when they're given hormone-based treatments. Once again, acupuncture seems to help.

***Scientific evidence:*** One study found that nearly 90% of patients with breast or prostate cancers who were given acupuncture had a reduction in hot flashes of nearly 50% that lasted at least three months.

### How to Stay Safe

Virtually all oncologists and respected cancer centers in the US now support the use of complementary therapies, such as acupuncture and massage, to help cancer patients cope with nausea, pain, anxiety and other symptoms. These and other complementary therapies are used in addition to conventional treatments.

***To find an evidence-based complementary oncology program:*** Look for a comprehensive cancer center at the National Cancer Institute's website, Cancer.gov/research/nci-role/cancer-centers/find.

***Very important:*** When seeking complementary care, it's vital that the practitioner (including massage therapists, acupuncturists, etc.) be properly trained to work with cancer patients. Getting therapy at a comprehensive cancer center helps ensure that.

***Also crucial:*** Cancer patients should always talk to their doctors before taking any supplements (herbs, vitamins, etc.). They can sometimes interfere with chemotherapy and other cancer treatments. For more on specific supplements, go to Memorial Sloan Kettering's website, MSKCC.org/aboutherbs.

---

## Better Brain Cancer Treatment

Stereotactic radiosurgery, which precisely targets radiation to a few small tumors, results in less damage to the patient's short-term memory and thinking skills than whole-brain radiation, a recent study of about 200 brain cancer patients concluded. The current method of radiation to the entire brain may be more appropriate for patients with large or more widespread tumors.

Paul Brown, MD, radiation oncologist, Mayo Clinic, Rochester, Minnesota.

---

## New Scan for Esophageal Cancer

A new computer scan spots early-stage esophageal cancer nearly as effectively as top medical specialists. Early detection is important because these cancers are often missed—and five-year survival from late-stage cancer is less than 5%.

*Endoscopy* (journal).

---

## NSAID Fights Cancer

A new cancer fighter may be on its way. *Recent study:* Use of the prescription nonsteroidal anti-inflammatory drug (NSAID) *diclofenac* (Voltaren) was associated with less growth and spread of esophageal, breast, ovarian, lung and other cancers after surgery. Diclofenac was also reported to improve response to chemotherapy and radiation.

***If you have cancer:*** Ask your doctor about this drug.

Pan Pantziarka, PhD, coordinator, Repurposing Drugs in Oncology, London.

# The Cancer-Carb Connection

Barry Boyd, MD, MS, a medical oncologist and founder and former director of the Integrative Medicine Program at Greenwich Hospital-Yale Health Systems, where he is currently the director of Cancer Nutrition. He is author of *The Cancer Recovery Plan.* DrBarryBoyd.com

More bad news for carb lovers. The same refined, low-fiber foods that contribute to obesity, diabetes and other serious conditions are now believed to increase one's risk for cancer—and to worsen outcomes in those who already have it.

***Alarming new finding:*** In a study recently published in *Cancer Epidemiology, Biomarkers & Prevention*, people who ate the most *high-glycemic* (blood sugar–spiking) carbohydrates—foods such as white bread, white rice and russet potatoes—were 49% more likely to be diagnosed with lung cancer than those who ate the least.

Even though this isn't the first study to link "junk" carbohydrates to cancer, the evidence has now gotten strong enough that more and more medical experts are advising us to take a very close look at the quality of the carbs that we eat.

## What's the Link to Carbs?

Dietary carbohydrates are a critical driver of blood sugar (glucose) levels and must be tracked by people with diabetes to keep their blood glucose levels steady.

We have known for a long time that people with diabetes are more likely to get cancer than those who do not have diabetes. More recently, we've learned that even in the absence of diabetes, many people are "prediabetic," with elevated blood glucose and insulin (the blood sugar–regulating hormone)—due to poor diet, a lack of exercise and other causes. Prediabetes makes people more likely to develop cancer...and puts them at greater risk for poor outcomes when they do.

***Recent finding:*** A variety of cancers, such as breast, colorectal, endometrial and pancreatic, seem to be affected by high glucose and high insulin. It is clear that a "Western-style" diet—typically loaded with high-GI foods—creates some of the conditions that make it easier for cancers to thrive. *What happens...*

- **High-GI foods trigger an increase in insulin,** which results in a rise in *insulin-growth factor* (IGF-1). Both insulin and IGF-1 will promote the growth of cancer cells and inhibit their natural death.
- **Obesity,** particularly when there is excess fat in the belly area, is strongly associated with prediabetes. People with obesity have more inflammation, oxidative stress and estrogen—all of which increase cancer risks.

## Self-Defense

Unless you already have diabetes or are at a high risk of developing it (for example, you are overweight or obese with belly fat* and/or have a sedentary lifestyle), I don't advise too much emphasis strictly on total carbohydrate intake or GI food ratings. I focus more on the quality of carbohydrates and, in practice, find that people who try to track the GI of all the foods they eat tend to give up healthy eating altogether because it becomes too much work.

Also, high-GI foods are just one part of the equation. Vegetarians (who generally eat low-GI foods) tend to have a lower risk for cancer. But is it because of their carbohydrate choices or because they're also more likely to be physically active and have lower body weights? The evidence isn't clear.

***My advice:*** Follow an overall strategy that both controls blood glucose and may help you prevent/manage cancer. *Key steps...*

*Abdominal obesity is defined as a waist measurement of 35 inches or more in women.

• **Limit weight gain through a prudent diet and physical activity.** You don't have to avoid all high-GI foods, but you should limit them. Consider eating plans (such as the Mediterranean diet) that emphasize whole grains, legumes, vegetables and other low-GI foods. Such diets have been linked to reduced risk for cancer-promoting obesity, diabetes and elevated blood glucose levels. Regular exercise has also been linked to a reduced risk and improved survival in many cancers—in part, by reducing insulin.

• **Avoid processed foods as much as possible.** They tend to be high in added sugar, which raises blood glucose very quickly.

***One of the worst:*** Sugared soft drinks, which typically have the equivalent of 10 teaspoons of sugar per serving!

• **Cut back on red meat.** It is among the main sources of saturated fat in the American diet. Even if you mainly eat healthy carbohydrates, too much saturated fat increases the risk for insulin resistance (when the body becomes less sensitive to the hormone's effect, triggering the release of more insulin to compensate) and cancer.

• **Improve your gut health.** A healthy intestinal "flora" can help prevent obesity, along with preventing both insulin resistance and inflammation. It's another argument for eating low-GI carbs—they tend to be high in fiber and act as prebiotics, foods that promote the growth of healthy intestinal bacteria.

• **Ask about *metformin* (Glucophage).** It's a diabetes drug that reduces insulin resistance, decreases the production of glucose by the liver and lowers insulin levels. It's also less likely to cause weight gain than other diabetes medications. One large study found that it can reduce overall cancer risk by 31% in people with diabetes.

But it is not a miracle drug. Research has shown that lifestyle changes are more effective than metformin at preventing diabetes.

### For Those with Cancer

If you have cancer, try your best to stay active and eat well—during and after treatments. It's common for cancer survivors to deal with stress by overindulging in comfort foods. But research shows that those who maintain a healthy weight, are physically active and eat nutritious, low-GI carbs will be less likely to have a cancer recurrence.

## Better Surgery for Bladder Cancer

A surgical technique called narrow band imaging (NBI) has been found to reduce recurrence for patients with early-stage bladder cancer. NBI's vision-enhancement technology allows surgeons to see and remove more tumors than in the traditional "white light" procedure.

***Details:*** In a study of 965 patients, only 5.6% of those low-risk patients who underwent NBI surgery had tumors recur within 12 months, compared with 27.3% in the traditional surgery group.

Richard Bryan, MBChB, PhD, senior research fellow, University of Birmingham, UK.

## Sunshine and Cancer

Michael F. Holick, PhD, MD, a professor of medicine, physiology and biophysics at Boston University School of Medicine. He is author of *The Vitamin D Solution: A 3-Step Strategy to Cure Our Most Common Health Problems.*

It's a gorgeous summer morning, so you step outside to enjoy a touch of sun while sipping your morning coffee. But wait... what about sunscreen?

According to some medical organizations, any sun exposure is a serious risk factor for melanoma and other skin cancers. For this reason, Americans often are advised to get vitamin D only from foods and/or supplements. But not all medical experts agree with that advice.

Michael F. Holick, PhD, MD, is a leading expert on vitamin D and a firm believer that avoiding all sunshine can pose health risks that may be worse than those from sensible sun exposure.

His advice on finding the sweet spot for just the right amount of sun exposure...

## A Common Deficiency

Vitamin D is one of the most common nutrition deficiencies in the US. More than half of older adults are deficient—in part because the body's ability to synthesize vitamin D from sunlight declines with age.

***Those with dark skin fare worst:*** Research has found that 40% of Hispanics and a staggering 84% of African-Americans over age 50 were vitamin D deficient.

Only a few foods (such as salmon, sun-dried mushrooms, cod-liver oil and, to a much lesser extent, egg yolks) contain vitamin D, so most Americans rely on fortified foods (such as milk and some breakfast cereals). Taking a vitamin D supplement helps, but it isn't the same as sunshine. The vitamin D produced by sunshine enters the bloodstream slowly and maintains its health-promoting biological activity for at least twice as long as supplemental D.

## Dangers of Low Vitamin D

Humans have evolved to depend on sunshine. So what happens when you never go outside without wearing sunscreen—or rarely go outside at all? When used properly, a sunscreen with an SPF of 30 reduces vitamin D production by 97%. *Important health risks now being linked to low vitamin D levels...*

- **Multiple sclerosis.** You're five times more likely to get this disease if you live in North America or Europe than in the tropics. In the US, prevalence of this disease in northern states such as Maine, Minnesota and Washington is nearly double that found in sunnier areas.

- **Cancer.** There isn't conclusive proof that people with low vitamin D have an increased risk for cancer. But there's persuasive evi-

## Melanoma Updates

**Check here for skin cancer.** When checking your skin for changes (in the size, color and/or shape of moles or for any that bleed), don't forget to examine the bottoms of your feet.

***Recent finding:*** In a study of more than 100 melanoma patients, the deadly skin cancer was found to often be more advanced when it developed on the soles of the feet, possibly because this area is not examined as often as skin exposed to the sun.

***Also:*** Repeated skin damage due to walking was identified as a possible trigger for melanoma on the soles of the feet.

Ryuhei Okuyama, MD, professor of dermatology, Shinshu University School of Medicine, Matsumoto, Japan.

**Drug for long-term melanoma survival.** *Pembrolizumab* (Keytruda)—one of the medications used to treat former president Jimmy Carter—helps the immune system fight cancer cells.

***Recent finding:*** 40% of the patients given Keytruda were alive after three years, and 15% showed no sign of cancer. The drug is given intravenously every three weeks.

***Among the more common side effects:*** Fatigue, itchiness, rash.

Caroline Robert, MD, PhD, chair of dermatology, Institut de Cancérologie Gustave Roussy, Villejuif, France, and lead author of a study of 655 patients, presented at the 2016 meeting of the American Society of Clinical Oncology.

**Drug to stop cancer spread.** Melanoma, the most dangerous form of skin cancer, quickly spreads to other parts of the body.

***In development:*** A drug that reduces cancer-cell migration by 85% to 90%.

*Molecular Cancer Therapeutics.*

dence from population and observational studies that people with sufficient vitamin D are 30% to 50% less likely to develop breast, colorectal or other cancers than those with vitamin D deficiencies.

• **Heart disease.** Vitamin D deficiency is associated with increased heart attack risk. People who live in sunny climates are also less likely to have high blood pressure.

Other health problems linked to vitamin D deficiency include osteoporosis, diabetes and depression.

## The Real Cancer Risk

Dermatologists have long used the "C" word to warn people about the sun. It's true that chronic sun exposure increases one's risk for basal and squamous cell carcinomas.

While these "nonmelanoma" skin cancers are a significant health problem, they're fortunately among the easiest to cure and are rarely fatal. Meanwhile, the noncancer health risks from low vitamin D, such as those described earlier, generally outweigh the risks from these cancers.

Melanoma is another story. A frequently fatal cancer that results in some 10,000 deaths in the US each year, melanoma is strongly linked to sunburns. People who get only short-term and occasional sun exposure don't face the same risk. In addition, melanoma often develops on parts of the body with little (or no) sun exposure, such as the buttocks.

## A Sensible Compromise

***Let me be clear:*** I do not recommend sunbathing or tanning. I advise most adults to get just enough sun (without sunscreen) to help produce a vitamin D blood level of at least 30 ng/mL, as measured by a 25-hydroxy vitamin D blood test. The rest of the time, you should use sunscreen and wear a hat and other protective clothing. *My approach...*

• **Follow the "no sunburn" rule.** The amount of vitamin D produced by your body depends on such factors as the season, time of day, your geographic location and your pigmentation. I advise my patients to spend about one-half the time in the sun that it would ordinarily take them to get a mild sunburn. This should be done between 10 am and 3 pm (when the angle of the sun's rays maximizes vitamin D production).

During this time, expose your arms and legs to the sun (without sunscreen). Together, your limbs account for about half of your body's surface area. Exposing them to sun (with the rest of your body covered) should gradually increase your vitamin D level over four to eight weeks and then stabilize it.

• **Keep close track of the time.** While one's sun "dose" is highly individual, people with dark skin will usually be able to expose their skin to sunshine for up to 30 minutes, three times a week. If you're fair, five to 10 minutes is likely enough.

• **Use sunscreen the rest of the time.** I recommend using sunscreen with an SPF 30 rating whenever you're not getting your controlled sun dose.

***Important:*** Be sure to use sunscreen on your face anytime you're outdoors. Very little vitamin D is produced via sun exposure to your face...and too much sun on your face, which gets sun whenever you're outdoors, will cause wrinkles and increase your risk for skin cancer.

• **Take a supplement.** Even if you enjoy regular "sun sessions," there will be times (particularly in the winter) when your body won't produce enough vitamin D. To ensure consistent adequate levels of vitamin D, a supplement (typically 2,000 IU daily for adults) will make up the difference. To determine your optimal dose of a vitamin D supplement, ask your doctor for advice. He/she may recommend a 25-hydroxy vitamin D blood test to check your body's vitamin D level.

***Important:*** If you have had skin cancer or are at increased risk (due, for example, to family history)...or have a medical condition or take medication that increases your sun sensitivity, ask your doctor about appropriate sun exposure and the best ways to maintain adequate vitamin D levels.

## Self-Tanner Safety

The only safe tan comes from a topical self-tanner. A real tan raises risk for skin cancer—especially if you use indoor ultraviolet tanning beds. And so-called tanning pills should never be used. They are not FDA-approved and can cause liver and retinal damage.

Most self-tanning products contain dihydroxyacetone (DHA), a nontoxic chemical that darkens the top layer of skin. Self-tanners are available as creams, lotions, sprays or wipes. For best results, exfoliate with lotion or pads containing 10% glycolic acid for three days before applying the self-tanner. This will help even out the top layer of skin and provide better absorption of DHA. If you're using a spray, cover your nose and mouth to avoid ingesting it.

Your tan should last for a week or so before it naturally fades. You will still need to use broad-spectrum sunscreen when outdoors, since faux tans will not protect your skin.

Neal Schultz, MD, a dermatologist in private practice in New York City.

## Talk Therapy Fights Chemo Brain

About half of patients who get chemotherapy develop chemo brain, which causes them to have trouble following conversations or remembering steps needed to complete a project. In a small study, a specially developed form of cognitive-behavioral therapy called memory and attention adaptation training (MAAT) led to reduced memory problems and better processing speed. Patients who received MAAT also reported less anxiety about mental issues two months after the sessions ended.

Study of 47 breast cancer survivors by researchers at Eastern Maine Medical Center, Bangor, and Lafayette Family Center, Brewer, Maine, published in *Cancer*.

## Cancer + Cancer

One in 12 cancer patients will develop a second unrelated cancer (not a metastasis of the original malignancy), a recent study of two million adults found.

***Details:*** Those with bladder cancer were at greatest risk for an unrelated cancer—most often lung cancer.

***Possible reason:*** People with bladder cancer often have risk factors for other types of cancer, such as smoking and exposure to workplace chemicals.

***If you have any type of cancer:*** Be sure your doctors monitor for other cancers.

Nicholas Donin, MD, urologic oncology fellow, David Geffen School of Medicine at UCLA.

# Chapter 3

# LUNG HEALTH AND ALLERGIES

## Another Menopause Side Effect: Shortness of Breath?

As if hot flashes and night sweats weren't enough, a recent study suggests that a woman's lung function seems to decline during menopause.

As their periods stop, women could find themselves becoming short of breath, said study author Kai Triebner, a graduate student in epidemiology at the University of Bergen in Norway.

"Women are living longer and, therefore, many years beyond menopause," Triebner said. "Our study highlights the importance of maintaining respiratory health long after the menopausal transition."

### Study Details

The researchers found two aspects of lung function in particular that declined in menopausal and postmenopausal women.

These functions were forced vital capacity—a measurement of the total volume of air the lungs can exhale after taking the deepest breath possible...and forced expiratory volume in one second (FEV1)—a measurement of how much air a person can forcefully blow out in one second. The reductions in performance, the study authors said, are beyond those that would be expected from aging.

The decline in forced vital capacity was equivalent to the damage caused by smoking 20 cigarettes a day for 10 years. The reduction in FEV1 was similar to what a pack-a-day smoker experiences over two years, the researchers said.

The findings were based on an analysis of more than 1,400 European women who were 25 to 48 years old when they joined the study. The researchers tracked them for 20 years.

Not surprisingly, smokers showed a steeper rate of lung function decline, the study found.

The researchers reported their findings in the *American Journal of Respiratory and Critical Care Medicine.*

### Possible Explanation

Hormonal changes related to menopause may play a role in lung function decline since they can lead to systemic inflammation and the bone-thinning disease osteoporosis. Os-

Kai Triebner, graduate student in epidemiology, University of Bergen, Norway.

American Thoracic Society, news release.

teoporosis can compress the height of the chest vertebrae, limiting air intake, the researchers said.

## Implications

"The decline in lung function may cause an increase in shortness of breath, reduced work capacity and fatigue," Triebner said. "Symptoms depend upon how much lung capacity is reduced, and a few women may actually develop respiratory failure as a result of this decline."

"Women, and their physicians, should be aware that respiratory health might decline considerably during and after the menopausal transition," Triebner said. "This could mean that they experience shortness of breath already with low physical activity."

For more information about menopause, visit the website of the U.S. National Institute on Aging, NIA.nih.gov/health/publication/menopause.

---

# Secrets to Managing COPD

Dawn Fielding, RCP, AE-C, a licensed respiratory therapist and certified COPD and Asthma Educator based in West Haven, Utah. She is executive director of the Chronic Lung Alliance, a nonprofit organization involved in education and research related to chronic lung disease. She is also author of *The COPD Solution*.

---

If you are living with chronic obstructive pulmonary disease (COPD), the simple act of breathing can feel like you're pushing a boulder uphill.

And COPD has recently replaced stroke as the third leading cause of death for women in all categories, according to the Centers for Disease Control and Prevention.

***What you may not know:*** Because your ability to breathe is affected by everything in your life—including your thoughts and emotions—few disorders have as strong a mind-body connection as COPD.

While most doctors talk to their patients with COPD about inhalers, oxygen therapy and sometimes even surgery, the additional approaches described here will help ensure the best possible results for those who have this disorder.

## The COPD Spiral

With COPD (which includes chronic bronchitis and/or emphysema), air can't flow easily into and out of the lungs because of a blockage in the airways, typically caused by excess mucus, inflammation or dysfunctional lung tissue.

Being unable to breathe is a primal terror. The constant worry and anxiety that accompany this fear push the body into a stress reaction that makes breathing even more difficult, triggering more fear and stress. The key is to break the spiral and create a steadier breathing environment.

In addition to proper breathing techniques that should be practiced regularly—such as pursed breathing (as though you're whistling) and belly breathing, which strengthens muscles that assist with breathing—try these simple steps...

***SECRET #1:*** **Change your thoughts.** When you have a negative thought—such as *I can't do this anymore because of my COPD*—your brain registers the emotion behind it and reacts by signaling the body to produce stress hormones and to speed up your respiration rate and blood pressure.

This is helpful in an emergency...say, if you fear an oncoming car and your body reacts to avoid a collision. But in the absence of an actual threat, the response can be physically harmful by lowering your body's natural defenses and sapping your energy levels.

***What helps:*** Positive statements reduce anxiety, help you cope and tell your brain that it's OK to relax.

***What to do:*** When you find yourself becoming stressed, stop! Break that cycle of anxiety by repeating a phrase, such as those below, to set your brain on a positive track...

- **"No more negativity...I'll just focus on what I can do."**
- **"One day at a time. I got through yesterday. I'll get through today."**

Positive thinking and deep breathing lower blood pressure, slow heart rate and make more oxygen available for breathing.

***SECRET #2:*** **Watch what you eat.** Food choices are a surprisingly important factor in controlling COPD symptoms.

***Here's why:*** Breathing is a process that involves the exchange of carbon dioxide (CO2) and oxygen in the blood.

A person with COPD has a less efficient oxygen-CO2 exchange process. Anything that increases the amount of CO2 in blood (whether it's stress or a certain type of food, such as soda or sugary food products) revs up your breathing rate—which worsens COPD.

What to do...

- **Cut back on foods that increase levels of CO2 in the blood.** The worst offenders are carbonated beverages (even fizzy water)...and anything made with refined sugar or white flour (everything from cakes and cookies to certain breads and pastas).
- **Avoid caffeinated beverages, including coffee, tea and colas.** Caffeine "wakes up" your nervous system, causing your body to work faster, accelerating your breathing rate. Whenever possible, replace soda and other caffeinated beverages with water. Why water? It helps thin mucous secretions and transports nutrients throughout our bodies. For variety, choose flavored waters (such as those infused with lemon or mint).

***SECRET #3:*** **Do the right exercises.** For people with COPD, breathing alone is so physically taxing that it's crucial to also improve physical stamina.

In a recent study of people with COPD in *Respiratory Medicine*, researchers compared the benefits of specific types of exercise. All the study participants did cardiovascular exercise (such as walking and biking) twice a week for three months, but one group added more strength training (including weight training for the upper and lower body) than the other group.

***Result:*** People who did the most strength training had much stronger muscles throughout the body, which resulted in more efficient breathing.

In addition to doing upper-body exercises, such as bicep curls, try the following three times a week...

- **Leg lifts.** This exercise targets large muscle groups that allow us to move about freely.

***What to do:*** While sitting in a chair, straighten one leg and lift, foot flexed, as high as you can while keeping your back straight. Hold that position for a count of five, then lower your leg. Repeat five times with each leg. Don't worry if you cannot hold your leg up for very long—your strength will improve over time.

***Also:*** Aerobic exercise is crucial—try to get at least 2,000 steps a day (use a pedometer or fitness tracker) while going about your daily activities, including getting the mail, going shopping, etc. Try to exercise when your energy levels are high...and check with your doctor about the best time to take your medications when exercising.

## Make Peace with COPD...

People with COPD can experience a wide range of troubling emotions, including denial, guilt, anger and depression. If you believe that you need help coping, consider joining a support group.

The American Lung Association (ALA) sponsors Better Breathers Clubs across the US. These groups are led by a trained facilitator and offer educational presentations as well as emotional support.

To find a local group, call the ALA at 800-LUNGUSA...or look online at Lung.org (under "Support & Community," click on "Better Breathers Club").

## COPD Linked to Falls

Having chronic obstructive pulmonary disease (COPD) could significantly increase the risk of falling, according to a recent study of 73 adults.

***Why:*** People with COPD often don't get enough exercise, which can lead to loss of balance, and they're more likely to have other risk factors linked to falling, such as low blood oxygen levels.

***If you have COPD:*** Talk to your doctor about ways to reduce your risk of falling, such as exercises to improve balance and using a cane.

Cristian Oancea, MD, PhD, lecturer in pulmonary rehabilitation, Victor Babes University of Medicine and Pharmacy, Timisoara, Romania.

## 5 Mistakes to Avoid If You Have Asthma

Gailen D. Marshall, MD, PhD, the R. Faser Triplett Sr. MD Chair of Allergy and Immunology at The University of Mississippi Medical Center in Jackson. His major research interests include factors affecting asthma risk and the effectiveness of integrative approaches to clinical care for asthma and other immune-based diseases. Dr. Marshall is in his third term as editor in chief of the *Annals of Allergy, Asthma & Immunology.*

Whether it's the wintertime pleasure of sitting next to a crackling log in the fireplace...or the summertime thrill of cooling off in a swimming pool, many of our most treasured seasonal pastimes can mean big trouble for some people.

***Hidden threat:*** If you or a family member is among the 24 million Americans coping with asthma, such seemingly harmless activities could be a mistake.

Asthma, which inflames and narrows the airways, is serious business. Half of all adults with asthma have poorly controlled or even uncontrolled asthma, meaning they are at increased risk for sudden worsening of symptoms, which can lead to complications—such as persistent breathing difficulties and even death.

That's why it is imperative for asthma sufferers to avoid common missteps that may prevent them from properly controlling their condition. *Among the biggest mistakes...*

***MISTAKE #1:*** **Not seeing the right doctor.** Too many asthma patients—and even some doctors—fail to recognize the crossover component between asthma and allergies. For about one-third of adult asthma patients, acute episodes and poor control can be triggered by allergies to common substances such as mold, dust, pollen and animal dander. When the immune system of an asthma patient mistakes these substances for a foreign intruder, allergy antibodies (known as IgE) are produced and make their way to the lungs, often leading to an asthma attack.

An internist or a family doctor can manage asthma cases that flare up only occasionally. But for people with severe and persistent asthma (marked by repeated episodes of coughing, wheezing and/or difficulty breathing that take multiple medications to control), the best doctor is often an allergist, who can perform testing to determine whether a patient's asthma triggers are allergy-based.

***My advice:*** Consider seeing an allergist if you have persistent asthma symptoms (described above) that limit everyday activities or you've ever had a life-threatening asthma attack. If an allergist is not available in your area, ask your doctor for a referral to a pulmonologist (a lung function specialist).

***MISTAKE #2:*** **Not getting treated for allergies.** To pinpoint allergies that may be contributing to their asthma, patients should undergo allergy testing as soon as possible after an asthma diagnosis.

Unfortunately, some asthma patients who learn they indeed have allergies don't get allergy shots, a form of immunotherapy that can reduce sensitivity to these triggers. Until this step is taken, repeated bouts of severe asthma symptoms are likely.

A relatively new treatment, sublingual immunotherapy (in which an allergen in tablet form is taken under the tongue) may be an option for certain allergy sufferers. If you're interested, talk to your doctor.

***MISTAKE #3:* Missing less obvious triggers.** Asthma triggers include anything—whether a true allergen or other irritant—that can aggravate symptoms. While most people already know about many of their own asthma triggers, such as strenuous exercise, rapidly breathing in cold air, certain medications, including nonsteroidal anti-inflammatory drugs like aspirin, *ibuprofen* or *naproxen*, or even strong emotions, many other triggers fly under the radar. What are some of these less obvious irritants?

• **Household plants.** Asthma attacks can be precipitated by mold spores that are often found in the soil of many household plants.

***My advice:*** Mold-sensitive patients should minimize indoor plants and keep them out of rooms in which they spend a lot of time, such as the bedroom. If you want to have some plants in your home, you may want to try English ivy, a peace lily or a rubber plant. These plants have been found in research to reduce airborne toxins, including mold spores.

***Note:*** Keep English ivy, peace lily and the Indian rubber plant out of the reach of pets and children—these plants can be toxic if consumed.

• **Wood smoke.** Most people realize that cigarette and cigar smoke are irritants, but wood smoke is often overlooked, even though it too can trigger an asthma flare-up.

***My advice:*** If you have asthma, avoid exposure to wood smoke from fireplaces, grills and open fires to avoid worsening symptoms.

• **Chlorine.** A dip in the pool can be invigorating and even help build lung function, but it can also take your breath away if the water is highly chlorinated. While not a true allergy, chlorine sensitivities can trigger chest tightness, coughing and wheezing.

***My advice:*** If you have asthma, limit your exposure to freshly chlorinated pools—especially hyper-chlorinated public pools—and shower thoroughly afterward. If possible, swim in a saltwater pool.

Also, if chlorinated pools make your symptoms worse, be careful about using household cleaning products that contain bleach—only use these products in areas that are well-ventilated.

• **Candles and air fresheners.** Pleasant aromas from scented candles and air fresheners can irritate nasal passages and contribute to an asthma attack.

***My advice:*** To prevent a possible allergic reaction, it's best to avoid scented candles and air fresheners.

***MISTAKE #4:* Not getting a flu shot.** Getting an annual flu shot is especially important for asthmatics, who are at increased risk for dangerous flu complications, such as pneumonia. It's best to get the flu shot in October, but it's still helpful to get it up until March. Pneumonia vaccines, which can be given anytime during the year, are also recommended for people with asthma.

***MISTAKE #5:* Not recognizing flare-up symptoms.** It's crucial that people with asthma watch for subtle warning signs—such as increasing shortness of breath while exercising or restless sleep—that indicate their asthma may be veering out of control.

***Rule of thumb:*** Asthma is considered poorly controlled if wheezing or other symptoms occur more than twice a week or if you awaken more than twice a month with asthma symptoms. Other red flags include needing to use "rescue" inhalers, such as albuterol more than twice a week...requiring oral corticosteroids to treat severe attacks...and/or changing activity patterns (such as avoiding stairs, etc.).

• **Spices.** Powdered spices such as cumin, mustard and paprika don't just make for yummier food—they can also exacerbate asthma if inhaled. This can also happen with flour, powdered sugar and other products that are finely ground.

***My advice:*** Whenever possible, avoid using finely ground ingredients. Fresh herbs and spices are much less likely to be inhaled.

If you do need to use powdered ingredients, try putting on a fiberglass painter's mask when doing your food preparations.

## Lungs That Smell

Newly discovered olfactory receptors in lung tissue trigger smooth muscle contraction/relaxation.

***Takeaway:*** Scent molecules could affect drug treatments for asthma or other lung conditions.

*Frontiers in Physiology.*

## Beware of Adult-Onset Asthma

Adults who develop asthma are 57% more likely to have a heart attack, stroke, heart failure, angina or other cardiovascular condition than adults without asthma, according to a recent study. It's unknown how asthma is linked to cardiovascular disease, but inflammation may be a factor. Symptoms of adult-onset asthma include persistent dry cough, shortness of breath and wheezing.

Matthew Tattersall, DO, assistant professor of medicine, University of Wisconsin School of Medicine and Public Health, Madison.

## Hidden Smoking Danger

Liz Williams, project manager for the Berkeley, California-based nonprofit Americans for Nonsmokers' Rights. No-Smoke.org

Far too many people still smoke—and often do so in their cars, subjecting others inside the vehicle to the dangers of secondhand smoke...even if the window is open.

***Latest development:*** Virginia is the latest of eight states and several municipalities (plus Puerto Rico) to enact laws that prohibit car-smoking when children are present. Similar legislation has been proposed in 12 other states.

"Car occupants exposed to secondhand smoke breathe air at levels much higher than what the EPA considers hazardous," notes Liz Williams, project manager for the Berkeley, California–based nonprofit Americans for Nonsmokers' Rights (No-Smoke.org).

***Why it matters:*** Nonsmokers who breathe secondhand smoke have a 25% to 30% increased risk for heart disease...20% to 30% increased risk for stroke...and 20% to 30% increased risk for lung cancer.

***What you may not realize:*** Thirdhand smoke—the sticky, smoky residue that clings to walls and other surfaces—can persist for years, according to research. Children are especially at risk because they can ingest tobacco residue just by touching contaminated surfaces (such as flooring and walls) and putting their hands in their mouths.

If a smoker has ever lived in your home, you might need to replace furniture, carpets and drapes to remove the ashtray smell. Washing walls might help.

***Better:*** "Encapsulating" tobacco residues with a fresh coat of paint.

***Bottom Line:*** Always insist on smoke-free environments, whether it's a public place or someone's home or car.

## Catch COPD Early

Many smokers and former smokers have COPD symptoms well before they are diagnosed with the disease. The symptoms of chronic obstructive pulmonary disease (COPD) include shortness of breath, coughing and difficulty exercising. If you have these symptoms and are a smoker or a former smoker, see your doctor without delay. COPD is the third-leading cause of death in the US.

Study of 2,723 current or former smokers led by researchers at University of Michigan Women's Health Program, Ann Arbor, published in *The New England Journal of Medicine.*

# Sneezing and Wheezing Could Mean a Dust Mite Allergy

Michael L. Lewin, MD, an allergist who has been practicing for 30 years. He has offices in New York City and Wilton, Connecticut, and is a faculty member of Weill Cornell Medical College in New York City. LewinAllergy.com

More than half of all Americans test positive for at least one kind of allergen. But there's one culprit that often gets overlooked by allergy sufferers.

***What you may not realize:*** Dust mites, which thrive in warm, humid weather, are one of the most common household triggers for allergies and asthma. Dust mites are tiny, eight-legged creatures that are too small to be seen by the naked eye, but they can wreak havoc if you are allergic to them.

Dust mites lurk in beds, carpets, draperies and upholstered furniture and surfaces. Their primary food source is human skin cells that we shed naturally. In fact, each of us sheds enough cells each day to feed one million dust mites. And depending on its age, a mattress can harbor up to 10 million dust mites! *What you need to know to protect yourself...*

## Are Dust Mites to Blame?

Allergies to dust mites are caused not by the mites themselves, but rather by their waste particles and dead body parts. Since we are constantly exposed to dust mites, those of us who have a dust mite allergy are likely to experience year-round symptoms. These can include sneezing...runny nose...red, itchy or watery eyes...stuffy nose...postnasal drip...and cough. (Eczema and asthma symptoms can be triggered or exacerbated by contact with dust mites.) Because dust mite allergy symptoms are so similar to those caused by other common allergens, such as pollen, some patients fail to recognize when the ubiquitous little creatures are the cause of their allergy symptoms or worsening symptoms due to another allergy.

***If you have a dust mite allergy:*** You may notice that your symptoms are worse when you're in bed or when you first wake up in the morning. That's because of the high concentration of dust mites in mattresses and bedding. Your symptoms may also flare up when you're dusting or vacuuming—droppings can easily become airborne...or when the temperature and humidity are higher than usual.

## Easy Tests

There are a few testing methods that can determine whether you are allergic to dust mites.

***The easiest is a skin-prick test:*** A drop of dust mite antigen is placed on the skin...the doctor lightly scratches your skin through the drop...and then watches to see if you develop redness, swelling or itching within about 20 minutes.

If you cannot have a skin test (some skin conditions and medications make the test unreliable), your doctor might recommend a blood test that looks for antibodies that are produced in response to specific allergens.

## Avoidance First

As a first step to treating a dust mite allergy, it's a good idea to follow the strategies below to reduce the load of dust mites in your home. You can't eliminate them entirely, but reducing their number may be enough to lessen or eliminate symptoms. *To start...*

- **Cover your bedding.** Your bed has more dust mites than any other area in the house.

***What helps:*** Cover your mattress, box spring, pillows and comforters with dust mite encasings. These encasings work by creating a barrier between you and the dust mites. These products, which are available online, are made of microporous fabrics with a pore size that is too small to be permeated by dust mites.

- **Hot-water washes.** Once a week, be sure to wash your bedding (sheets, blankets, mattress covers, pillowcases, etc.) in water that's 130°F or hotter. It will kill mites as well as their eggs.

• **Vacuum frequently.** Avoid wall-to-wall carpeting since it provides a large area for dust mites to inhabit. Vacuum your rugs, carpeting, drapes and other upholstered or fabric-covered surfaces once a week. A vacuum fitted with a HEPA filter will help prevent allergy-causing particles from getting stirred up in the air you breathe.

• **Steam clean.** A steam cleaner that produces superheated steam will kill mites and deactivate the allergy-causing proteins in their droppings. Consider steam cleaning carpets, drapes, upholstery, etc., once or twice a year.

• **Keep humidity low.** Because dust mites thrive in warm, humid environments, keep your humidity levels below 50%. Use a dehumidifier if necessary during the more humid months of summer. You can place it in the room(s), including the bedroom, where you spend the most time. To keep an eye on the humidity levels in your home, you can purchase a hygrometer online for less than $10.

• **Use a HEPA filter air purifier.** House "dust" contains copious amounts of skin cells and mites and their droppings, but you can reduce allergy symptoms by using a filtering mechanism to remove airborne particles. Portable HEPA units filter all the air in a room, trapping particles as they pass through. You can also consider a full-house filter for your HVAC system.

## For Additional Help

If the steps above don't alleviate your symptoms, you may want to consider either over-the-counter or prescription medications such as antihistamines, nasal sprays or eye drops. If medication—plus environmental control—still doesn't give you adequate relief from your symptoms, you should consider allergen immunotherapy.

Allergen immunotherapy is the process by which the body builds immunity to allergens such as dust mites. This is accomplished by administering small, incremental doses of dust mite (or other antigens), prompting the immune system to respond by decreasing the body's reactivity to these substances.

Allergen immunotherapy can be administered by subcutaneous injections (commonly called allergy shots)—given in a doctor's office (usually weekly in the beginning, then once every few weeks for maintenance) for three to five years.

A newer method is sublingual immunotherapy—allergy drops. Allergy drops are made of the same antigens as allergy shots but are formulated into drops that are placed under the tongue.

Once you have been tested and your allergies have been identified, your doctor can prepare your allergy drops based on your test results. Allergy drops are an effective, safe and convenient way to treat allergy symptoms. Once your drops have been formulated, you take the first dose at your doctor's office and then continue treatment at home daily for three to five years.

# Dry Eye Linked to Seasonal Allergens

Dry eye—a condition of red, watery, gritty-feeling eyes—peaks each year in April, the same month as pollen. Dry eye affects about 20% of women and 10% of men. The correlation between dry eye and the peak in pollen may mean that people with dry eye would benefit from allergy-prevention approaches in addition to current treatments, such as artificial tears.

***Examples:*** Wearing goggles outside when doing yard work...using air filters indoors.

Study of 3.4 million visits to Veterans Affairs eye clinics between 2006 and 2011 by researchers at Bascom Palmer Eye Institute, University of Miami, Florida, published in *Ophthalmology*.

## Allergen Alert If You Travel

If you have allergies, ask a hotel about its fragrance use before booking a room, advises travel expert Peter Greenberg. Many hotels pump fragrances into common areas and even individual rooms. If you are concerned, choose a different hotel.

Peter Greenberg, travel editor for *CBS News*, Studio City, California, and author of *The Best Places for Everything*.

## Nosebleeds and Spicy Food

Can hot, spicy food cause nosebleeds? It could. Food that contains capsaicin (a compound that gives chili peppers their spice) or allyl isothiocyanate (found in horseradish and hot mustard) irritates and inflames the mucous membranes in the nose, mouth and eyes, causing the nose to run and eyes to water.

This irritation can be good for nasal congestion, since it can temporarily relieve stuffed-up sinuses. Some nasal sprays even contain capsaicin. But when nasal membranes are thin and dry, this irritation can cause them to crack and bleed. Consult your doctor if you have frequent nosebleeds (more than once a week)—this may signal the need for an adjustment in the dosage of a blood thinner or an underlying condition, such as kidney disease.

Murray Grossan, MD, otolaryngologist, Tower Ear, Nose & Throat, Los Angeles, and author of *The Whole Body Approach to Allergy and Sinus Health*.

## Chronic Nosebleed Relief

Salt spray may relieve chronic nosebleeds. People with hemorrhagic telangiectasia (HHT) have as many as two nosebleeds a day.

***Recent finding:*** People with HHT who sprayed a saline solution into their noses twice daily for 12 weeks got as much relief from nosebleeds as those who used *bevacizumab*, estriol or *tranexamic acid*. Nosebleeds in HHT are not very different from common nosebleeds, so saline spray might help those as well.

Kevin J. Whitehead, MD, associate professor of internal medicine at University of Utah School of Medicine, Salt Lake City, and leader of a study of 121 people with HHT, published in *JAMA*.

## How Yoga Helps a Cold

If you hate taking decongestants when you have a cold, yoga can help you breathe easier.

A calming technique known as alternate nostril breathing can ease congestion and may help kick-start the immune system.

***What to do:*** Sit up tall. Take your right hand and curl down your index and middle fingers into your palm. Press your ring finger over your left nostril and inhale for a count of four through your right nostril. Then close off your right nostril with your thumb so that both nostrils are closed. Hold your breath for a count of four. Release your ring finger and let all of your air out through your left nostril during a count of four. Reverse sides, and keep repeating for three to five minutes. Stop if you become uncomfortable at any time. If you have a chronic condition such as asthma or high blood pressure, check with your doctor before trying any special breathing techniques.

Tara Stiles, founder, Strala Yoga, based in New York City. StralaYoga.com

## Fatal Wind Instruments

Bagpipes, trombones and other wind instruments can harbor organisms that trigger "bagpipe lung," a potentially fatal lung infection.

***Recommended:*** Clean instruments frequently and let them drip-dry between uses.

*Thorax.*

# A Lonely Heart Could Worsen a Cold

Angie LeRoy, psychology graduate student, Rice University, Houston.

Chris Fagundes, PhD, assistant professor, psychology, Rice University, Houston.

Rice University and the American Psychological Association, news releases.

A cold is never fun, but it's even more misery for folks who feel lonely, recent research suggests.

"We think this is important, particularly because of the economic burden associated with the common cold," said study coauthor Angie LeRoy, a psychology graduate student at Rice University in Houston.

"Millions of people miss work each year because of it. And that has to do with how they feel, not necessarily with how much they're blowing their noses," she said.

## The Study

For the study, LeRoy and Rice psychologist Chris Fagundes, PhD, used nose drops to deliberately infect a group of 159 volunteers with the cold virus. The participants were all unmarried and ranged from 18 to 55 years of age.

Each also filled out standard psychological questionnaires aimed at assessing their feelings of social isolation.

According to LeRoy, "Research has shown that loneliness puts people at risk for early death and other physical illnesses. But nothing had been done to look at an acute but temporary illness that we're all vulnerable to —the common cold."

In their recent research, the investigators tracked the mental and physical health of the volunteers as they were quarantined—often with a nasty cold—in hotel rooms for a period of five days, and for some time afterwards.

## Study Findings

Would each participant's mental state affect whether they caught the cold, or their symptoms?

First off, three-quarters of the participants did go on to develop a cold. But whether or not the participants were lonely didn't seem to play a role in cold acquisition, the findings showed.

However, even though the study couldn't prove cause-and-effect, there was a difference in terms of symptoms.

Dr. Fagundes and LeRoy found that people who said they had less "social support" had cold symptoms that were more severe compared with people who felt more socially included.

And this was true regardless of the size of an individual's social network, the study authors said.

The findings were published in *Health Psychology.*

## Implications

"This paper is about the quality of your relationships, not the quantity," LeRoy explained. "You can be in a crowded room and feel lonely. That perception is what seems to be important when it comes to these cold symptoms."

The findings echo those of prior studies linking loneliness with physical ills, the researchers said.

"Previous research has shown that different psycho-social factors—like feeling rejected or feeling left out or not having strong social bonds with other people—do make people feel worse physically, mentally and emotionally," LeRoy said.

Dr. Fagundes added that feeling alone is a form of mental stress, and stress is known to exacerbate illness. "Anytime you have an illness, it's a stressor, and this phenomenon would probably occur," he said.

## Recommendation

LeRoy's advice? Do what you can to get more socially active.

"If you build those networks—consistently working on them and your relationships—when you do fall ill, it may not feel so bad," she said.

For more on loneliness, visit the website of *Psychology Today* at PsychologyToday.com/basics/loneliness.

---

### A Powerhouse Snack

A handful of nuts every day can do more than lower risk for heart disease and cancer.

***Recent finding:*** Adults who ate 20 g (about one-quarter cup) of either plain or salted walnuts, almonds, cashews, peanuts or other nuts every day cut their risk of dying from respiratory disease by nearly half and from diabetes by about 40%.

***Possible reason:*** The antioxidants and nutrients in nuts that promote cardiovascular health also help fight other conditions.

Dagfinn Aune, PhD, postdoctoral research fellow, Imperial College London, UK.

---

# What's Really Causing That Annoying Cough?

Jonathan P. Parsons, MD, MSc, FCCP, professor of internal medicine at The Ohio State University College of Medicine and director of the Multidisciplinary Cough Clinic and the OSU Asthma Center at The Ohio State University Wexner Medical Center, all in Columbus.

The occasional cough is nothing more than your body's normal lung maintenance—a quick spasm that expels mucus or other irritants from the airways.

On the other hand, a cough that sounds unusual or is unpredictable (for example, there's no identifiable trigger or the cough occurs at different times of day)...severe...or long-lasting suggests that something else is going on—but what?

***Surprising finding:*** A recent study published in *Annals of Family Medicine* found that a cough from a cold or the flu sticks around longer—for about 18 days, on average—than the one-week threshold that most people consider normal.*

But a cough's duration is not the only clue to its cause. While it's not surprising that infections such as pneumonia or whooping cough would lead to coughing, there are other conditions that most people wouldn't expect. *For example...*

- **Asthma.** People with asthma assume that they'll have moments of wheezing or breathlessness. But for some patients, a persistent cough is the only symptom.

***What to watch out for:*** A wheezy-sounding cough that is usually worse at night. Frequent wheezing and/or coughing means that inflamed airways have narrowed, and it's a hallmark of poorly controlled asthma. Your doctor might recommend spirometry (a simple test that measures your lung capacity) or other lung tests to assess how well—or how poorly—you're doing.

***My advice:*** If you have a wheezy cough but have never been diagnosed with asthma, see your doctor. If you know that you have asthma and find that you're using a "rescue" inhaler—a fast-acting bronchodilator that quickly relieves coughing and other symptoms—more than twice a week, see your doctor. You probably need to work harder to reduce flare-ups. This may include adjusting medication, avoiding pollen and air pollution, reducing stress and other measures.

- **Gastroesophageal reflux disease (GERD).** Most GERD patients suffer from both heartburn and coughs, but about one-third experience only a cough or unexplained sore throats. A GERD-related cough occurs when a surge of stomach acid reaches the voice box (the larynx). The irritation and inflammation that result from the acid can lead to a persistent, raspy cough.

**Note*: Be sure to see your doctor if a cough lasts for more than three to four weeks.

***What to watch out for:*** The cough sounds "barky" rather than wheezy. It gets worse when you lie down...after heavy meals...and/or when you consume certain trigger foods or drinks, such as spicy dishes, alcohol, chocolate, onions or citrus. You might also notice that your voice is more hoarse than it used to be.

***My advice:*** For relief, take an over-the-counter (OTC) acid-suppressing drug such as *omeprazole* (Prilosec) or *ranitidine* (Zantac). Such a drug is unlikely to cause side effects and often is effective—although it might require long-term use (eight to 12 weeks) before your symptoms improve, so you should be monitored by a doctor.

***Also important:*** Medication usually doesn't work unless you also make lifestyle changes. For example, don't eat large meals late at night. In fact, you should avoid food altogether for at least three hours before going to bed. Propping up your upper body with pillows also can prevent stomach acid from going upstream while you sleep.

- **Postnasal drip.** When there's a persistent drip of mucus from the sinuses, you're going to periodically cough. Typically, allergies are to blame. People with hay fever often have congestion and postnasal drip. The mucus can irritate the throat as well as the larynx and cause a nagging cough.

***What to watch out for:*** A seasonal cough. If you mainly cough during the spring, summer and/or fall, an allergy-related cough is likely. This cough could sound barky and will probably get worse at night due to mucous drainage. It might be accompanied by other allergy symptoms such as a tickling in the throat, itchy eyes, sneezing, etc.

***My advice:*** Reduce drainage by taking a daily OTC nonsedating antihistamine such as *loratadine* (Claritin) or *cetirizine* (Zyrtec).

Nasal steroid sprays are another effective alternative. They start working within hours, although it may take several days—or even weeks—to get the full benefit. Some brands (such as Flonase) are available in OTC versions.

- **ACE inhibitor drugs.** Patients who take these blood pressure–lowering drugs—such as *lisinopril* (Zestril), *captopril* (Capoten) and *enalapril* (Vasotec)—are told that they may experience occasional dizziness. They aren't always warned, however, about the nasty cough that can result in up to 20% of patients taking them.

***What to watch out for:*** A throat tickle followed by a nagging, dry cough that begins anywhere from a few weeks to a year after starting the medication.

***My advice:*** You can keep taking the drug if the cough isn't bothering you (and you're successfully managing your blood pressure). Switching to a different ACE inhibitor may help if you have a mild cough. Patients with severe coughs from ACE inhibitors are often advised to switch to a different drug class altogether—usually an angiotensin-receptor blocker (ARB) such as *losartan* (Cozaar) or *valsartan* (Diovan). They work like ACE inhibitors but without the cough.

### When a Cough Is COPD or Cancer...

A chronic cough (persistent or episodic) may be the first symptom of two of the most serious lung conditions—lung cancer and chronic obstructive pulmonary disease (COPD), a lung disease that includes emphysema and chronic bronchitis. Both diseases are more common in people who smoke, once smoked or have had significant secondhand smoke exposure than in nonsmokers.

***Important:*** Even though people who have never smoked are less likely than smokers to get COPD or lung cancer, it can still happen. Don't take chances. Anyone who has a cough for more than three to four weeks should see a doctor. And call your doctor anytime you cough up blood.

---

## Allergy Medication Alert

Sedating antihistamines, such as Benadryl and Vistaril, can worsen symptoms of restless legs syndrome, a neurological condition. Nonsedating antihistamines, such as

Claritin, don't appear to worsen symptoms as much—perhaps because they don't cross the blood–brain barrier as easily.

William Ondo, MD, director, Movement Disorders Clinic, Houston Methodist Neurological Institute.

## Recover Faster from a Cold

Zinc acetate lozenges can shorten the common cold by almost three days, according to a recent analysis. Don't exceed 100 mg of elemental zinc per day.

Harri Hemila, MD, department of public health, University of Helsinki, Finland, and lead author of an analysis published in *British Journal of Clinical Pharmacology.*

# Vitamin D Can Halt Asthma

Patients who took vitamin D supplements every day had an average of 37% fewer asthma attacks that required oral corticosteroids. Vitamin D also cut the likelihood of emergency department visits/hospitalizations by 50%.

***Important:*** Vitamin D should not be used as a substitute for regular asthma medications.

***Editor's note:*** The RDA for vitamin D is 600 IU. If you are age 70 or older, 800 IU.

Christopher Griffiths, PhD, deputy director for research at Centre for Primary Care and Public Health, Blizard Institute, Barts, and The London School of Medicine and Dentistry.

# Thunderstorms Can Trigger Asthma Attacks

Norman H. Edelman, MD, senior scientific adviser for the American Lung Association. He is professor of preventive medicine, internal medicine, and physiology and biophysics at State University of New York at Stony Brook.

Eight people in greater Melbourne, Australia, died as a result of a freak thunderstorm in November 2016, and thousands more were hospitalized. The victims were not struck by lightning—they suffered asthma attacks. The Melbourne incident, which occurred when pollen and humidity were high, was not an isolated event. There is strong evidence that thunderstorms can increase the risk for asthma attacks. One study published in *Thorax* found that asthma-related visits to emergency rooms in the Atlanta, Georgia, area increased following thunderstorms.

The most likely explanation for "thunderstorm asthma" is that these storms can cause pollen already in the air to burst into tiny particles that are very easy to inhale deeply into the lungs. These tiny particles can be especially dangerous for people prone to allergy-induced asthma. When you have allergy-induced asthma, the pollen that can trigger, say, hay fever also can trigger an asthma attack.

An alternate theory proposes that downdrafts of cold air associated with thunderstorms might increase pollen concentrations low in the atmosphere, where the pollen is then more likely to be inhaled.

***What to do:*** If you have allergy-induced asthma, ask your doctor whether you should take special precautions when thunderstorms begin. For example, he/she might recommend taking an extra dose of an asthma-control medicine such as an inhaled corticosteroid...and/or remaining indoors as much as possible during the day following a thunderstorm.

# A Patch for Peanut Allergies

A skin patch may help fight a peanut allergy. Nearly half of the participants who wore a patch that delivered small amounts of peanut protein to their bodies for one year were able to consume at least 10 times more peanut protein at the end of the year than they were able to tolerate at the start of the study.

Study of 74 children and young adults led by researchers at US National Institute of Allergy and Infectious Diseases, Bethesda, Maryland, published in *Journal of Allergy and Clinical Immunology.*

## Lookout for Allergens When You Tattoo

Allergies to tattoos are common, reports Johanna S. Youner, DPM. Allergic reactions, such as swelling, redness and a rash or bumps, can be caused by substances in tattoo pigments such as dichromate (green), cobalt (blue), cadmium (yellow) and mercury salt (red). And pigments contaminated with nickel sulfate also can cause allergic reactions. Choose inks or colors that do not contain these substances—ask the tattoo artist.

Johanna S. Youner, DPM, a certified laser specialist in private practice in New York City.

## Third-Hand Smoke

Smoking deposits toxins on carpets, clothing and other surfaces. This third-hand smoke has been linked to liver and lung damage and could increase the risk for type 2 diabetes.

*PLOS ONE.*

## Sleep Apnea Alternative

A customized oral appliance that moves the jawbone slightly forward during sleep helps keep the airway open and may work better for some adults who cannot tolerate a continuous positive airway pressure (CPAP) mask and machine.

***Recent finding:*** Nearly 100 adults with mild- to-moderate sleep apnea who wore this type of mouth guard nightly showed improvement in sleep apnea and snoring.

***If you've been diagnosed with sleep apnea:*** Ask your doctor whether an oral appliance would be appropriate. If so, a dentist can custom-fit one. Most devices cost about $2,000 and may be covered by insurance.

Karl Franklin, MD, senior lecturer, Umea University, Sweden.

### Foods That Help Prevent Lung Cancer

Apples, tomatoes and oranges provide antioxidants that help nourish the lungs. Carrots, yellow squash and dark, leafy greens provide antioxidants called carotenoids that protect lung tissue. Water helps flush out toxins. Whole-soy foods contain phytoestrogens that may have a protective effect.

***Still the number-one recommendation:*** Do not smoke.

DrWeil.com

## What Is It? Snoring or Sleep Apnea?

National Institutes of Health/National Heart, Lung and Blood Institute...National Sleep Foundation... American Sleep Apnea Association...*Merck Manual*... University of Maryland Medical Center.

It's the middle of the night and once again you've been awakened by your partner's snoring. Or perhaps your husband has complained about your nighttime noises. Is it simple snoring—or life-threatening sleep apnea? *Here's how to tell these tricky terms apart...*

### Snoring 101

When the airways of your mouth, nose and throat relax during sleep, they get narrower. The tissues then vibrate as you breathe. *Result*: Snoring.

Just about everyone snores, at least sometimes. Temporary snoring can happen when your airways are narrowed by any upper-respiratory infection, including a cold or sinusitis, as well as by allergies. Drinking alcohol can relax the muscles of the throat and soft palate and lead to occasional snoring as well. So can some medications, such as tranquilizers, sleeping pills, antihistamines and beta-blockers. Pregnancy's hormonal changes, which relax muscles, can bring it on, too.

If you snore more than occasionally, however, you might have an enlarged uvula (the dangling tissue at the back of your mouth), which partially blocks the airflow. If you're overweight, you may have some extra tissue at the back of your throat that narrows the airway. And some people just naturally have a thicker soft palate or a deviated septum in the nose, which leads to snoring. Sleep position also can contribute—when you sleep on your back, gravity pulls your relaxed throat muscles down and partially blocks your airway.

## Sleep Apnea Signs

Snoring, even on a regular basis, doesn't mean you have sleep apnea. But it does mean that you should be on the lookout for these apnea signs...

- Constant, extremely loud snoring
- Gasping or choking
- Pauses in breathing
- Sudden awakenings with a snort
- Excessive daytime sleepiness
- Morning headaches

If you have sleep apnea, your breathing repeatedly stops while you sleep, sometimes for one minute or even longer. Each time you stop breathing, your sleep is disrupted but not enough to consciously wake you up. The poor quality of your sleep can increase the risk for high blood pressure, stroke, heart disease and type 2 diabetes. Extreme sleepiness during the daytime, another symptom, can lead to falling asleep while driving—and thus, car crashes. *There are two main types of sleep apnea...*

- **Obstructive sleep apnea (OSA),** the most common type, usually is caused by soft tissue at the back of your throat collapsing and blocking the airway. Your blood oxygen level drops, and your brain wakes you just enough to get you breathing again—even if you're not consciously aware that you've actually woken up momentarily. If you have OSA, you have five or more of these mini-awakenings every hour during sleep.
- **Central sleep apnea,** where your breathing repeatedly stops and starts while you're asleep, is much rarer. It happens because your brain isn't sending the right signals to the muscles that control your breathing. Sometimes central sleep apnea is caused by a condition such as heart failure, but often the reason is unknown. (Some people have mixed sleep apnea—a combination of the obstructive and central sleep apnea.)

***Bottom line:*** Losing even a small amount of weight, not smoking, skipping alcohol within four hours of bedtime, sleeping on your side and even doing anti-snoring throat exercises can help with a snoring problem, including sleep apnea. But if you think you or your bed partner might have sleep apnea, see your primary care doctor, who can evaluate you and, if needed, refer you to a sleep specialist. If you are diagnosed with this condition and the approaches above don't fix it, you may want to try an oral device that keeps your airways open or go with the medical gold standard, a continuous positive airway pressure (CPAP) machine.

# Toxic Metals Found in E-Cigarette Liquid

Johns Hopkins Bloomberg School of Public Health, news release.

Centers for Disease Control and Prevention. CDC.gov

*HealthDay* news service.

Electronic cigarette liquids can contain high levels of toxic and potentially cancer-causing metals, a recent study suggests.

"We do not know if these levels are dangerous, but their presence is troubling and could mean that the metals end up in the aerosol that e-cigarette users inhale," said study leader Ana Maria Rule, PhD, of Johns Hopkins Bloomberg School of Public Health in Baltimore. Dr. Rule is an assistant scientist in the department of environmental health and engineering.

### Pregnant Women Should Not Vape to Quit Smoking

Electronic cigarettes come in different sizes and shapes, including pens, mods (types modified by the user) and tanks. Most e-cigarettes contain a battery, a heating device and a cartridge to hold liquid. The liquid typically contains nicotine, flavorings and other chemicals. "Vaping" is the act of inhaling or exhaling the vapor produced by an e-cigarette.

According to a recent survey out of the University of Maryland, more than 40% of pregnant women surveyed believe that e-cigarettes are less harmful than tobacco cigarettes. Only 57% of the women believed that e-cigarettes contain nicotine. And fewer than two-thirds of the women surveyed thought that e-cigarettes could be addictive.

According to the Centers for Disease Control and Prevention, e-cigarettes and other products containing nicotine are not safe to use during pregnancy. Nicotine is a health danger for pregnant women and developing babies and can damage a developing baby's brain and lungs.

And there is not enough evidence to show whether or not e-cigarettes help women (and other individuals) quit smoking, according to the CDC.

Several vaping products are being marketed specifically to women.

### Johns Hopkins Study Details

Dr. Rule and her colleagues analyzed the liquid of five brands of so-called first-generation e-cigarettes, which resemble traditional cigarettes. (Newer e-cigarettes look like small cassette recorders with mouthpieces.)

The researchers found liquids in those brands contained the heavy metals cadmium, chromium, lead, manganese and nickel. These metals are toxic when inhaled, the researchers said.

In first-generation e-cigarettes, the cartridge of liquid is stored in close contact with the heating coil. When heated, the liquid creates the aerosol, or vapor, that users inhale. The researchers believe this heating coil is the main source of the dangerous metals.

"Perhaps regulators might want to look into an alternative material for e-cigarette heating coils," Dr. Rule said in a Hopkins news release.

The researchers did not examine the possible presence of the five metals in the aerosol.

### Current Regulations

Currently, the U.S. Food and Drug Administration requires e-cigarette makers to submit ingredient lists and information about potentially harmful ingredients, including four of the five metals detected in this study—nickel, lead, chromium and cadmium.

The agency has studied but not yet issued proposed rules on e-cigarette labeling.

The findings were published recently in the journal *Environmental Research*.

The U.S. National Institute on Drug Abuse has more about e-cigarettes at DrugAbuse.gov.

## Fireworks Can Harm Your Lungs

Fireworks produce particles that can travel deep into the respiratory system, causing coughing, shortness of breath and even heart attack or stroke. On average, the air is worst on July 4 from 9 pm to 10 pm local time until about noon on July 5.

Study by researchers at National Oceanic and Atmospheric Administration's Air Resources Laboratory, College Park, Maryland, published in *Atmospheric Environment*.

# Chapter 4

# STROKE RISKS, SYMPTOMS AND HELP WITH RECOVERY

## Study Finds Stroke Care Faster for Men Than Women

Male stroke patients are more than twice as likely as female patients to receive clot-busting stroke treatment within 30 minutes of hospital arrival, a recent study reports.

This means men who suffer a stroke are less likely to face long-term disability, since every minute counts when it comes to treatment with the clot-buster known as tissue plasminogen activator, or tPA, said lead researcher Archit Bhatt, MD. He's a neurologist with the Providence Brain and Spine Institute in Portland, Oregon

To have any effect, tPA must be administered within 4.5 hours of the onset of stroke. The drug works by dissolving blood clots that have blocked the flow of blood to the brain, causing what's called an ischemic stroke.

Standard treatment protocols call for administration of tPA within 60 minutes of arrival at the hospital, but Dr. Bhatt and his colleagues decided to evaluate the chances of receiving "ultrafast" treatment within a half hour of arrival.

"Studies have shown that 60 minutes is good, but for every 15-minute reduction in treatment time, the patient's health outcomes improve," Dr. Bhatt said.

### Study Details

To evaluate how often ultrafast treatment is occurring, the researchers reviewed nearly 2,700 stroke patients treated at one of 26 hospitals in the Pacific Northwest between 2009 and 2015.

Only about 4% of patients had tPA treatment times under a half hour, Dr. Bhatt said.

Three factors appeared to make a difference in whether or not stroke patients received ultrafast treatment...

- Men were 2.2 times more likely than women to get ultrafast treatment.
- People arriving by ambulance were 4.7 times more likely to get the fast treatment than stroke patients driven to the hospital.
- Weekday arrivals were nearly twice as likely as those arriving during the evening or weekends to get ultrafast treatment.

Archit Bhatt, MD, MPH, neurologist, Providence Brain and Spine Institute, Portland, Oregon.

Daniel Lackland, DrPH, professor, neurology, Medical University of South Carolina.

International Stroke Conference, Houston.

The advantages of arrival by ambulance are obvious, Dr. Bhatt said. Medics treating stroke patients are communicating with the hospital during the ambulance ride, making sure that resources and specialists are available by the time they hit the door.

"When you arrive by ambulance, the biggest advantage is that your assessment starts before you are even in the hospital," Dr. Bhatt said.

It also makes sense that stroke victims would receive more prompt treatment during weekdays, when hospitals are fully staffed and more nimble, Dr. Bhatt added.

But the disparity between men and women proved to be a head-scratcher, Dr. Bhatt said.

Stroke patients must receive a brain scan before getting tPA, to make sure their stroke is caused by a blood clot, but women are undergoing these scans about as promptly at men, Dr. Bhatt said.

Men also aren't more likely to arrive by ambulance than women, and aren't more likely to arrive on a weekday, he added.

### Reasons for the Disparity

Daniel Lackland, a professor of neurology with the Medical University of South Carolina, said he believes there is a real disparity between men and women when it comes to quick stroke care.

Lackland suspects that wives might be better at detecting stroke symptoms in their husbands and pushing them to get prompt care.

"I think that may play a major role," Lackland said. "It's not the male stroke victim—it's the others doing what they're supposed to do and bringing the man in for treatment."

The fact that women tend to suffer strokes later in life than men might be another factor, although it could not be assessed using the data available in this study, Dr. Bhatt said.

Women are also more likely to live alone, he said.

"If you are in the emergency department and you don't have anybody with you, it takes longer to identify the next of kin and try to get the history of the patient and why the patient is here," Dr. Bhatt said.

Steps could be taken to better prepare emergency response for older women living alone, Dr. Bhatt said. For example, these women could be provided better 911 alert systems that are easy to activate during a medical emergency.

"Calling an ambulance has to be a first priority when you are experiencing stroke-like symptoms," Dr. Bhatt said.

---

## Take Control of Your Stroke Risk

Victor C. Urrutia, MD, an associate professor in the department of neurology at The Johns Hopkins University School of Medicine and director of the Comprehensive Stroke Center/Stroke Prevention Clinic at The Johns Hopkins Hospital, both in Baltimore.

If you've ever needed strong proof that you can dramatically influence whether you're struck by a serious medical condition, here's some eye-opening news.

***Stunning research finding:*** When it comes to stroke, the fifth-leading cause of death in the US (fourth cause of death for women), 90% of your risk is due to factors that you can control, according to a study published in *The Lancet*.

***New development:*** To incorporate the latest scientifically proven actions that minimize risk for stroke—both ischemic (caused by a blood clot) or hemorrhagic (due to bleeding)—the American Stroke Association has updated its guidelines.

### The Stroke-Fighting Plan

Main steps that reduce one's odds of having a stroke...

***STEP 1:*** **Test your blood pressure at home.** It's long been known that lowering high blood pressure (hypertension) is the best way to prevent strokes. Unfortunately, not enough is being done to effectively fight hypertension.

Part of the problem is that most people get their blood pressure checked only when they see a doctor. However, blood pressure readings can fluctuate widely throughout the day and from one day to the next—you might have normal pressure in the doctor's office and higher pressure at home...or vice versa.

***Important finding:*** Use of an automated digital upper-arm cuff to measure blood pressure at home helps. A recent study that looked at 450 patients with hypertension found that 72% of those who home-tested achieved good control, compared with 57% of those who did not test at home. Even if you haven't been diagnosed with hypertension, you may want to consider occasional home-testing. Ask your doctor for advice.

***Latest thinking:*** With home-testing, you can see daily changes and identify trends over time that you can discuss with your doctor. It's also a good way to track the effects of medications and/or dose changes. At first, your doctor might advise that you check your blood pressure a few times at different times of the day. After you have steady control, once a day (or even weekly) is usually enough.

***STEP 2:* Don't focus so much on LDL "bad" cholesterol.** Until recently, doctors depended on LDL targets when prescribing statins and/or choosing drugs or doses. A desirable reading was generally considered to be below 100 mg/dL...for very high-risk patients with existing cardiovascular disease, a reading below 70 mg/dL was considered optimal.

***A better approach:*** The decision to take a statin—or increase (or decrease) your dose if you're already on one—should be based less on a specific LDL target and more on a patient's 10-year risk of having a stroke or heart attack, according to the new guidelines. Doctors are now advised to use risk calculators (such as CvRiskCalculator.com) before writing prescriptions or changing statin doses. The calculator also takes into account such factors as diabetes and HDL "good" cholesterol levels.

***Important:*** High-sensitivity C-reactive protein (hs-CRP) levels can also help guide treatment.

For people who have not yet had a stroke or heart attack, there is some disagreement about relying solely on such calculators. For now, anyone who has a greater than 7.5% risk of having a stroke in the next 10 years and is between the ages of 40 and 75 will probably need a statin—regardless of his/her LDL level. People with very high LDL (190 mg/dL or higher) will also benefit from taking a statin.

***STEP 3:* Don't be afraid to take a blood thinner.** Most strokes are caused by blood clots in blood vessels in the brain. *Warfarin* (Coumadin), the most widely prescribed drug for preventing clots, can reduce stroke risk by about 65% in people with atrial fibrillation, a common heart arrhythmia. But it's a tricky drug to use because it requires frequent blood tests to check/correct the dose...can cause bleeding if it's not carefully monitored...and intake of vitamin K, which affects blood clotting, needs to be carefully controlled. For these reasons, some people refuse to take it.

The updated guidelines include three additional drugs—*apixaban* (Eliquis), *rivaroxaban* (Xarelto) and *dabigatran* (Pradaxa). They work as well as warfarin, without the need for dietary changes or frequent blood tests. However, they're more expensive than warfarin and have their own limitations (they can't be used by some patients with kidney disease, for example). Bleeding is still a risk with new anticoagulants.

## Stroke-Depression Link

Depressed women have a 29% greater stroke risk than women who are not depressed.

***Possible reason:*** Depression is linked to increased inflammation, which raises stroke risk.

***Also:*** People with depression may not exercise regularly, use prescribed medications consistently or take other steps that help prevent strokes. The study looked only at women, but the findings likely apply to men as well.

Kathryn Rexrode, MD, associate professor of medicine at Harvard Medical School. She is senior author of a study of 80,574 women, published in *Stroke*.

***Bottom line:*** Don't let your concerns about side effects stop you from taking one of these drugs if you need it. Any anticoagulant can potentially cause bleeding, but the stroke-prevention benefit far outweighs the risks.

***STEP 4:*** **Go Mediterranean!** For years, "DASH"—short for "Dietary Approaches to Stop Hypertension"—has been the go-to diet for lowering blood pressure and reducing stroke risk. For the first time, the new guidelines encourage patients to consider a Mediterranean diet, which includes plenty of fish, fresh fruits, vegetables and nuts, along with olive oil and the occasional (optional) glass of wine.

***Game-changing research:*** An influential Spanish study, known as PREDIMED, randomly assigned participants into dietary groups that included people who followed a low-fat diet...and others who followed a modified Mediterranean diet that emphasized an increased intake of walnuts, almonds and hazelnuts.

***Results:*** The Mediterranean group had a lower stroke risk than the low-fat diet group. Based on these findings, the new guidelines advise patients to consider the Mediterranean diet, including a daily one-ounce serving of walnuts, hazelnuts or other unsalted nuts.

***STEP 5:*** **Take migraines seriously.** For reasons that aren't clear, women age 49 and under who suffer migraine-with-aura (a migraine accompanied by visual disturbances such as flashing lights and blind spots) are more than twice as likely to have a stroke (during the headache or at any time) as those without such migraines. For those who also smoke and take oral contraceptives, the risk is 10 times higher.

It's not known whether migraine medication will help prevent stroke in these women.

***What does matter:*** Giving up smoking is critical. Migraineurs-with-aura who smoke and take birth control pills may also want to talk to their doctors about other forms of contraception. In men, migraine-with-aura does not significantly affect stroke risk.

# Marijuana Can Cause Heart Attack and Stroke

According to a recent finding, hospital patients ages 18 to 55 who had used marijuana had a 26% increased stroke risk and 10% higher heart failure risk than ones who did not use it. The study did not say how much marijuana patients used or for how long they had been using it. But the analysis—adjusted for common cardiovascular risk factors such as hypertension, diabetes and smoking—found that marijuana appears to be an independent risk factor for cardiac problems.

Aditi Kalla, MD, a cardiology fellow at Einstein Medical Center in Philadelphia and leader of an analysis of 20 million health records at more than 1,000 US hospitals in 2009 and 2010.

# A Woman's Weight Has Complex Link to Stroke Risk

Mitchell Roslin, MD, chief, obesity surgery, Lenox Hill Hospital, New York City.

Richard Libman, MD, vice chairman, neurology, Long Island Jewish Medical Center, New Hyde Park, New York.

Gillian Reeves, MD, professor of statistical epidemiology, University of Oxford, England.

*Neurology*, news release.

Excess weight may put women at increased risk for the most common form of stroke, but at lower risk for a less common stroke type, recent research shows.

***Still, experts say the overall message remains the same:*** Keep trim to help keep stroke at bay.

## The Study

Specifically, the British study of more than 1.3 million women found that overweight and obese women were more likely to suffer an ischemic stroke, where blood flow is blocked to the brain. According to the American Stroke

Association, it is by far the leading form of stroke, accounting for about 87% of cases.

The study found that overweight and obese women were somewhat less likely to have a bleeding, or hemorrhagic, stroke, which comprises about 13% of cases.

The study was led by Gillian Reeves, MD, of the University of Oxford in England. Her team tracked the 12-year health history of British women who averaged 57 years of age.

During that time, rates of ischemic (the blockage type) stroke were 1% among obese women and 0.7% among women with a healthy weight.

On the other hand, rates of bleeding stroke were 0.4% among obese women and 0.5% among women with a healthy weight.

The study was published in the journal *Neurology*.

## Implications

"While the results of this study may appear contradictory or somewhat confusing, the take-home message is that overall, obesity causes more harm than good," said Richard Libman, MD, who reviewed the findings. He's vice chair of neurology at Long Island Jewish Medical Center in New Hyde Park, New York.

"Our findings add to the growing body of evidence that different types of stroke have different risk profiles," Dr. Reeves said.

Dr. Libman called the study "well done," noting that prior studies have also found that race plays a role in the relationship between weight and stroke risk.

"For Europeans in general, consisting mostly of whites, the risk of stroke due to blockage increases with greater obesity, while the risk of stroke due to bleeding decreases with greater obesity," he said. However, "in Asians, the risk of both types of stroke seems to increase with obesity."

And just because excess weight may confer a tiny benefit in lowering bleeding stroke risk, that's no reason to pile on the pounds, Dr. Libman said.

"As weight increases, the risk of having any type of stroke outweighs any apparent

## Beware of These Stroke-Risk Boosters

**Get tested for anemia.** Stroke patients with anemia (a lack of healthy red blood cells) were nearly twice as likely to die in the year after their stroke as those without anemia, a study of 30,000 stroke survivors found.

***Possible reason:*** People with anemia may have lower oxygen delivery to the brain.

***If you've had a stroke:*** Make sure you are tested for anemia and receive treatment, such as iron supplements.

Phyo Myint, MD, chair of old age medicine, University of Aberdeen, Scotland.

**Weight gain/loss stroke risk.** Yo-yo dieting raises stroke risk in people who already have coronary artery disease (CAD). In a five-year study of people with stable CAD, the 20% with the highest weight variability—meaning that they lost and regained the most weight—had 117% higher risk for heart attack and 136% higher risk for stroke, compared with those with the lowest weight variability. This does not prove cause and effect, but it points to the importance of not only losing weight but also keeping it off.

Sripal Bangalore, MD, associate professor, NYU Langone Medical Center, New York City, and leader of a study of 9,509 women and men, published in *The New England Journal of Medicine*.

**Caring for an ill spouse raises stroke risk.** Caregivers who said that they were stressed by taking care of a chronically sick or disabled husband or wife had a 95% greater stroke risk than noncaregivers whose other risk factors were similar.

***Self-defense:*** Family caregivers of ill or disabled patients should have their own health evaluated and speak with a doctor about ways to reduce stress.

Analysis of data on more than 6,000 people by researchers at University of Alabama at Birmingham, presented at a recent American Heart Association meeting.

benefit of increasing obesity on the risk of stroke due to bleeding," he said.

Mitchell Roslin, MD, is chief of obesity surgery at Lenox Hill Hospital in New York City. He said that, as in many health issues, "not every obese person has the same risk."

But Dr. Roslin noted that obesity is strongly tied to heart risk factors such as diabetes and high blood cholesterol levels.

For more information on stroke, visit the American Academy of Family Physicians website, FamilyDoctor.org, and search "stroke."

# Stroke Risk Can Rise with Pregnancy-Linked Disorder

*Stroke*, news release.

Several factors raise the risk of pregnancy-related stroke in women with preeclampsia, a recent study suggests.

Preeclampsia is a condition marked by high blood pressure and protein in a pregnant woman's urine. It affects between 3% and 8% of pregnancies. Women with preeclampsia are at increased risk for stroke during and after pregnancy, though pregnancy-related strokes are rare.

"Preeclampsia is a very complex disorder that's not completely understood. Our study sought to discover if there are clues that may help identify the women with preeclampsia who are at the highest risk for pregnancy-related stroke," said lead author Eliza Miller, MD, a vascular neurology fellow at New York-Presbyterian Hospital/Columbia University Medical Center.

## Study Details

Researchers looked at nearly 89,000 women who developed preeclampsia between 2003 and 2012. Of those, about 200 had a pregnancy-related stroke.

Women who had a pregnancy-related stroke were seven times more likely to have severe preeclampsia or eclampsia, according to the study. They were three times more likely to arrive at the hospital with infections; a history of high blood pressure before developing preeclampsia; or blood clotting disorders.

The study was published in the journal *Stroke*.

"We were looking for risk factors that could be prevented or treated," Dr. Miller said. She added that a link between stroke risk and urinary tract infections (UTIs) was interesting, because UTIs are not only treatable but also preventable.

## Look Out for Neurological Symptoms

Women who develop preeclampsia should be alert for warning signs, even after the baby is born, Dr. Miller advised.

"Women with preeclampsia should take any neurological symptoms, such as severe headache, very seriously, especially during the postpartum period. This needs to be a major focus of future stroke research in women," Dr. Miller said.

The U.S. National Institute of Child Health and Human Development has more on preeclampsia and eclampsia at NICHD.nih.gov/health/topics/preeclampsia/.

# The "Silent" Stroke Trigger

Walid Saliba, MD, medical director of the Center for Atrial Fibrillation and director of the Electrophysiology Lab at Cleveland Clinic. His research has been published in many journals, including *Circulation: Arrhythmia and Electrophysiology* and *American Journal of Cardiovascular Drugs*.

When it comes to preventing stroke and heart-related disorders such as heart failure, it's crucial to identify and properly treat "AFib"—short for atrial fibrillation, the most common type of abnormal heart rhythm. Unfortunately, a significant number of the estimated three million Americans who have AFib don't even realize it.

***Now:*** With new diagnostic and treatment approaches, one's chances are greater than ever that this potentially dangerous condition can be spotted and stopped—if you receive the right tests and medical care. *What you need to know...*

## When AFib Is Silent

If you have AFib, it's possible to experience a range of symptoms including a quivering or fluttering heartbeat...a racing and/or irregular heartbeat...dizziness...extreme fatigue...shortness of breath...and/or chest pain or pressure.

But AFib can also be "silent"—that is, symptoms are so subtle that they go unnoticed by the patient. Silent AFib is sometimes an incidental finding during a physical exam when the doctor detects an irregular heartbeat. It may also be suspected in patients with nonspecific symptoms such as fatigue or shortness of breath—especially in those with a family history of AFib or a condition such as high blood pressure or diabetes that increases risk for AFib. But whether the symptoms are noticeable or not to the patient, the risk for stroke and potentially heart failure remains just as high, so AFib needs to be diagnosed.

***To check for AFib:*** The standard practice has been to perform an electrocardiogram (ECG) for a few minutes in the doctor's office to record the electrical activity driving the heart's contractions. But if AFib episodes are intermittent, the ECG may be normal.

When AFib is suspected based on symptoms such as dizziness and/or palpitations or racing heartbeat, but the ECG is normal, doctors have traditionally recommended monitoring for 24 to 48 hours. This involves wearing a small device that is clipped to a belt, kept in a pocket or hung around your neck and connected to electrodes attached to your chest. But this approach, too, can miss occasional AFib episodes.

***What works better:*** Longer-term monitoring. Research published in *The New England Journal of Medicine* found that AFib was detected in five times more patients when they were monitored for 30 days instead of only 24 hours. Guidelines from the American Heart Association now recommend AFib monitoring for 30 days within six months after a person has suffered a stroke with no known cause.

***New option:*** With a doctor's supervision, mobile ECG devices (about the size of a cell phone) can now be used periodically to record 30-second intervals of your heart rhythm. Ask your doctor for details.

## Getting the Right Treatment

AFib almost always requires treatment. Besides the danger of stroke, the condition tends to worsen if left alone—symptoms become more troublesome, and normal rhythm is harder to restore.

There are numerous options depending on other risk factors, your treatment goals and your own preference. Treatment is chosen based on frequency and severity of symptoms and whether the patient already has heart disease. *Examples...*

- **Prevent stroke.** To keep clots from forming, many patients need blood-thinning medications (anticoagulants). The old standby, *warfarin* (Coumadin), is effective but requires regular blood tests and dietary restrictions.

In recent years, a new generation of easier-to-use anticoagulants has appeared, including *dabigatran* (Pradaxa), *rivaroxaban* (Xarelto) and *apixaban* (Eliquis). These newer drugs have no dietary restrictions and do not require routine blood tests. However, all anticoagulants carry the risk for bleeding, which is harder to stop with the newer drugs.

Some patients at otherwise low risk for stroke may need only low-dose aspirin (such as 81 mg daily).

- **Slow down a rapid heart rate.** This is usually done with a beta-blocker like *atenolol* (Tenormin) or a calcium channel blocker like *amlodipine* (Norvasc) or *diltiazem* (Cardizem).

- **Normalize heart rhythm.** Anti-arrhythmic drugs, such as *amiodarone* (Cordarone), *flecainide* (Tambocor) and *dofetilide* (Tikosyn), are available. However, these are powerful drugs, with potentially serious side effects (such as dizziness and uncontrollable shak-

### What to Do If You Have a Stroke...

**Statin remedy.** Take a statin drug as soon as possible after an ischemic stroke to reduce risk for infection or further strokes.

***Recent finding:*** infection risk was reduced by 58% in ischemic (blockage) stroke patients who got statins upon hospital admission or early in their stays, compared with similar patients given statins later or not at all.

Douglas L. Weeks, PhD, director of research at St. Luke's Rehabilitation Institute and an adjunct professor at Elson S. Floyd College of Medicine and Washington State University's School of Biomedical Sciences, all in Spokane.

**Aspirin for a ministroke.** Take aspirin immediately after a ministroke to cut the risk for a fatal or disabling stroke over the next few weeks by up to 80%.

***Ministroke symptoms:*** Muscle weakness, especially on only one side, trouble speaking, numbness/tingling, confusion and/or balance problems. Symptoms may last only a few minutes.

***If you suspect a ministroke:*** Get to the ER, and take a regular-strength, 325-mg aspirin.

Peter Rothwell, MD, PhD, professor of clinical neurology and founder and head of Centre for the Prevention of Stroke and Dementia, University of Oxford, UK.

ing), that can worsen rhythm abnormalities and must be used cautiously.

• **Ablation.** Another option to normalize heart rhythm and reduce stroke risk is known as ablation. With this procedure, the doctor threads a series of catheters up a vein to the heart to destroy the tiny group of cells that generate electrical impulses that cause fibrillation.

The procedure may have to be repeated but may be a good alternative to lifelong drug treatment. Ablation used to be saved for patients who didn't respond to drugs, but it's being offered as first-line therapy nowadays for those who want to avoid lifelong medication.

***New procedure:*** Just last year, the FDA approved a procedure that can sharply reduce AFib stroke risk—left atrial appendage occlusion places a plug in a tiny sac of the atrium where 90% of clots form.

Each of these procedures, which eliminates the need for long-term blood thinning, carries a small risk for serious complications, such as stroke, and is best performed in a hospital that has experience with the surgery and the resources and expertise to provide emergency backup if needed.

• **An anti-AFib lifestyle.** The best way to cut your odds of developing AFib is to modify risk factors. If you have high blood pressure or sleep apnea, get effective treatment. If you're obese, lose weight. Exercise regularly. If you have AFib, these steps will make your treatment work better—and reduce symptoms.

## Eat Eggs to Slash Stroke Risk

Eating up to one egg each day cut stroke risk by 12%—without increasing risk for heart disease—a recent study of more than 300,000 adults has found.

***Theory:*** Eggs are rich in antioxidants (shown to reduce inflammation) and protein—both of which help lower blood pressure, an important risk factor for stroke.

***Important:*** The new Dietary Guidelines for Americans eliminates restrictions on dietary cholesterol and notes that eggs are an inexpensive source of important nutrients.

Dominik D. Alexander, PhD, MSPH, principal epidemiologist, EpidStat Institute, Ann Arbor, Michigan.

## Blood Test Predicts Second Stroke

If you've had one ischemic stroke (due to a blocked blood vessel), a common blood test could help your doctor predict whether you'll have another. Stroke patients who had elevated blood levels of C-reactive protein (CRP), an enzyme routinely checked to measure risk of developing heart disease, were more likely to have a second stroke than those with the lowest levels, recent research found. Elevated CRP also indicates higher risk for a first stroke.

Stephen Williams, PhD, assistant professor of neurology, University of Virginia School of Medicine, Charlottesville.

# A Grapefruit a Day Helps Keep Stroke Away

Kathryn M. Rexrode, MD, MPH, physician, division of preventive medicine, Brigham and Women's Hospital, and associate professor of medicine, Harvard Medical School, both in Boston.

Mmm, citrus. There's nothing like a refreshing orange, a tangy tangerine or a sweet pink grapefruit. It really does taste like sunshine.

But these juicy fruits aren't just delicious—they may actually help you ward off a stroke, according to recent research.

And you may be surprised to hear that it's not because of the vitamin C...

## Focusing on Flavonoids

Many studies have shown the health benefits of eating fruit, including studies that have shown that people who eat five or more servings of fruits and vegetables have a 25% lower risk for stroke (both ischemic and hemorrhagic) compared with those who eat three or fewer servings. Researchers have suspected that flavonoids, antioxidant compounds found in many fruits and vegetables, are one key to their power since they reduce inflammation and improve blood vessel function.

But there are six different types of flavonoids found in foods, and each has a subtly different chemical structure. Given the variety, researchers from England, Italy and the US wanted to learn which specific flavonoids and which fruits or vegetables, in particular, are most beneficial for preventing stroke.

To learn more about the study, we spoke with one of the authors—Kathryn M. Rexrode, MD, MPH, a physician in the division of preventive medicine at Brigham and Women's Hospital and associate professor of medicine at Harvard Medical School, both in Boston.

## The Flavonoid That Came Out on Top

The researchers used information from 70,000 women who were followed for 14 years as part of the Nurses' Health Study. Every two years, the participants completed questionnaires that covered their medical histories and lifestyles. And every four years, the women completed food questionnaires, which asked how much of certain foods and drinks they consumed and how often they consumed them.

The women's diets were analyzed for the six different types of flavonoids, and their medical histories were reviewed for the number and type of strokes that the women had. What they found was that high consumption—more than about 63 milligrams per day of a certain subclass of flavonoids called flavanones (the amount found in about one to two servings of citrus per day)—was associated with a 19% reduced risk for ischemic stroke (the type caused by a clot, not by a bleed), compared with low flavanone consumption (under 13.7 milligrams per day). And this was after adjusting for other stroke risk factors, such as smoking, age, body mass index and others. The other five flavonoids studied reduced stroke risk, too, but not by as much (only by 4% to 13%).

Dr. Rexrode said that one reason that the flavanones may have been associated with decreased risk for ischemic stroke is that flavanones may inhibit platelet function and clotting factors. The researchers didn't study whether citrus affected risk for hemorrhagic stroke, but Dr. Rexrode said that it's unlikely that eating citrus would lead to an increased risk for hemorrhagic stroke. She said that it takes a relatively small amount of clotting to cause an ischemic stroke, but, on the other hand, it takes a relatively large amount of excessive bleeding to cause a hemorrhagic stroke.

Although this study, which was published in *Stroke*, looked only at women, Dr. Rexrode said that there is no reason to think that these findings wouldn't apply to men, too.

## Pick Your Citrus

Dr. Rexrode said that you can get all the flavanones you need (about 63 milligrams) from eating one or two servings of citrus each day. Whole fruits are always better than juices or smoothies, she said, because the bulk of the flavanones are found in the inner membranes of the fruit and the pith or white part of the fruit. The pith is generally removed when the fruit is juiced or cleaned for smoothies.

The USDA provides information about the amount of flavanones in every 100 grams of edible fruit, so to save you the trouble of weighing your fruits, here are estimates of the flavanone content for some common citruses:

**Grapefruit** (one-half of a four-inch diameter) have 47 milligrams.

**Oranges** (25⁄8 inch diameter) have 42 milligrams.

**Tangerines** (2½ inch diameter) have 18 milligrams

Dr. Rexrode doesn't recommend supplements—she said sticking to whole fruit is best. And don't overdo it on citrus, or else your stomach or teeth might suffer from the acid. Just a serving or two a day is all you need!

# Being Bilingual Is Good for Recovery

Stroke patients who speak more than one language recover better than similar patients who speak only a single language. Bilingual patients were more likely to recover cognition fully after a stroke than single-language speakers.

Study of 608 patients led by researchers at National Institute of Mental Health and Neurosciences, Bangalore, India, and University of Edinburgh, UK, published in *Stroke.*

# New Treatment for Stroke Recovery

New treatment improves hand movement after a stroke. Therapists often use electrical stimulation to elicit contractions in weakened hand muscles. In the new therapy, the patient uses a sensor-equipped glove on the unaffected hand. When he opens his "good" hand, the other one receives corresponding stimulation—strengthening the muscles and possibly changing neural connections. Moderately impaired patients who used the glove showed more than twice the improvement of patients using stimulation on the weaker hand.

Jayme Knutson, PhD, senior staff scientist at Metro Health Medical Center, Cleveland.

# Chapter 5

# PRESERVE YOUR BRAIN

## Women Are More Resilient to Effects of Alzheimer's Genes

Certain gene variants are known to raise a person's risk of Alzheimer's disease. But a recent study finds that even in people carrying this DNA, factors such as gender and physical or mental activity can affect that risk.

The study tracked dementia rates for 642 people aged 53 to 95 at the start of the study. All carried at least one of two types of DNA linked to higher Alzheimer's disease risk—the APOEe4 or CLU CC gene variants.

Carrying the APOEe4 variant "confers a risk of developing Alzheimer's disease of up to 10 to 14 times compared to that of non-carriers," explained Luca Giliberto, MD, who reviewed the findings.

He's an investigator in Alzheimer's disease at the Feinstein Institute for Medical Research in Manhasset, New York.

But Dr. Giliberto stressed that "having a [genetic] risk factor does not mean you will get the disease." And that's what the recent study found—especially for people with certain characteristics.

Led by Kirstie McDermott, of the University of Alberta in Edmonton, Canada, the researchers tracked the Alzheimer's gene carriers for nine years.

The study found that gender appeared to matter. While about 47% of men showed signs of decline in their memory level and stability over the study period, that number was approximately 32% for women.

This "memory resilience" over time was also found to be improved for both sexes in people who had higher education, better muscle tone, or who engaged in "challenging, everyday" intellectual activities, such as playing bridge, for example.

For women, specifically, having healthy lungs, a good walking speed and an active social life—things such as volunteering and visiting family and friends—were also linked to maintaining a healthy memory, the study found.

Luca Giliberto, MD, PhD, neurologist, Northwell Health's Neuroscience Institute, Manhasset, New York, and investigator physician, Litwin-Zucker Research Center for the Study of Alzheimer's Disease, Feinstein Institute for Medical Research in Manhasset, New York.

Ezriel (Ed) Kornel, MD, director, Neurosciences, Orthopedic and Spine Institute, Northern Westchester Hospital, Mount Kisco, New York.

Alzheimer's Association's International Conference, news release.

***One factor seemed specific to men in keeping dementia at bay:*** Avoiding depression.

Dr. Giliberto wasn't surprised by the findings.

"Conducting an active lifestyle, higher education and physical activity are all reasonable predictors of better aging," he said. "Thus, it is not surprising that their effect would also be evident in carriers of genetic risk for Alzheimer's disease."

Ezriel Kornel, MD, directs the Neurosciences, Orthopedic and Spine Institute at Northern Westchester Hospital in Mount Kisco, New York.

"What all of this means, in a nutshell, is that if you take care of yourself physically, mentally and participate in your community, you are more likely to maintain a well-functioning memory," even if you carry Alzheimer's-linked DNA, Dr. Kornel said.

# Don't Panic If You Draw a Blank: How to Quickly Check Your Brain Health

Majid Fotuhi, MD, PhD, a neurologist and medical director, NeuroGrow Brain Fitness Center, McLean, Virginia. He is also author of *Boost Your Brain.*

Starting in their 40s, many people begin to have lapses in remembering names, occasional difficulty in finding a word and/or slowness in thinking speed (such as mentally adding numbers). Such occasional forgetfulness commonly occurs as we get older and is not necessarily a sign of dementia, as many people fear.

However, memory lapses that occur several times every day could be a sign of an underlying health problem and should be evaluated.

Many health conditions, including depression, thyroid problems and dehydration, can affect memory. Too much stress, too little sleep or a deficiency of vitamin B-12 can make someone forgetful, too.

Many medications, including tricyclic antidepressants, antihistamines and drugs that treat high blood pressure and cholesterol, can also cause memory loss. Your doctor may be able to prescribe other drugs that don't have this side effect.

Signs that memory lapses may be more serious include becoming lost in familiar places, asking the same question repeatedly and getting confused about time, people and places. If any of these signs occur, consult a neurologist.

You can quickly check your brain health with the free risk calculator developed by neurological researchers. Go to TheNeurocore.com/brain-fitness-risk-calculator. The good news is that many people can boost their brain health and performance within weeks.

# The Groundbreaking Alzheimer's Prevention Diet

Richard S. Isaacson, MD, director of the Alzheimer's Prevention Clinic, Weill Cornell Memory Disorders Program at Weill Cornell Medicine and NewYork-Presbyterian. He is coauthor of *The Alzheimer's Prevention & Treatment Diet: Using Nutrition to Combat the Effects of Alzheimer's Disease.*

As head of the renowned Alzheimer's Prevention Clinic at Weill Cornell Medicine and NewYork-Presbyterian, Richard S. Isaacson, MD, is on top of the latest research on Alzheimer's disease. Groundbreaking studies show that proper diet can make a real difference not only in slowing the progression of the disease but also in preventing it.

Here, Dr. Isaacson explains how we can change our eating habits to fight Alzheimer's. His recommendations are not specifically designed for weight loss, but most overweight people who follow this eating plan will lose weight—important because obesity more than triples the risk for Alzheimer's.

## Fewer Calories

The Okinawa Centenarian Study (an ongoing study of centenarians in the Japanese prefecture of Okinawa) found that these long-lived people typically consume fewer calories (up to 1,900 calories a day) than the average American (up to 2,600 calories).

Lowering calorie intake appears to reduce beta-amyloid, particles of protein that form brain plaques—the hallmark of Alzheimer's disease. A 2012 study at the Mayo Clinic found that people who overate had twice the risk for memory loss...and those who consumed more than 2,142 calories a day were more likely to have cognitive impairment.

I generally advise my patients to try to have fewer than 2,100 calories a day. I can't give an exact number because calorie requirements depend on body type, activity level, etc. Many of my patients tend to consume less than 1,800 calories a day, which may be even more protective.

***Bonus:*** Calorie restriction also lowers insulin, body fat, inflammation and blood pressure, all of which can reduce the risk for cognitive impairment. It even improves neurogenesis, the formation of new brain cells.

## Less Carbs, More Ketones

Glucose from the breakdown of carbohydrates is the fuel that keeps the body running. But you don't need a lot of carbs. Ketones, another source of fuel, are healthier for the brain.

When you restrict carbohydrates, the body manufactures ketones from stored fat. On occasion, a "ketogenic diet" is recommended for some patients with Alzheimer's disease because ketones produce fewer wastes and put less stress on damaged brain cells. There's some evidence that this diet improves mild cognitive impairment symptoms (and theoretically may slow further damage).

We previously found in our clinic that patients consumed an average of 278 grams of carbohydrates daily before their first visits. We recommend reducing that slowly over the nine weeks of the diet plan to 100 to 120 grams of carbohydrates daily. (One sweet potato has about 23 grams.) The USDA SuperTracker website (SuperTracker.USDA.gov) gives carbohydrate amounts and other nutritional information for specific foods. Eat healthful carbohydrates such as beans and whole grains in moderation. Unlike refined carbs, they are high in fiber and can help to reduce insulin resistance and improve blood sugar control—which reduces risk for Alzheimer's.

## Fasting

Some trendy diets recommend extreme fasts. With the Alzheimer's prevention diet, you'll fast—but mainly when you wouldn't be eating anyway, during sleep!

Several times a week, you'll go without food (particularly carbohydrates) for more than 12 hours. After 12 hours, the body starts making ketones. This type of fast, known as time-restricted eating, reduces inflammation, improves metabolic efficiency and improves insulin levels, insulin sensitivity and brain health.

***How to do it:*** Eat an early supper—say, at about 5 pm. You won't eat again until after 5 am the next day. Your eventual goal will be to fast for 12 to 14 hours five nights a week.

## More Protein

The Institute of Medicine recommends getting 10% to 35% of calories from protein—go for the higher end. On a 2,000-calorie diet, that's about 175 grams. (Five ounces of cooked salmon has about 36 grams of protein.)

The amino acids in protein are important for memory and other brain functions. Protein-rich foods often are high in B vitamins, including folic acid and vitamins B-6 and B-12. The Bs are critical because they reduce homocysteine, an amino acid linked to poor brain performance and an increased Alzheimer's risk.

***Which protein:*** Chicken, fish, nuts, legumes and eggs all are good choices. I recommend limiting red meat to one weekly serving because of potential associated health risks, including an increased risk for certain cancers...and because too much saturated fat (see below) can be a problem.

***Helpful:*** Aim for four to eight eggs a week. They're high in selenium, lutein, zeaxanthin and other brain-healthy antioxidants.

## Limit Saturated Fat

A large study found that people who eat a lot of foods high in saturated fat—rich desserts, red meat, fast food, etc.—may be up to 2.4 times more likely to develop Alzheimer's disease.

Saturated fat limits the body's ability to "clear" beta-amyloid deposits from the brain. It also raises cholesterol and increases the risk for cardiovascular diseases—and what's bad for the heart also is bad for the brain.

Consuming some saturated fat is healthful—it's only in excess that it causes problems. The American Heart Association advises limiting it to about 5% to 6% of total calories. I recommend a little more—up to 10% of your daily calories. On a 2,000-calorie diet, the upper limit would be about 20 grams. (One ounce of cheese can have as much as eight grams.)

## Fish, Turmeric and Cocoa

Studies have shown that a few specific foods can fight Alzheimer's...

- **Fish.** A UCLA study found that adults who regularly ate foods high in omega-3 fatty acids (the healthful fats in fish) had a lower risk for mental decline. Other research has shown that low blood levels of DHA (a type of omega-3) are linked to smaller brain volume and lower scores on cognitive tests.

***My advice:*** Eat one serving of fatty fish (such as wild salmon, mackerel and sardines) at least twice a week.

- **Turmeric.** In India, where people use the spice turmeric frequently, the risk for Alzheimer's is lower than in the US. This doesn't prove that turmeric is responsible (genetic factors, for example, also could be involved), but other evidence suggests that it's protective. Turmeric contains the compound curcumin, which has potent antioxidant and anti-inflammatory effects.

***My advice:*** Use the spice in recipes—don't depend on supplements—because curcumin is fat-soluble and absorption is enhanced by the fat in foods.

- **Cocoa.** The flavanols in cocoa improve memory and other cognitive functions. They also have been linked to reduced blood pressure and improved insulin resistance.

***My advice:*** Buy chocolate bars or cocoa powder that lists purified cocoa flavanols on the label.

---

# Memory Can Fade After Menopause

North American Menopause Society, news release.

Middle-aged women can remember more than men their own age, but recent research suggests that memory may fade as estrogen levels drop during menopause.

Memory loss is a common age-related complaint, affecting up to 75% of older people, the study's authors explained. The researchers noted that many women going through menopause report being more forgetful, though they still outperform men on memory tests.

"Brain fog and complaints of memory issues should be taken seriously," said JoAnn Pinkerton, MD, executive director of the North American Menopause Society (NAMS).

"This study and others have shown that these complaints are associated with memory deficits," she said in a society news release.

The study by Harvard Medical School researchers was led by Jill Goldstein, PhD, a professor of psychiatry and medicine. It included 212 men and women, between 45 and

55 years old. For the study, Dr. Goldstein's team used memory and thinking tests to rate the memory, executive function, word processing and verbal intelligence of these adults.

The study found that women who had gone through menopause had worse memory than those who had not gone through menopause. A drop in estrogen levels among older women was associated with lower rates of learning new information and recalling memories, the researchers said.

Memory storage and consolidation, however, weren't affected, the study authors said.

The study findings were published in the journal *Menopause*.

The U.S. National Institute on Aging provides more information on age-related memory changes at NIA.NIH.gov/health/publication/forgetfulness.

## Don't Worry About Brain Fog

"Brain fog" during menopause is normal and not a sign of cognitive decline, reports Emily Goard Jacobs, PhD. Women's handling of certain memory tasks declines as levels of estradiol (a form of estrogen) fall. This explains why up to 60% of women going through menopause complain of a kind of brain fog—forgetfulness, trouble concentrating and difficulty thinking clearly.

***Helpful:*** Exercise, and ask your doctor about short-term hormone therapy.

Emily Goard Jacobs, PhD, assistant professor, psychological and brain sciences, at Neuroscience Research Institute, University of California, Santa Barbara. She led a study of brain changes before and during menopause, published in *The Journal of Neuroscience*.

## It May Not Be Alzheimer's After All

Marc E. Agronin, MD, vice president for behavioral health and clinical research at Miami Jewish Health and an adult and geriatric psychiatrist and affiliate associate professor of psychiatry and neurology at the University of Miami Miller School of Medicine. Dr. Agronin is also author of *How We Age*. Marc Agronin.com

People joke about having the occasional "senior moment," but the humor partly deflects an unsettling concern: What if this memory lapse—forgetting an appointment, calling someone by the wrong name, losing your car in the parking lot, etc.—marks the beginning of an incurable mental decline? Not so fast.

Some middle-aged adults (defined roughly as ages 40 to 65) do develop early-onset Alzheimer's or other forms of dementia, but it's rare. Their flagging memories are much more likely to have simpler—and very treatable—explanations. If you have memory or other cognitive changes, it's critically important to seek early diagnosis and treatment before more serious problems ensue...or the changes become irreversible.

### Forgetfulness Happens

The fear of mental decline makes sense for older adults. While the prevalence of Alzheimer's disease and other types of dementia is nearly 10% at age 65, it jumps to up to half of those age 85 and older.

However, many patients in their 50s and 60s are convinced that the mildest mental slips mean that the worst is just around the corner. This is usually not the case.

Once you reach your mid-40s, your brain processes information more slowly. Memories are more transient than they used to be. Forgetting facts or incorrectly recalling details becomes more common. These are normal changes.

If you've noticed that you're more distracted or forgetful than usual, ask your doctor to perform a general checkup to rule out any obvious medical issues, such as a vitamin B-12 deficiency or a thyroid problem. If nothing is uncovered, it's still possible that something other than dementia is causing your cognitive symptoms. *Possible suspects*...

• **Medications.** If you're taking codeine or another opioid medication for pain, you expect to be a little fuzzy. But some of the drugs that affect memory aren't the ones that most people are aware of—or think to discuss with their doctors.

***Examples:*** Cholesterol-lowering statins. A small percentage of people who take these drugs describe mental fuzziness as a side effect. The benzodiazepine class of sedatives/antianxiety drugs (such as Valium, Xanax, Halcion, etc.) can also cause cognitive problems and frequently affect memory. The mental effects are amplified when you take multiple drugs—say, one of these medications for sleep and another for daytime anxiety.

Don't overlook the possibility that some over-the-counter drugs—decongestants and antihistamines are common offenders—can also cause mental fuzziness.

***Dr. Agronin's advice:*** Pay attention (and tell your doctor) if your cognitive symptoms seem to get worse after starting a new medication. You might need to change drugs or take a lower dose.

• **Mental health.** When you meet people at a party, do you remember their names? Or are you so nervous about making a good impression that their names don't register?

Anxiety and stress cause distraction, and it's impossible to form memories when you're not paying attention. Some people become so worried about memory problems that every slip causes them to freeze up and quit paying attention to what's happening around them. It becomes a self-fulfilling prophecy.

Depression is also linked to cognitive lapses, especially since it interferes with concentration...interest in activities...and sleep—all essential factors for good memory.

***Dr. Agronin's advice:*** If you notice that your memory has good days and bad ones—and some days when it's horrible—it's reasonable to suspect that the problem is benign and you might just be going through an emotionally difficult time.

Talk to your doctor about what may be bothering you emotionally. If there's a problem with stress, anxiety or depression, get a referral to a mental health provider for a more thorough evaluation to assess your mood, thinking and behavior.

***Important:*** Your doctor or a mental health professional should also talk to you about potential alcohol or recreational drug abuse, which can have a significant impact on cognition.

All of these conditions can be treated with medication, therapy and/or a variety of lifestyle changes, such as getting more exercise and practicing relaxation techniques.

• **Obstructive sleep apnea.** It's a common sleep disorder, particularly among those who are overweight. A blocked airway during sleep impedes the flow of oxygen to the brain. This can occur dozens or even hundreds of times a night. Diminished nighttime oxygen can impair memory and concentration. Patients with sleep apnea also have a higher risk for stroke and heart disease.

***Warning signs:*** Gasping, snorting or loud snoring during sleep...a dry mouth in the morning...morning headaches...and/or difficulty staying alert during the day.

The good news is that obstructive sleep apnea can be overcome almost completely with the use of a continuous positive airway pressure (CPAP) machine, a small bedside device that delivers mild air pressure through a hose to help keep the airways open. These machines can be noisy, and the mask or nose piece that connects to the air hose can be somewhat uncomfortable—but CPAP does work. And it's definitely preferable to a lifetime of brain fog.

• **Adult ADD.** People associate attention deficit disorder (ADD) with children, but it also affects 2% to 4% of adults—and most are never diagnosed. It's a lifelong neurobiological disease that makes it difficult to focus or pay attention.

People with ADD are easily distracted... may have a history of work problems...and often don't follow through on tasks at home. It's easy to confuse these symptoms with cognitive impairments.

ADD is usually diagnosed by taking a history from the patient and family members. If the patient then responds to medication such as *methylphenidate* (Ritalin), he/she is considered to have ADD.

## The New Alzheimer's "Prescription"

Dean Sherzai, MD, a neurologist and director of the Alzheimer's Disease Prevention Program at Cedars-Sinai Medical Center in Los Angeles. For more on brain health, follow him on Facebook at Team Sherzai.

Every now and then, researchers announce yet another "breakthrough" drug to halt mental declines or clear away the sticky brain plaque (beta-amyloid) that's the hallmark of Alzheimer's disease.

Unfortunately, the enthusiasm tends to fade as limitations of these drugs become apparent. The handful of medications that help ease the cognitive symptoms of Alzheimer's (such as memory loss and confusion) do not stop the disease's progression (see medication choices at the end of this article).

***What most people don't realize:*** Even though medication plays a role in treating Alzheimer's symptoms, certain lifestyle changes actually can slow the progression of Alzheimer's disease by 30% or more—something that is impossible with even the newest drugs.

To learn more, we spoke with Dean Sherzai, MD, one of the country's leading authorities on Alzheimer's disease.

### The Neuro Approach

When I treat a person at risk for dementia or newly diagnosed with this disease or mild cognitive impairment (a condition that often precedes Alzheimer's), I recommend a set of lifestyle changes I call NEURO. This stands for Nutrition...Exercise...Unwind...Restful sleep ...and Optimize mental/social activities.

People who practice each of these steps—and who also address health conditions, especially high blood pressure and diabetes, that increase the risk for and symptoms of Alzheimer's—can significantly slow the disease from progressing. Regardless of whether the person is also taking an Alzheimer's medication, these lifestyle steps are crucial.

What you need to know about the five-step NEURO approach...

***STEP 1:*** **Nutrition.** With few exceptions (see next page), I don't often recommend individual vitamins, antioxidants or other supplements—the totality of your diet is more important because healthy foods contain a complex mix of nutrients that work together to give maximum benefit.

***Best choice:*** A Mediterranean-style diet. This diet includes lots of fruits, vegetables, whole grains, beans, fatty fish and monounsaturated fats (such as olive oil). Research has shown that a version of this diet that emphasizes certain brain-healthy foods (such as berries and leafy-green vegetables) is especially effective.

***Important findings:*** In a study that was published in *Archives of Neurology*, researchers tracked nearly 1,400 people—482 of whom had already been diagnosed with mild cognitive impairment—for an average of more than four years. They found that those with this condition who were most careful about following a Mediterranean diet were 48% less likely to develop full-fledged Alzheimer's disease than those who were more lax in their eating habits. And those who were still healthy at the start of the study were 28% less likely to develop symptoms in the first place.

Will supplements help when you are already eating well? Maybe—but the evidence isn't conclusive. *Supplements to consider...*

- **Vitamin B-12.** I've found that Alzheimer's patients with B-12 blood levels even at the lower end of the normal range (typically around 180 ng/L) sometimes have fewer cognitive symptoms when they take B-12 supplements.

• **Omega-3s.** Increasing blood levels of omega-3 fatty acids might help as well.

• **Vitamin D.** If vitamin D levels are low, a supplement may improve symptoms and help slow Alzheimer's progression.

***STEP 2:*** **Exercise.** Exercise can slow progression by about 30% or more. Exercise works on multiple levels—it stimulates growth factors that maintain neurons (brain cells)...and increases circulation of blood in the brain, which promotes healthy cognitive function.

***My advice:*** Get 30 minutes of exercise five or more times weekly.

***What works well for some people:*** Riding a recumbent bike while watching TV.

***STEP 3:*** **Unwind.** People who experience a lot of stress are up to two-and-a-half times more likely to develop Alzheimer's disease than those who have less or who deal with it more effectively.

Why? No one's sure, although it seems likely that the stress-related surge in cortisol and other hormones is harmful to the brain.

Exercise and volunteering are great stress reducers. Some people manage stress by keeping busy with hobbies...practicing yoga...and/or enlisting help from friends/relatives to deal with daily responsibilities. Do what works best for you—and make stress reduction a priority.

***STEP 4:*** **Restful sleep.** Many Alzheimer's patients don't sleep well. Experts once assumed that poor sleep was merely an Alzheimer's symptom. But recent research suggests that a lack of restful sleep may play a role in the development and progression of the disease.

***Important finding:*** A study in *JAMA Neurology* that looked at 70 older adults found that those who got less than five hours of sleep a night had higher brain levels of beta-amyloid than those who slept more than seven hours. Researchers speculate that poor sleep impairs the body's ability to clear beta-amyloid or other toxic molecules from the brain.

***Also:*** Sleep apnea, a very common (and underdiagnosed) condition in which breathing intermittently stops and starts during sleep, reduces brain oxygen and is strongly linked to Alzheimer's.

If you frequently snore or snort during sleep, or you're tired in the morning despite having what you thought was a good night's sleep, your doctor might suggest a sleep study that measures brain waves and blood oxygen levels to detect apnea and other sleep disorders.

***STEP 5:*** **Optimize mental/social activities.** People who stay mentally busy with hobbies, for example, and do other stimulating activities (such as playing challenging video games that require memory, problem-solving, hand-eye coordination, etc.) have smaller declines in memory and other cognitive functions...less Alzheimer's-related brain damage...and slower disease progression. They have a deeper "cognitive reserve," the neural connections (and brain size) that can forestall future impairments.

Once people start doing these new activities, it's both motivating and rewarding because the positive changes—including improved cognitive functioning—can occur within a matter of weeks.

## Medication Choices for Alzheimer's

The drugs that are FDA-approved for treating Alzheimer's disease affect brain chemicals and can improve memory, alertness and concentration. *The two classes of these medications...*

• **Cholinesterase inhibitors (Aricept, Exelon and Razadyne).** These drugs block an enzyme that breaks down acetylcholine, a neurotransmitter that's vital for memory, language, learning and other cognitive functions. There are no serious side effects, but some patients may experience nausea, vomiting, diarrhea or other problems. If this occurs, an Exelon patch can be used.

• **N-Methyl-D-Aspartate (NMDA) receptor blocker (Namenda).** This drug affects glutamate, another brain chemical. It's approved for treating moderate-to-severe Alzheimer's, but it can also help patients with milder forms of the disease. In some patients, Namenda, which may cause side effects such as dizziness and/or headache, works best when combined with Aricept or another cholinesterase inhibitor.

# Postmenopausal Women at High Risk for High Blood Pressure and Dementia

Costantino Iadecola, MD, professor, neurology and neuroscience, Weill Cornell Medical College, New York City.

Sam Gandy, MD, PhD, director, Center for Cognitive Health, Mount Sinai Hospital, New York City.

*Hypertension*, online.

High blood pressure, particularly in middle age, might open the door to dementia, the American Heart Association warns in a recent scientific statement.

## Equal Opportunity Offender

Dementia affects some 30 million to 40 million people worldwide. That number is expected to triple by 2050, as the world's population ages and treatments remain elusive, the association noted.

And, according to the American Heart Association, many people erroneously believe that high blood pressure is a man's problem, but it's an equal opportunity offender, affecting women as much as men. In fact, postmenopausal women 65 and over are actually more likely to have high blood pressure than men.

"People with high blood pressure tend to have more dementia," said statement author Costantino Iadecola, MD. He is a professor of neurology and neuroscience at Weill Cornell Medical College in New York City.

Whether controlling high blood pressure ("hypertension") reduces the odds of developing dementia, however, has not been scientifically proven, he said.

## Hypertension's Link to Dementia

"There are a lot of small observational studies that looked at people who were treated for blood pressure and, generally, there was an improvement in cognition [thinking skills]," Dr. Iadecola said.

"However, what we really need is a trial that specifically addresses the link between hypertension and cognition. What we need is a big trial to really narrow this down," he suggested.

High blood pressure is "the worst possible thing for the brain," Dr. Iadecola said. First, high blood pressure damages the blood vessels in the brain and leads to hardening of the arteries. Second, it affects tiny blood vessels and the brain's ability to control blood flow, which is essential to keep it working normally, he explained.

Most of the trials that the committee reviewed did not deal directly with the effects of high blood pressure on dementia, so it was impossible to come up with clear recommendations for doctors on how to treat patients with the condition, Dr. Iadecola said.

One of the problems is that years may elapse between the time high blood pressure is diagnosed and dementia starts. Long-term studies addressing questions—such as when to start treatment to protect the brain, the ideal blood pressure to achieve, and which medications can help—are badly needed, he said.

The SPRINT-MIND trial, a study designed to evaluate treating high blood pressure to stall dementia, may give the answers to some of these questions, Dr. Iadecola said. Results of that trial are expected to be available late 2017, early 2018, the authors of the report noted.

## Recommendation

Until then, Dr. Iadecola recommends treating high blood pressure on a patient-by-patient basis to protect brain, heart and kidneys.

"Although scientifically we don't have evidence, treating blood pressure is going to be important. It not only saves the brain, but also the heart and the kidney. So in the absence of evidence, the best thing to do is to control blood pressure," Dr. Iadecola suggested.

The American Heart Association statement was published online in the journal *Hypertension*.

## Expert Commentary

According to Sam Gandy, MD, PhD, director of the Center for Cognitive Health at Mount Sinai Hospital in New York City, controlling blood pressure during midlife probably reduces risk for dementia in late life. "My instinct is to say that this is certainly true, but there is a qualification," he added.

"If hypertension is allowed to smolder along untreated through midlife, then initiating blood pressure control in late life may not show benefit, or may even be harmful," Dr. Gandy said.

It's becoming clear that dementia begins in midlife, and by the time the symptoms emerge, the patient is 70 or 80 or more, "and the horse is out of the barn, so closing the door at that point is just way, way too late," he explained.

"My guess is that we eventually will begin amyloid brain scans around age 50 and repeat them every two to five years," Dr. Gandy said.

"We are working hard on dementia, but we haven't made a meaningful dent. And that will probably hold until we realize that, at 65, it may be too late to have any impact on the dementia outcome. We might eventually have to begin interventions as early as age 45," he suggested.

For more information on high blood pressure and dementia, visit the Alzheimer's Association website, ALZ.org, and search "blood pressure."

# BP Meds Could Cut Alzheimer's Risk

People with mild thinking and memory difficulties who took an angiotensin-converting-enzyme (ACE) inhibitor, such as *captopril* or *lisinopril*...or an angiotensin-receptor blocker (ARB), such as *losartan* or *valsartan*...were less likely to develop Alzheimer's disease than similar patients taking other hypertension drugs. More research is needed, but if you are taking a medication for high blood pressure, ask your doctor if switching to an ACE or ARB drug is appropriate.

Analysis of the medical records of 784 patients with high blood pressure and mild cognitive impairment by researchers at Emory University, Atlanta, presented at the Alzheimer's International Conference 2015, Washington, DC.

# Fluctuating Blood Pressure Linked to Cognitive Decline

Blood pressure fluctuations may accelerate mental decline. People whose systolic blood pressure (top number) varied significantly between doctor visits showed faster mental deterioration than those whose pressure stayed within the normal range. Variability in diastolic blood pressure (bottom number) was associated with more rapid declines in thinking skills only among people ages 55 to 64 but not among people ages 65 and older. This recent research adds to the mounting evidence that blood pressure changes may have significant health consequences.

***Recommendation:*** Keep blood pressure stable and within normal ranges.

Study of 976 people by researchers at Rutgers Cancer Institute of New Jersey, New Brunswick, published in *Hypertension*.

# Animal Study Hints at Gene Therapy's Possible Promise for Alzheimer's

Magdalena Sastre, PhD, senior lecturer, department of medicine, Imperial College London.
David Reynolds, PhD, chief scientific officer for Alzheimer's Research UK, Cambridge, England.
Imperial College London, news release.

Gene therapy might one day offer a way to prevent and treat Alzheimer's disease, recent research in mice suggests.

## The Study

Scientists at Imperial College London used a modified virus to deliver a gene called PGC1-alpha into the brain cells of mice. Previous research suggests this gene may prevent the formation of a protein called amyloid-beta peptide.

It's the main component of amyloid plaques, the sticky clumps of protein in the brains of Alzheimer's disease patients. These plaques are thought to be associated with brain cell death.

These very early findings could lead to a way of preventing Alzheimer's or stopping it in the early stages, according to study senior author Magdalena Sastre, PhD.

Alzheimer's is the most common type of dementia. It causes memory loss, confusion, and changes in mood and personality. There is no cure.

The study was published in the journal *Proceedings of the National Academy of Sciences.*

"There are many hurdles to overcome, and at the moment the only way to deliver the gene is via an injection directly into the brain," Dr. Sastre said in a college news release.

It's also important to note that therapies that look promising in mice often don't work in humans.

"However, this proof-of-concept study shows this approach warrants further investigation," she added. Dr. Sastre is a senior lecturer in the department of medicine.

## Expert Commentary

David Reynolds, PhD, chief scientific officer for Alzheimer's Research UK, said studies like this one are important because current treatments do not stop progression of Alzheimer's damage.

"This research sets a foundation for exploring gene therapy as a treatment strategy for Alzheimer's disease, but further studies are needed to establish whether gene therapy would be safe, effective and practical to use in people with the disease," Dr. Reynolds said in the news release.

For more on Alzheimer's disease, visit the U.S. National Institute on Aging, NIA.NIH.gov, and search "Alzheimer's disease fact sheet."

# Trouble Navigating New Surroundings May Indicate Alzheimer's

Difficulty navigating new surroundings may be an extremely early sign of Alzheimer's.

***Recent finding:*** Study participants were tested on their ability to remember how to navigate a maze on a computer. People with preclinical Alzheimer's—based on analysis of fluid from around their brains and spinal cords—had significantly more trouble creating a map of the maze than people without the cerebrospinal markers.

Study of 71 people by researchers at Washington University School of Medicine, St. Louis, published in *Journal of Alzheimer's Disease.*

## Early Alzheimer's Sign?

Difficulty identifying certain smells, such as lemon or smoke, could signal Alzheimer's disease 10 years before the onset of memory loss, according to a recent study of older adults.

***Why:*** Alzheimer's can cause brain circuits to lose memory of certain smells.

***Self-defense:*** If you or a loved one has difficulty identifying familiar smells, talk to your doctor about screening for Alzheimer's disease.

Mark Albers, MD, PhD, assistant professor of neurology, Harvard Medical School, Boston.

## Watch Out for Apathy

Apathy may be an early sign of Alzheimer's. Families should watch older loved ones for emotional apathy and other behavioral changes such as suspicion or paranoia... greater-than-usual agitation or aggression... and loss of socially appropriate behavior. If new and sustained, these behaviors may be signs of mild behavioral impairment, an early indicator of Alzheimer's disease and other dementias.

Zahinoor Ismail, MD, FRCPC, a neuropsychiatrist and assistant professor of psychiatry and neurology at Hotchkiss Brain Institute, University of Calgary, Canada.

## Calcium Supplements-Dementia Link

Calcium supplements may increase dementia risk.

***Recent finding:*** Women over age 70 with a history of stroke who regularly took calcium supplements had nearly seven times higher risk for dementia than other stroke survivors. If you had a stroke, ask your physician whether the risk from calcium supplements outweighs the benefit.

Silke Kern, MD, PhD, a neuropsychiatric researcher at Sahlgrenska Academy, University of Gothenburg, Sweden, and coauthor of a study of 700 women, published in *Neurology*.

### Anxiety and Alzheimer's

Moody, anxious middle-aged women are twice as likely to develop Alzheimer's as other women. Women with a neurotic personality style, defined as being easily distressed and exhibiting anxiety, jealousy or moodiness, have double the risk for Alzheimer's. These personality traits do not trigger Alzheimer's—more research is needed to understand the association.

Study of 800 women over 38 years by researchers at University of Gothenburg, Sweden, published in *Neurology*.

## Too Busy? It's Good for Your Brain!

Study titled "The Busier the Better: Greater Busyness Is Associated with Better Cognition," by Sara B. Festini, PhD, Denise C. Park, PhD, and Ian M. McDonough, PhD, The University of Texas at Dallas, The University of Alabama, Tuscaloosa, published in *Frontiers in Aging Neuroscience*.

When you have too much to do, you might dream of spending time up a lazy river. But if you want to keep your brain sharp and your memory strong, you're better off staying busy.

Really busy—so busy that you feel like you have so many things to do that you can't possibly get them all done. So busy that you wish the day were longer. So busy that you sometimes stay up later than you want to in order to get everything done.

That's the surprising conclusion of a recent study of men and women ages 50 to 89. Researchers at the University of Texas at Dallas studied 330 participants who filled out a "busyness" questionnaire and then measured that against memory and brain function scores. *Results...*

- **The busiest ones processed information faster,** reasoned better, could remember more at one time and had a better recall of important moments in their own lives.
- **The strongest association was for "episodic" memory**—remembering specific times and places.
- **While participants in their 50s and 60s tended to be busier than those in their 70s and 80s,** the cognitive benefits of busyness remained a strong association at any age. "Our findings," the authors conclude, "offer encouragement to maintain active, busy lifestyles throughout middle and late adulthood."

It's an observational study, to be sure, so it doesn't prove cause and effect. Plus, the researchers note, it's well-established that chronic high stress levels can impair cognitive function, including memory—so there's no point to being so busy that you want to tear your hair out.

But it may be time to stop envying the lucky old sun, who keeps rolling around heaven all day. It's good to stay busy—at any age.

---

# Think Fast! Can a Brain Game Prevent Dementia?

Cynthia R. Green, PhD, a practicing clinical psychologist and founder and president of Total Brain Health and TBH Brands, LLC, a brain-health and memory fitness consulting service in Montclair, New Jersey. Her most recent book is *Your Best Brain Ever: A Complete Guide & Workout.* TotalBrainHealth.com

Paper based on "Advanced Cognitive Training for Independent and Vital Elderly" (ACTIVE) study, presented at the Alzheimer's Association International Conference 2016.

---

If the latest news about "brain games" and dementia makes your head spin, that's understandable. Claims and refutations have made this field an intellectual roller coaster.

Not long ago, ads implying that online games designed to sharpen cognitive skills can help prevent dementia flooded the Internet, radio and TV. Then the Federal Trade Commission ruled that these claims were essentially bogus.

Now a recent study claims that a certain kind of brain game is, in fact, associated with a reduced risk of developing Alzheimer's. It's been touted as a significant finding in *The New Yorker*, and *Time* ran an article with the headline "The Best Way to Delay Dementia Without Drugs."

A little investigation, however, made us skeptical. Is it really time to invest your time—and money—in these programs to protect yourself from dementia?

## Teasing Out an Alzheimer's Link

Cynthia R. Green, PhD, founder of the brain-health consulting service Total Brain Health in Montclair, New Jersey, and founding director of the Memory Enhancement Program at Mount Sinai School of Medicine in New York City, has already looked closely at the matter.

The recent research, presented at the Alzheimer's Association International Conference, provided a new analysis of data from University of South Florida, Indiana University and The Pennsylvania State University based on an ongoing study called "Advanced Cognitive Training for Independent and Vital Elderly" (ACTIVE). That study looked at men and women over age 65 who showed no evidence of dementia when they enrolled.

One kind of brain game stood out, researchers found. Over the course of 10 years, the men and women who had training in something called "speed of processing" were about one-third less likely to develop cognitive impairment or dementia compared with those who didn't have this kind of training. Since there was no actual measurement of dementia in the study, researchers used a statistical analysis to indirectly pick up evidence of dementia.

***Here's what speed-of-processing games train you to do:*** Process visual information faster. For example, you may be asked to click on an icon of a bird in a flock that looks different from the other birds—and then do so faster and faster while the background gets more and more complicated. The goal is to speed up your brain's ability to process information.

A one-third reduction in dementia risk is an exciting finding, right? Yes...but it's too soon to conclude that think-fast brain games are proven dementia protectors, says Dr. Green. As she explains in her blog post, "Think Fast! Should Processing Speed Challenges Be Part of Your Brain Health Plan?," the study hasn't been subject to peer review in a medical journal yet and wasn't even designed to study dementia—the goal of the study was to determine whether cognitive interventions (e.g. "brain games") can help adults keep their cognitive skills as they age. That's actually a different thing from identifying who is going to get Alzheimer's or another form of dementia. According to an article published in *MedPage Today*, "Watch Out for Brain Training Claims" (free subscription required), there may also be a conflict-of-interest issue because a close colleague of one of the study authors has had financial links to the company, Posit Science, that developed the speed-of-processing test that was studied.

Even so, Dr. Green is decidedly enthusiastic about training our brains to think and act faster. She believes that learning new ways to speed up the brain's processing ability is an important tool in your brain-training toolbox. Why? Because there is growing evidence that this kind of practice can help you stay sharper as you age—it's a core skill that enables many other mental abilities, including memory and learning. "The rate at which we 'think through' information is critical to everyday intellectual performance," she writes. Games and activities that teach you to process information against the clock, she writes, "may help us maintain our processing speed as we grow older." Honing visual speed-of-processing skills is also key to being able to drive safely as you get older, which helps you stay independent longer.

Those are all good things—even if they don't prevent dementia.

## How to Think Faster

Dr. Green has several suggestions to enhance your ability to think faster...

- **Play games against the clock.** They can be board games, electronic games—anything that you time. Now try to do it faster!

- **Play online games with friends,** such as Word Streak with Friends (free, available for both iOS and Google Play), which challenges everyone playing to make as many words as possible with a set amount of letters before the time runs out.

- **Do anything faster.** Whether it's prepping vegetables for dinner, folding the laundry or doing new dance steps—try timing yourself and see how you can improve your time.

Dr. Green has nothing against "Double Decision," the speed-of-processing game developed by Posit Science's program that is available along with other games by subscribing to BrainHQ, which is a version of the computer program used in the ACTIVE study. You may decide that it's worth $96 a year.

But there are many ways to learn how to think faster every day, for free—and doing so is only part of an overall lifestyle that's good for brain health.

# Rosacea May Increase Alzheimer's Risk

Women with the common skin disorder rosacea are at higher risk for Alzheimer's disease. Rosacea patients (both men and women) are 25% more likely, on average, to develop Alzheimer's disease than those without rosacea. The increase is greatest among women, who had a 28% greater risk. Rosacea is also more frequently diagnosed in women (according to the National Rosacea Society). It is not known whether rosacea actually causes Alzheimer's, but the presence of rosacea in elderly people may aid in early detection and treatment.

Alexander Egeberg, MD, PhD, associate professor of dermato-allergology, Herlev and Gentofte Hospital, University of Copenhagen, Denmark, and leader of a 15-year study of 82,439 rosacea patients, published in *Annals of Neurology.*

Rosacea.org

## How Often Is Alzheimer's Misdiagnosed?

Two in 10 cases of Alzheimer's may be misdiagnosed, says Melissa Murray, PhD.

***Reason:*** There is no medical test that can definitively diagnose Alzheimer's. Instead, diagnosis is based on symptoms. Men seem to develop Alzheimer's at an earlier age than women, who typically develop it in their 70s or later...and men's symptoms may be behavioral or involve motor problems, while women's are more likely to involve memory issues.

Melissa Murray, PhD, is assistant professor of neuroscience at Mayo Clinic, Jacksonville, Florida, and leader of a study of the brains of more than 1,600 people, presented at a recent Alzheimer's Association International Conference.

## Cocoa Could Be a Brain Booster

People with impaired blood flow in the brain who drank two cups of flavonol-rich cocoa per day for one month did better on memory tests than similar people who drank flavonol-poor cocoa. Choose chocolate with at least 35% cocoa or cocoa solids.

Study of 60 people led by researchers at Brigham and Women's Hospital, Boston, and the VA Boston Healthcare System, published in *Neurology.*

## Low Blood Pressure Alert

Risk for dementia is 15% higher among those with orthostatic hypotension (a condition in which blood pressure falls suddenly upon standing, resulting in dizziness and/or light-headedness), according to a 24-year study of more than 6,000 older adults.

***Theory:*** These brief periods of hypoxia, or lack of oxygen, may cause long-term damage to brain tissue.

***If you have orthostatic hypotension:*** Talk to your doctor about drinking more water, wearing compression stockings and/or taking medication to raise blood pressure.

M. Arfan Ikram, MD, PhD, professor of neuroepidemiology, Erasmus University Medical Center, Rotterdam, the Netherlands.

## Probiotics for Brainpower

When 52 patients with Alzheimer's disease took a probiotic supplement containing four billion units of Lactobacillus and Bifidobacterium, they showed improvement in memory and other cognitive test scores after 12 weeks.

***Possible explanation:*** These probiotics may decrease inflammation in the brain.

***If a loved one has Alzheimer's disease:*** Talk to his/her doctor about a probiotic supplement.

Mahmoud Salami, PhD, professor of neurophysiology, Kashan University of Medical Sciences and Health Services, Iran.

# Sharpen Your Memory with Music

Galina Mindlin, MD, PhD, assistant clinical professor of psychiatry at Mount Sinai Hospital in New York City. She is coauthor of *Your Playlist Can Change Your Life: 10 Proven Ways Your Favorite Music Can Revolutionize Your Health, Memory, Organization, Alertness, and More.* BrainMusicTreatment.com

Imagine yourself giving a toast, making a speech or delivering a big presentation at work—only to forget midway through what you wanted to say. If the mere thought makes you cringe, you'll be intrigued by a process that reveals how to use music to improve your recall. The best part is that whatever type of music appeals most to you is what will be most effective—so you don't have to suffer through music you find boring or annoying.

Because music permeates all areas of the brain, it has a tremendous capacity to deposit any memories you attach to it in assorted locations. This embeds them deeper into your brain and makes it possible to retrieve them from multiple memory banks.

You may remember the buzz back in the 1990s when a small study reported that listening to a Mozart piano sonata produced a temporary improvement in spatial reasoning skills. These modest findings were blown out of proportion in the popular press, which disseminated the exaggerated idea that "Mozart makes you smart." Subsequent research has shown that music can indeed have cognitive benefits, but it's not about Mozart. In fact, my method works with any type of music—country, classical, reggae, rock, rap, pop, opera or whatever—provided you enjoy it. The more you like the music, the more it activates brain networks and functions that amplify and sustain the effects you are working toward, such as increased concentration and alertness.

## Choosing Your Music

So, getting back to memorizing that toast, speech or presentation, here's what you do. *First, create three lists of musical selections…*

**1. Calming songs.** On this list, include songs that you know from experience make you feel relaxed and balanced because they are associated with pleasurable, peaceful events from your past. For instance, one song might remind you of a blissful solitary stroll in the woods…another might bring back memories of a glorious sunset sail.

***Tip:*** Research shows that songs with a slower tempo of 100 beats per minute (BPM) or less tend to bring on relaxation and calm.

***Examples:*** "New York, New York" sung by Frank Sinatra or "American Pie" by Don McLean.

**2. Fast-paced "activating" songs.** Activating songs are mentally energizing. They might remind you of a time when you zoomed through a challenging task, celebrated an accomplishment or won a race. Generally, songs that work well in this category have a tempo of 130 BPM or faster—for instance, "Beat It" by Michael Jackson or "Jailhouse Rock" sung by Elvis Presley. Such rhythms tend to boost motivation and endurance.

**3. Medium-paced activating songs.** Here, select songs that recharge your batteries yet have a slightly slower tempo, typically 100 to 130 BPM. Examples include "Stayin' Alive" by the Bee Gees or the Beatles' "Lady Madonna." These types of songs help your brain lock in whatever you're trying to commit to memory.

Choose half a dozen or more selections for each list.

***Reason:*** Feelings shift from day to day. For example, you might normally feel relaxed by a song you and your husband slow-danced to at your wedding—but if you two just had an argument, that song might upset you today. Assess your current emotions each time you use your playlists, selecting the songs that feel appropriate for the particular moment.

Once you've selected your songs, create your three playlists on your iPod or record the songs onto CDs or cassettes.

## Putting Your Playlist to Work

Now you're ready to use your music to enhance your ability to memorize whatever it is that you want to commit to memory. *Follow these steps in order...*

- **Listen to one or more calming songs to prepare your brain to be receptive to learning.** As you listen, recall as vividly as possible the relaxing, positive memories associated with each song. Continue listening until you reach that state of relaxed mental alertness.
- **Play fast-paced activating songs to shift your brain into remembering mode.** Again, as you listen, visualize in detail the upbeat memories linked with that music. Continue listening until you feel energized and ready to approach your task.
- **Turn the music off and focus on what you want to remember.** For instance, read your speech aloud from start to finish, moving around or gesturing as you read—the sound of your voice and your physical movements provide additional anchors that help cement the speech in your memory.
- **When you finish rehearsing, listen to one or more mid-tempo activating songs.** This serves as a mental cool-down to further fix the material in your mind.

For maximum effect, use this technique daily. The amount of time you spend depends on the material you're trying to remember, but generally the music portion of the activity takes about 10 to 15 minutes per session.

***Key:*** Remember to have fun with this—it should not be a chore, but instead a source of enjoyment.

### Surprising Traffic Danger

Dementia is more common in those who live within about 165 feet of a major road.

***Reasons:*** Noise, pollution and disturbed sleep may damage the brain.

*The Lancet.*

## Arthritis Drug May Prevent Alzheimer's

*Etanercept* is an injectable drug given to patients with rheumatoid arthritis (RA) to block tumor necrosis factor (TNF), a protein that promotes inflammation. TNF also is elevated in Alzheimer's patients.

***Recent finding:*** RA patients were more likely to have Alzheimer's disease than people in the general population, and RA patients treated with etanercept were less likely to have Alzheimer's disease than ones treated with another RA drug.

Richard C. Chou, MD, PhD, assistant professor of medicine at Geisel School of Medicine, Dartmouth College, Hanover, New Hampshire, and leader of a study that analyzed data from more than eight million subjects, published in *CNS Drugs*.

## Crafty Brain Helpers

Doing crafts may have health benefits. Rhythmic, repetitive movements and focused attention, as in knitting, can reduce stress and improve mood. This is in addition to the satisfaction of completing a project. Older people who knit or do quilting also may have a lower risk for mild cognitive impairment, which can lead to dementia. And activities such as these can help distract people from chronic pain.

Studies in *British Journal of Occupational Therapy* and *The Journal of Neuropsychiatry & Clinical Neurosciences*, and a study presented to The British Pain Society.

## Make Your Brain Younger

Older adults who did regular moderate-to-intense exercise like running or swimming laps had the memory and other cognitive skills of someone a decade younger than those who were sedentary or did light exercise such as gardening, a recent study of 900 older adults found.

***Possible reason:*** Exercise boosts blood flow to the brain and enhances brain cell connections. It also lowers risk for high blood pressure, elevated cholesterol and diabetes—all of which can impair cognitive function.

Clinton Wright, MD, scientific director, Evelyn F. McKnight Brain Institute, University of Miami.

## New Hope for Parkinson's Patients

Low-dose *nilotinib* (Tasigna), a drug currently approved for treating leukemia, increases dopamine and reduces toxic proteins in Parkinson's patients. The drug also caused improvements in cognition/motor function.

An investigational drug (MSDC-0160) may be the first to actually slow Parkinson's disease progression. The drug appears to reduce the inflammation and death of nerve cells. Human studies are scheduled to begin late 2017.

*Journal of Parkinson's Disease.*
*Science Translational Medicine.*

### Sniff This to Boost Memory

Need to remember to make a phone call or take your medication? A whiff of rosemary oil could help.

***Recent study:*** 150 people over age 65 performed memory tasks either in a rosemary-scented room or in a room without scent. The aroma of rosemary significantly improved both mood and prospective memory (the ability to remember planned events and tasks).

***Why:*** The herb contains compounds that boost the area of the brain involved in memory.

Mark Moss, PhD, head of psychology, Northumbria University, Newcastle upon Tyne, UK.

## Time for Your Cognitive Checkup

Malaz A. Boustani, MD, the Richard M. Fairbanks professor in aging research at the Indiana University Center for Aging Research and founding director and chief innovation and implementation officer at the Sandra Eskenazi Center for Brain Care Innovation, both in Indianapolis. He is the recipient of the 2012 American Geriatrics Society Outstanding Scientific Achievement for Clinical Investigation Award. AgingBrainCare.org

One of your favorite actors appears on the screen, but you can't put a name to the face. Or you walk into the kitchen for—well, you walked in there for something, but you can't remember what.

Sound familiar? If so, you are probably at least middle-aged. These and other memory hiccups usually reflect nothing more than normal brain changes, but how can you be sure? It's a legitimate concern because up to 76% of cases of cognitive impairment aren't spotted by primary care physicians during the mild-to-moderate phases.

***Recent development:*** You may have heard about the "annual wellness visit" that the Affordable Care Act has added as a new Medicare/Medicaid benefit. As you might imagine, this free checkup includes standard tests (such as blood pressure), a review of screening tests, etc. But this exam also includes a thorough assessment to detect memory problems or other cognitive impairments. Some private insurance policies may also cover this type of exam.

***Why it's important:*** People with Alzheimer's or other forms of dementia are typically diagnosed three to five years after they've developed impairments. The cognitive checkup offers the chance for earlier detection of a problem and the opportunity to develop an effective plan for coping with symptoms of cognitive impairment.

## What the Exam Includes

During the annual wellness visit, your doctor will start with a general health assessment. If you're like most adults, you probably have one or more health issues—such as high blood pressure or diabetes—that increase the risk for cognitive impairments. Certain medications can also cause cognitive problems.

The exam (combined with subsequent tests) can also help identify reversible causes of cognitive declines, such as thyroid problems, low vitamin B-12 and depression.

After that, the exam will include...

- **Personal stories.** Your doctor will ask how your life is going. This is your chance to discuss any changes you might have noticed—maybe it's getting harder to balance your checkbook...perhaps you're forgetting to take medications (or you're taking them at the wrong times). Buttoning clothing might be harder...possibly you've slipped and fallen in the bathroom...or maybe you've felt depressed lately. Such self-reported observations can raise important red flags.

- **A conversation with a family member/close friend.** It's common for patients with cognitive changes to be unaware (or only partly aware) of how much they're affected. You may think that you're on top of daily details, but someone else in your life might notice that you keep missing appointments or taking wrong turns on your drive home. A different perspective is helpful.

***My advice:*** I strongly encourage patients to bring someone with them to their wellness visits whether they suspect cognitive problems or not. The doctor or a member of the medical team may interview the person separately so that he/she can speak freely. If you and your companion say that your memory is good, there's a strong likelihood that everything's fine...and that you won't need further testing for another year.

## Possible Problem Areas

If you have noticed changes in your memory or daily routines, your doctor will ask focused questions.

***Examples:*** "During the last 12 months, have you noticed that confusion/memory loss is happening more often or getting worse?" "Did you need help from others during the last week in performing daily activities, such as grooming, walking or getting dressed?"

Problems in any of these areas could mean that you need...

- **Cognitive testing.** If your doctor suspects (based on the above discussions) that you might have some degree of cognitive impairment, commonly used tests include the Memory Impairment Screen (MIS)...the General Practitioner assessment of Cognition (GPCOG)...or the Mini-Cog. Each can be administered by a medical staff member in less than five minutes.

***Example:*** The MIS is a verbally administered word-recall test. You might be asked to read four words—for example, checkers, saucer, telegram and bus—out loud. Then you'll be told to think of categories (such as "games") and come up with words that fit in each category. After a few minutes, you'll be asked to remember the four words you read earlier. You may also be asked to spell a word (such as "world") backward...or count back from 100 by sevens.

Patients who "fail" a test may have cognitive impairments—or they could simply be having an off day. Further evaluation by a neurologist, geriatrician or other specialist will be recommended.

## What's Next?

If the wellness visit and subsequent testing point to a cognitive decline, you'll need appropriate follow-up.

***Recent research:*** The collaborative care model (a team approach to care) has been shown to be more effective than the standard one-doctor/one-patient approach. With the collaborative approach, a team of clinicians (which may include a primary care doctor and memory care doctor) led by a care coordinator (a registered nurse or a social worker) works with the patient and family to improve quality of care.

In a study of 153 patients with mild-to-moderate Alzheimer's, patients who received collaborative care had fewer behavioral/psychological problems and were more likely to be given effective drug treatments than patients receiving "standard" care with one doctor.

Many patients can live a relatively normal life with cognitive decline, but they'll need a lot of help along the way. A collaborative program is the best way to provide it.

***Note:*** All aspects of this care may not be covered by insurance.

## Get Up and Out to Fight Dementia

Being sedentary raises dementia risk so much that it matches the risk faced by people with genetic factors that make dementia more likely. Sedentary older adults without risk factors for dementia were just as likely to develop it as people with a genetic disposition caused by a variant of the apolipoprotein E genotype. Exact types of exercise that can protect against dementia are not yet known—but in general, a physically active lifestyle seems to help the brain work more effectively, reducing the chance of dementia.

Study of more than 1,600 Canadian adults over five years by researchers at McMaster University, Hamilton, Ontario, Canada, published in *Journal of Alzheimer's Disease.*

## New Treatment for Essential Tremor

Focused sound waves guided by MRI can be sent into the brain area called the thalamus to kill cells causing the tremor. The treatment is approved only for patients who are 22 or older and for whom standard medication therapy has not worked. Side effects, including numbness and tingling of the hands and face and difficulty walking, usually are transient.

Travis Tierney, MD, PhD, a pediatric neurosurgeon at Nicklaus Children's Hospital, Miami, Florida.

# Chapter 6

# PHYSICAL INJURY AND BONE HEALTH

## What to Do About Calcium and Your Bones

The calcium supplements that millions of Americans take for bone health may cause serious damage to the heart. That's the conclusion of the latest study examining the long-term risks of these supplements.

The research, published in *Journal of the American Heart Association*, found that people who supplement with calcium are more likely to develop arterial calcification than those who get their calcium from foods. Calcium that accumulates in the arteries can impair circulation and increase the risk for heart disease.

Yet an estimated 43% of Americans continue to supplement with calcium.

### What Your Bones Really Need

Calcium supplements have become a controversial topic. It is a fact that Americans don't get enough calcium. Only 42% meet the estimated average daily requirement of 1,000 milligrams (mg) to 1,200 mg (the exact amount depends on age and gender). It's a serious problem because both women and men need calcium—along with exercise, vitamin D and other nutrients—to prevent bone weakness and osteoporosis, a leading cause of disability and fracture-related deaths.

But supplements aren't the answer for many people. They may slightly increase bone density, but they do little to reduce your risk for bone fractures. In a recent analysis of studies published in *BMJ*, researchers concluded that "evidence that calcium supplements prevent fractures is weak and inconsistent."

The calcium that you get from food is different. It enters the body slowly and in small amounts. That's very different from the calcium rush that you get from supplements. Also, food delivers a "package" that includes calcium along with dozens of other minerals and nutrients, including vitamins, proteins, fiber, amino acids and, in the case of plant foods, phytonutrients. It seems likely that our bodies benefit from nutritional complexity. You don't get this from single-ingredient supplements.

---

Susan Levin, MS, RD, director of nutrition education for the Physicians Committee for Responsible Medicine, a Washington, DC–based nonprofit group dedicated to promoting preventive medicine, better nutrition and higher standards in research.

## Calcium in the Wrong Places

In the *Journal of the American Heart Association* study, researchers analyzed medical tests that were done on more than 2,700 people who participated in a large heart disease study. They were looking for coronary artery calcium, a heart disease risk factor.

Your calcium score (as measured by a heart CT scan) should be zero. But as people age, levels of calcium-based plaque tend to accumulate in the aorta and other arteries. These levels increase more in people who take calcium supplements.

The study found that people who supplemented with calcium were 22% more likely to have increased coronary calcium scores over a 10-year period than those who didn't supplement. It wasn't the amount of calcium that mattered most—it was the type. People who did not take supplements but who got a lot of calcium from foods (more than 1,400 mg daily) were 27% less likely than those who consumed the least amount of calcium from foods to have calcium scores that indicated an elevated heart risk.

Calcium deposits affect more than just the heart. A high calcium score also has been linked to increased risk for cancer including cancers of the prostate, lung, colon, breast, skin, blood, uterus and ovaries. It also has been linked to lung disease and chronic kidney disease.

***Example:*** A study published in *Journal of the American College of Cardiology: Cardiovascular Imaging* found that people with high coronary calcium scores were 70% more likely to develop kidney disease than those who had low scores.

***Caveat:*** None of the calcium/heart disease studies prove conclusively that supplements increase risks. The only way to know for sure would be to conduct a randomized, double-blind clinical trial in which some participants would take supplements and others wouldn't and then track their health over time. This type of study will probably never be done. The evidence linking calcium supplements and heart disease has become so persuasive that it would be unethical to give supplements to people who don't need them.

## When Calcium Makes Sense

We know that many Americans don't get enough calcium in their diets and that some of these people will never try to get more in their diets. Can supplements take up the slack? Perhaps—but this makes sense only for people who absolutely need to supplement. *Are you one of these people? Here's how to know...*

- **Get a workup first.** Calcium supplements should be treated as cautiously as prescription drugs. If you're worried about osteoporosis, talk to your doctor. Have your blood-calcium levels tested. If you're deficient, you might be advised to use supplements. Your doctor also should advise you on how to get more calcium in your diet and when to decide if you need supplements.

- **Focus on food.** Some people—particularly those who have already been diagnosed with osteoporosis or who are at high risk for it—might be advised to supplement despite the possible increase in heart risks. But most people can get more than enough calcium from foods if they make a conscious effort.

***Examples:*** One cup of low-fat yogurt has 415 mg of calcium...one cup of skim milk, 316 mg...one cup of boiled collard greens, 266 mg...one cup of white beans, 161 mg...and one cup of soy milk, 93 mg.

- **Consider all of the calcium in your diet.** The heart risks from supplemental calcium may be proportional to the dose. You don't want to take any more than you need to. Suppose that you're trying to get 1,200 mg of calcium in total each day. You're already getting some calcium from foods. Keep that in mind before choosing a calcium dose. Why take a high-dose supplement if you need only an extra 200 mg a day?

***My advice:*** Work with a nutritionist to help you find out how much calcium you actually consume in an average day. Or use the Internet—the USDA has a good calcium-content list at NDB.NAL.USDA.gov and click on "Food Search."

If you supplement, keep the doses low—your body can't absorb more than 500 mg at a time. Calcium carbonate has the highest amount of calcium (40% calcium) compared with calcium citrate (21% calcium). But citrate may be better tolerated by those with low stomach acids, which is common among people age 50 and older.

• **Get vitamin D and magnesium, too.** These help with absorption of calcium. Milk and many breakfast cereals are D-fortified. You also can get vitamin D from sunshine—between five and 30 minutes (depending on your skin type and age) twice a week is probably enough. Or your doctor may advise you to take a vitamin D supplement. There are different types of vitamin D (vitamin D-2, vitamin D-3). It doesn't matter which type you take—research has shown both types to be effective.

Magnesium helps with calcium absorption, too, but you don't need a magnesium supplement. You just need adequate magnesium in your diet. Magnesium is readily available in whole grains, nuts, seeds, beans and leafy greens.

• **Don't forget to exercise.** Physical activity slows the rate of bone loss in men and women with osteoporosis, and it's among the best ways to strengthen bones before they get weak. Weight-bearing exercises (such as walking, jogging and weight-lifting) are more efficient for strengthening bones than other types of workouts (such as biking or swimming).

***Recommended:*** 30 to 40 minutes of walking or other weight-bearing exercises most days of the week.

# Injected Drug May Help Women Fight Osteoporosis

Paul Miller, MD, Colorado Center for Bone Research, Lakewood, Colorado.

Caroline Messer, MD, director, Center for Pituitary and Neuroendocrine Disorders, Lenox Hill Hospital, New York City.

*Journal of the American Medical Association.*

An experimental drug appears to reduce the risk of bone fractures in postmenopausal women with osteoporosis better than a placebo and the currently available drug, a recent study finds.

## Osteoporosis Risk

A study based on 2010 U.S. Census data estimated that more than three million women between the ages of 50 and 69 have osteoporosis. A 60-year-old woman has a 44% lifetime risk of fracture due to low bone density.

## About the Study

In this phase 3 trial funded by the drug's maker, Radius Health, fewer women on the injectable drug *abaloparatide* had spine fractures (0.58%) than women receiving a placebo (4.22%) and slightly fewer than those taking a similar injectable drug, *teriparatide* (Forteo) (0.84%).

"If this gets approved, and there is no reason to think it won't, this will be the second drug available for the treatment of high-risk osteoporosis," said lead researcher Paul Miller, MD, of the Colorado Center for Bone Research.

Forteo has been in use for the past 16 years, he said. Abaloparatide works differently from Forteo and improves bone density more than Forteo, Dr. Miller said.

## Study Details

For the study, Dr. Miller and colleagues randomly assigned nearly 2,500 postmenopausal women with osteoporosis to receive injections of abaloparatide, Forteo or a placebo for 18 months. Their average age was 69.

Among the nearly 2,000 women who completed the trial, increases in bone mineral density were greater with abaloparatide than placebo, the researchers found.

In addition, fewer cases of hypercalcemia (abnormally high levels of calcium in the blood) occurred among women taking abaloparatide (3%) than Forteo (6%). Hypercalcemia can weaken bones, cause kidney stones and interfere with heart and brain function.

There were no differences among the groups in other serious side effects, such as nausea and heart palpations, Dr. Miller said. Previous animal studies with Forteo found a possible link to osteosarcoma, a serious but rare bone cancer.

Women taking abaloparatide also had fewer other types of fractures (2.7%) than those who got a placebo (4.7%) and slightly fewer than those on Forteo (3.3%), the researchers found.

Dr. Miller said many spine fractures are painless. Patients are often unaware they have happened until a doctor measures their height and finds they are up to an inch shorter than before, he said.

The report was published in the *Journal of the American Medical Association*.

## How the Drugs Work

Abaloparatide and Forteo are synthetic peptides that help grow and strengthen bone, Dr. Miller said.

Along with building bone density, they are the only ones that increase bone quality, he said. "Bone quality is an important aspect of bone strength—the ability to withstand a break," Dr. Miller said.

## Lower Costs

Dr. Miller predicts that when abaloparatide is on the market, it will compete with Forteo, driving down the price of both drugs.

"I am hoping that having a second drug available, that it will help reduce the cost," he said. "Forteo costs about $2,500 a month if you don't have insurance." Even if a patient is insured, monthly copays can range from $30 to $400. Forteo is covered by Medicare, Dr. Miller said.

## Expert Reaction

Caroline Messer, MD, director of the Center for Pituitary and Neuroendocrine Disorders at Lenox Hill Hospital in New York City, is eager for further research. There needs to be a large head-to-head trial between Forteo and abaloparatide, she said, to really see which drug is better.

"Everybody is going to want to know if this is inferior or superior to Forteo," she said, adding that this is an early study. "It shows more bone building and fewer fractures than Forteo, but whether it will replace that drug is still up in the air."

To learn more about osteoporosis, visit the American College of Rheumatology website, Rheumatology.org, and search "osteoporosis."

# BP Drug Protects Bones, Too

Blood pressure drug has a surprising benefit. Thiazide diuretics, commonly prescribed to lower blood pressure, decreased risk for hip and pelvic fractures by 21%, compared with ACE inhibitors and calcium channel blockers, a recent study of 22,000 older adults found.

***Possible reason:*** Thiazide diuretics, such as *chlorthalidone* and *indapamide*, lower calcium excretion in urine, which may slow bone loss.

***If you have thinning bones and/or an increased risk for fracture:*** Ask your doctor about taking a thiazide diuretic if you need blood pressure medication.

Joshua I. Barzilay, MD, endocrinologist, Kaiser Permanente, Duluth, Georgia.

## Menopause Before 40? Risk of Broken Bones May Be Higher

North American Menopause Society, press release. *Menopause.*

Women who undergo menopause before age 40 are more likely to get broken bones, and a recent study suggests calcium and vitamin D supplements won't eliminate the extra risk.

Researchers were disappointed by the finding because supplements and hormone replacement therapy have been thought to improve bone health.

The researchers were led by Dr. Shannon Sullivan, medical officer from the U.S. Food and Drug Administration. They examined the medical records of almost 22,000 women who took part in the Women's Health Initiative. This 15-year study, by the U.S. National Institutes of Health, reviewed the most common causes of poor health and death among postmenopausal women.

The study team found that those women who entered menopause before age 40 had a significantly higher risk of broken bones than those who did later, regardless of the treatments they tried. On average, women enter menopause around age 52.

The researchers said there's hope for other strategies, including earlier or longer treatment with calcium, vitamin D or hormones; different doses; or longer follow-up.

The study was published recently in *Menopause*, the journal of the North American Menopause Society.

"This study highlights the need for healthcare providers to take into consideration a woman's age at menopause onset when evaluating patients for fracture risk," said JoAnn Pinkerton, MD, the society's executive director.

"Women at risk for bone loss need 1,200 mg (milligrams) of calcium per day, with adequate vitamin D, and [are] encouraged to get as much as possible through diet due to concern that too much supplemental calcium may increase atherosclerotic plaque in women," she said in a society news release.

Dr. Pinkerton added that women with early menopause should ask their healthcare provider whether they are candidates for hormone therapy and discuss appropriate amounts of calcium, vitamin D and hormones.

## Pot Not Great for Bones

Heavy marijuana use may lower bone density. People who smoked marijuana very heavily—on at least 5,000 occasions in their lifetimes—had lower bone density and twice as much risk for broken bones as tobacco-cigarette smokers who didn't use marijuana. Moderate marijuana use, defined as an average of about 1,000 times in a lifetime, did not have an effect on bone health.

Study led by researchers at Center for Genomic and Experimental Medicine, University of Edinburgh, Scotland, published in *The American Journal of Medicine.*

### Simple Ways to Improve Your Balance

See how long you can stand on one foot with your eyes closed, and work on improving your time. Rise up on your toes 10 times with your eyes open and then 10 more times with them closed. Balance yourself on one foot for 10 to 15 seconds, then switch legs. Repeat 10 times, then do it again with your eyes closed. Walk in a straight line, placing the heel of one foot in front of the toes of the other foot.

***Caution:*** When doing these exercises, stand near a wall or some other support.

University of California, *Berkeley Wellness Letter.* BerkeleyWellness.com

# Girls and Women Vulnerable to Knee Injuries

Jo A. Hannafin, MD, PhD, orthopaedic director, Women's Sports Medicine Center, Hospital for Special Surgery, New York City.

Francesco Gallaro, MSPT, CSCS, a certified strength and conditioning coach and physical therapist in Norwalk, Connecticut.

There are many physiological and anatomical differences between men and women beyond the obvious ones—including, as it turns out, vulnerability to orthopedic injuries. It appears that how women are built leaves us—and our daughters—four times more likely to suffer knee injuries, especially to the anterior cruciate ligament (ACL) in the knee joint. Although the ACL is the smallest ligament in the knee, the fact that it is part of the connective structure between the femur (thigh bone) and tibia (shin bone) makes it critical to stability. A torn ACL can be painful and often requires surgery, followed by four to six months of physical therapy to regain proper functioning and return to sports. Recent research provides an improved understanding of how to protect yourself from the risk of injury—not to mention the resulting pain and cost for treatment.

## Research to Date

Research a few years ago revealed one major cause of ACL injury in women—after a jump, as in basketball or volleyball, females tend to land with straighter legs than males do, which puts more pressure on the ACL. Research also has shown that females often have an imbalance between the strength in their quadriceps muscles in the front of the thighs and the hamstring muscles in the back of the thighs. This alters knee functioning and may affect stability.

A more recent study on female knees comes from the University of Michigan, Division of Kinesiology, adding a subtle but important additional clue to the ACL/female injury issue. Researchers found that many women athletes maintain a knock-kneed position when landing after a jump. Knock-knees come about for several reasons. Some people (both male and female) are simply born this way—it is the anatomic alignment they were given. But often it is due to yet another muscle imbalance, this one between the inner (medial) and outer (lateral) thigh muscles. In this study, researchers determined that females—even those who are not knock-kneed—tend to activate the stronger outer thigh muscles in preparation for a landing. Without equally strong inner thigh muscles to provide balance, the knees rotate even further inward, increasing the risk to the ACL. Playing primarily one sport year-round or repeating the same exercise routines makes injury even more likely —repetition of one activity builds only the muscles the particular sport requires, and may create a strength imbalance. Cross training helps avoid this problem.

Not only jumping sports but any that involve torquing the knees—the twisting that is inherent in skiing, tennis or even ballroom dancing—puts pressure on the knee and increases risk of injury. This makes it important for all active women to pay special attention to their knee positioning and muscle strength balance.

To find out if your inner and outer thigh muscles are balanced, do a mini-squat on one leg (described under "Balance thigh muscles," next page)—if the bent knee goes toward the other knee rather than remaining pointed out straight, it shows weakness of the inner thigh muscles and the muscles of the hip and buttock that rotate the knee outward.

## Protect Yourself

Strengthening and balance training exercises to build up the muscles and paying close attention to how you jump, land and pivot can help you avoid such injury. For example, focusing on trying to land with knees that are slightly bent, or decelerating before switching directions when you're moving quickly (as in tennis) may help, according to a report by the *Journal of Athletic Training. Here are some suggestions...*

• **Wear the right shoes.** *Key:* Supportive shoes with a good, strong sole. Avoid flip-flops, sandals and fashion flats as these can aggravate problems in people who are flat-footed or who pronate excessively. Look for sandals with a built-in arch or use an arch support in your shoes.

• **Stand straight.** Pay attention to how you position your hips during all activities, including standing. You can get some sense of this by doing your exercises in front of a mirror, but if you are serious about sports, consider an assessment by a sports physical therapist.

• **Strengthen hips.** Strengthening hips also helps prevent injury. One way to do this is with hip abductions, says Francesco Gallaro, MSPT, CSCS, a certified strength and conditioning coach and physical therapist in Norwalk, Connecticut. These also serve to strengthen gluteus muscles. Do two or three sets of eight to 12 reps of standing resisted hip abductions, using a rubber band. Kick one leg from the midline of your body to the side in a backward diagonal direction. *Note*: Kick should be a smooth continuous motion. Try to complete the entire set without the foot touching the ground. Good hip strength prevents the knee from rolling inward into a knock-kneed position.

• **Balance thigh muscles.** To strengthen and balance the thigh muscles, include in a routine the one-sided mini-squat mentioned earlier. Keep the gluteus (the muscles of your buttocks) tight and pay close attention to activating muscles on both sides of the leg. To perform this exercise correctly, stand on one leg. Bending from the knee, lower your body down until your knee is bent to 45 degrees (you don't have to go all the way to a sitting position for it to be effective). Raise yourself back up. Do two or three sets of 10 repetitions, each leg.

• **Strengthen the hamstring** (for the quad-hamstring imbalances mentioned earlier). Gallaro suggests the deadlift. Stand on one leg, bend your body forward at the waist so you are at a 90-degree angle. Raise yourself back up—do three sets of eight to 12 reps. The leg not in contact with the floor should be straight and in proper alignment with your trunk. Try performing a set without letting your foot make contact with the ground. As you get stronger, you can do this exercise while holding weights.

• **Perform leg strengtheners.** Leg presses at the gym are also helpful—but with a strong caveat. It's important to maintain proper form, keeping your knees over your feet. Women tend to squeeze their knees—this further strengthens and trains the outside of the quad to do the work, leaving the inner thigh muscles getting weaker. Try placing a small ball between your knees when you are on the leg press.

• **Don't ignore your core.** Finally, try core strengthening exercises. Having strong pelvic and lower abdominal muscles, interestingly, helps to protect your knees. Pilates is good for this, of course, as are assorted core-exercise programs that employ large exercise balls.

---

## Concussions More Likely in Female Athletes

James Noble, MD, assistant professor, neurology, and Cecilia Davis-Hayes, medical student, Columbia University Medical Center, New York City.

Steven Broglio, PhD, director, NeuroTrauma Research Laboratory, and concussion lead, University of Michigan Injury Center, Ann Arbor.

American Academy of Neurology meeting, Boston.

---

Female athletes appear to be more likely than men to suffer concussions during their careers on the field, a recent study suggests.

The findings add to the existing evidence that female athletes may be more susceptible to concussions, even as attention has tended to focus on the risk to male football players.

"The more we look at concussion, the more we realize that women are at high risk," said study coauthor James Noble, MD. He's an assistant professor of neurology at Columbia University Medical Center in New York City.

Once a concussion occurs, however, the gender gap dwindles, the researchers found.

"For the most part, men and women experience concussion in about the same way," Dr. Noble said, "although men were more likely to report forgetfulness and women more likely to report sleep problems."

Concussions, especially among football players from high school to professional levels, have gotten intense attention in recent years.

In 2016, a study suggested that concussion diagnoses more than doubled from 2007 to 2014, with especially big jumps among children and teens. It's not clear, though, how much of the increase is due to increased awareness of concussions or a higher number of injured young people.

## Study Details

In the recent study, the researchers tracked more than 1,200 athletes from Columbia University from 2000 to 2014. More than 800 were male, and almost 400 were female.

The athletes all played sports believed to pose a higher risk of concussions.

For women, the sports included field hockey, soccer, basketball, softball and lacrosse, said study lead author Cecilia Davis-Hayes, a medical student at Columbia.

For men, the sports initially included just football but then also included wrestling, basketball and soccer, Davis-Hayes said.

The researchers found that 23% of the women and 17% of the men had at least one concussion during their college careers over the time of the study.

The difference "doesn't sound like much, but it's almost 50% more, meaning it's 50% more likely for women to get a concussion than men," Dr. Noble said.

Concussions in sports typically happen when athletes run into each other or hit the ground, Dr. Noble said. According to Davis-Hayes, lacrosse and soccer are especially physical sports for women with "a lot of contact on every play."

Levels of most concussion symptoms were similar among the men and women, although forgetfulness was more common for men (44% reported it, compared with 31% of the women). Women were more likely to experience insomnia (42%, compared with 29% of men).

The researchers found that it took an average of almost two weeks for the athletes to return to play, although Davis-Hayes said that's skewed because some players took especially long—months—to recover. The study didn't look at how the athletes were treated for their concussions.

The study also didn't take into account how long athletes played each sport. That means researchers don't know if the women or men were on the field for longer periods, potentially boosting their risk of concussion.

Why might women face a higher risk? It's not clear, Dr. Noble said, although he thinks it could be due to a variety of factors, such as differences in the bodies of men and women.

"Is there something about how the head moves in a woman versus a man?" he said.

## Expert Comment

Steven Broglio, PhD, director of the NeuroTrauma Research Laboratory at the University of Michigan, said the findings fit with other research.

"There are a multitude of studies that have shown that women participating in similar sports as men—like soccer, basketball, baseball/softball—report concussions at a higher rate. Concussions are not just a football or male injury," he said.

Dr. Broglio also noted that the recent study results suggest men and women recovered at the same speed. "Historically, we believed women took longer to recover from injury," he said, "but there is growing evidence suggesting this may not be the case."

The study authors said larger studies could offer more insight into the differences between the genders when it comes to concussion.

Learn more about concussion from the U.S. Centers for Disease Control and Prevention at CDC.gov/traumaticbraininjury/symptoms.html

## Is It a Concussion?

A concussion is typically diagnosed based on symptoms such as headache, blurred vision or confusion—sometimes hours or days after a head injury. If someone has taken a hard fall, can't recall events before or after a fall, loses consciousness (even briefly) or shows behavioral changes, take him to the emergency department, where he will undergo neurological tests, along with a CT scan or MRI to see if there is any injury to the brain. If symptoms continue, neuropsychological testing by a neuropsychologist who specializes in brain injury can accurately diagnose a concussion.

Diane Stoler, EdD, a neuropsychologist in private practice in Boxford, Massachusetts, and author of *Coping with Concussion and Mild Traumatic Brain Injury.*

## Sprain-Proof Your Ankles

Luke T. Donovan, PhD, ATC, an assistant professor in the department of kinesiology at The University of North Carolina at Charlotte, and past program director of the Post-Professional Athletic Training Program at The University of Toledo. His research interests include chronic ankle instability.

If you haven't sprained an ankle yet, it may be just a matter of time. About 25,000 Americans suffer from these painful injuries every day—that's a total of nine million such injuries each year.

But an ankle sprain is not that serious, right? We've all seen athletes limping off the field, only to return to the game soon after. You've probably done the same thing yourself. You take a wrong step...your foot turns...you hobble for a while...and you forget about it.

***What you may not realize:*** An ankle sprain can cause a lifetime of problems, including persistent ankle weakness, difficulty walking and even arthritis of the ankle. *What you need to know to protect yourself...*

### Lingering Damage

An ankle sprain occurs when a ligament (the band of tissue that connects bone to bone) stretches beyond its normal limits. The more a ligament stretches—or even tears—the more severe the sprain.

Most people who sprain an ankle never see a doctor. They assume that a little rest—along with an over-the-counter pain reliever and perhaps some ice packs—will take care of things. It's true that the immediate symptoms usually clear up quickly...within a matter of days or weeks. But what happens after that?

Studies have shown that more than 30% of people who sprain an ankle go on to develop chronic ankle instability. The joint feels as though it might "give" at any time. As a result, their health may suffer—they tend to exercise less...gain weight...and have more limitations in their daily movements. People who have sprained an ankle are also twice as likely to reinjure it.

To be clear, an ankle sprain does not cause high blood pressure or diabetes, for example, but it often does interfere with the types of activities that help prevent these and other serious chronic conditions. Ankle sprains have also been linked to a 13% to 16% increased risk for arthritic ankles.

### Sprain-Proof Your Ankles

The ankles are uniquely prone to injuries due to the mobility and wide range of motion of the ankle joint...and the fact that the ankles support the weight of your entire body.

For these reasons, it's wise for all adults—and especially those who have suffered previous ankle injuries (even if they were years ago)—to do a simple daily regimen of stretching, strengthening and balancing exercises.

Try to do all of the exercises below a few times a day—together, they take only about 10 minutes...

- **Stand on one foot.** This balancing exercise helps prevent ankle sprains by improving ankle muscle reflexes and proprioception, the body's ability to orient itself in space. I tell people to do the exercise when they're standing in line...talking on the phone...or even brushing their teeth.

***What to do:*** Simply stand on one foot near a chair or any other stationary object that you can grab on to if you lose your balance. Stand on one foot for about 30 seconds, then switch sides. Work up to a minute or two on each side.

***When it starts to feel easy:*** Close your eyes while you balance. Taking away the visual feedback forces the muscles and nerves to work harder.

- **Soft-surface stands.** To further improve ankle muscle function and your sense of balance, do one-legged stands (as described above) on a pillow, a foam pad or a balance disc (they're also called balance trainer balls and are available at sporting-goods stores and online).

The unstable surface forces your body to adapt to changes in balance and weight distribution. It makes your muscles more reactive, which can help you adjust to sudden changes in walking surfaces, posture, foot movements, etc.

- **Calf stretches.** The calf muscles connect to the Achilles tendon in the ankle. Stretching and strengthening the calves improves stability and range of motion.

***What to do:*** While facing a wall, stand back about one foot with your palms on the wall for support. Take one step back with your right foot and slightly bend your left leg. You'll feel the stretch in your right calf/ankle. Hold the position for about 10 seconds, then repeat on the other side. Perform the stretch three times on each side and work up to holding it for 30 seconds.

- **Ankle/calf raises.** As mentioned above, stronger calves and Achilles tendons improve ankle stability. This exercise strengthens both.

***What to do:*** While still facing a wall, with your palms on the wall for support, rise up on your toes as far as you can. Hold the stretch for a few seconds, then lower your heels to the floor. Repeat eight to 10 times. It's harder than it sounds! As your muscles get stronger, you can increase the difficulty by taking one foot off the floor when rising/lowering with the other foot.

- **Resistance exercises.** With an elastic resistance band, you can strengthen the ankle by moving it in its complete range of motion.

***What to do:*** While sitting in a chair, wrap an elastic resistance band under the ball of your foot. While holding the band tightly, move the foot/ankle up, down, left and right. Repeat a few times in each direction. Then perform on the other foot.

## When to Get Help

What if you think that you've actually sprained an ankle? First, see a doctor. You'll need an X-ray to determine whether you have a bone fracture, which typically requires the foot/ankle to be immobilized by a hard cast or boot.

If you have a sprain, don't try to simply "walk it off." The best thing you can do is keep weight off the ankle as much as possible until the pain and swelling are completely gone. An elastic bandage (such as ACE) can help minimize swelling.

During this time, you may also want to immobilize the joint with a brace (such as AirCast) for four to six weeks. Such braces are available online and at most drugstores for about $20 and up.

***Also helpful:*** To reduce pain and swelling, apply a cold pack (or ice wrapped in a towel) to the ankle for 20 minutes, once every hour for up to eight hours a day. Continue with this frequency for at least the first day after the sprain. After that, let pain be your guide—apply cold as long as the pain is severe and cut back as it eases.

***To help prevent long-term problems:*** I advise getting some form of rehabilitation—from a physical therapist or an athletic trainer—after the injury heals.

## Heal a Sprain at Home

Ankle sprain self-treatment works as well as supervised physical therapy. Patients who kept the ankle elevated and applied compression and ice, then gradually increased movement after a sprain did just as well in measurements of quality of life, pain, symptoms and function as patients who received up to seven sessions of physical therapy—including isometric resistance exercises, strength training and stretching. There was no difference between patients in the two groups at one, three or six months after the injury.

Study of 503 patients, ages 16 to 79, led by researchers at Queen's University, Kingston, Ontario, Canada, published in *BMJ Open*.

## Total Knee Replacements May Lead to Broken Bones

According to a Swedish study, people who have new knees are 19% more likely than others to experience spinal fractures and 4% more likely to break a hip.

***Possible reason:*** Patients become active before they are fully rehabilitated—which increases the risk of falling and breaking a bone.

***Self-defense:*** Ask your physician for balance exercises.

Sabrina Strickland, MD, a specialist in knee and shoulder surgery at Hospital for Special Surgery and associate professor of orthopedic surgery at Weill Cornell Medical College, both in New York City.

## After a Bone Fracture, Check Your Meds

Study titled "Patterns of Prescription Drug Use Before and After Fragility Fracture" by Jeffrey C. Munson, MD, Geisel School of Medicine, Dartmouth College, Lebanon, New Hampshire, and colleagues, published in *JAMA Internal Medicine*.

A broken bone can have devastating consequences for an older person. It can lead to functional decline and loss of independence—even increased risk for death. One of the biggest post-fracture health risks is getting another fracture. But few patients get the right care after a fracture to help them prevent future fractures, a recent study finds—and lots of people keep taking meds that increase fracture risk!

### The Drug Connection

It's not a secret that many drugs for conditions such as diabetes, depression, high blood pressure, insomnia and even GERD can contribute to increased fracture risk. But breaking a bone should be a loud wake-up call for doctors to reevaluate the meds a patient is taking.

Unfortunately, that isn't happening. A recent study from the Geisel School of Medicine at Dartmouth College looked at 168,000 Medicare recipients who had had bone fractures and found that four months after their fractures, more than 80% of them were still taking at least one medication known to increase risk for fracture. Even more alarming—more patients increased use of fracture-promoting drugs than decreased such use after their breaks!

The list of drugs most associated with fracture risk in the study included...

- **Oral steroids**
- **Proton pump inhibitors** (for peptic ulcers, GERD)
- **Thiazolidinediones** (a class of diabetes drug)

- **Diuretics** (for high blood pressure)
- **Hypnotics** (for insomnia)
- **Selective serotonin reuptake inhibitors** (antidepressants)
- **Antipsychotics**

Some of these drugs increase fracture risk because they increase the risk of falling—for example, hypnotics, antidepressants and even diuretics can make people dizzy. Others, such as proton pump inhibitors, decrease bone density—weakening bones.

***Bottom line:*** If you have had a fracture, be sure to discuss with your doctor whether any of the medications you are taking might either weaken your bones or make falls more likely. You may be able to take a different class of medication to accomplish the same purpose. You may also want to discuss whether you should take medications for osteoporosis, suggest the study authors.

You can also take steps—literally—to strengthen your bones and help keep you steady on your feet. Weight-bearing exercises, such as walking and lifting weights, can help strengthen your bones, while yoga and tai chi help improve balance—and prevent falls.

## Dents in Your Head

Alan M. Rapoport, MD, clinical professor of neurology, David Geffen School of Medicine at UCLA, Los Angeles, and immediate past president of the International Headache Society.

If you've given yourself a scalp massage recently, you may have felt a few dents in your skull. Should you be concerned?

Before birth, the skull forms in several pieces, which continue to grow and fuse together after birth. The adult skull isn't perfectly smooth, and most lines and dents are normal.

But changes to the skull sometimes need further evaluation, especially after head trauma or if a large or tender bump forms.

If you fall and hit your head, for example, you could have a skull fracture or scalp hematoma (a pooling of blood between the scalp and the skull).

Sometimes a fracture results in an irregular bone surface that can resemble a dent. Your doctor should check for a fracture if you've had a hard blow to the head, even if you have no pain, confusion or other symptoms.

Because falls are a major cause of skull injury in older adults, it is important to take preventive measures. Wear shoes with nonskid soles at home and keep clutter off the floor. Be sure to have an eye exam every year or two, and ask your doctor for alternatives if your medication increases risk for falls. Improve strength, balance and coordination with weight training and brisk walking several times a week.

***Also:*** A misshapen skull can result from rare bone disorders or cancer, so always contact your doctor if dents or swellings change in size or become hot and/or tender.

### Hands-Free Cell-Phones Are NOT Safe!

In a surprising finding, both handheld *and* hands-free cell phones caused a 40% increase in reaction time during a simulation of a pedestrian entering a crosswalk from the driver's peripheral vision compared with drivers not using a phone.

***Explanation:*** The cognitive power needed to hold a conversation can decrease the ability to process some visual information.

***Takeaway:*** Don't assume that hands-free calls are safe—stay off the phone altogether when driving.

Md. Mazharul (Shimul) Haque, PhD, senior lecturer, Queensland University of Technology, Brisbane, Australia.

## Sexual Assault on Airplanes Is on the Rise

Detective Kevin Coffey, a travel risk consultant and corporate trainer who is CEO of Los Angeles–based Corporate Travel Safety. CorporateTravelSafety.com

Sexual harassment and assault during air travel are on the rise. FBI investigations into in-flight sexual assaults increased by 45% in 2016 over the year before. More seats crammed into planes and fewer flight attendants are contributing factors.

It isn't fair to ask women to change their behavior to avoid this crime—that's close to blaming the victim—but women who wish to take steps to minimize the danger do have options. *These options are worth considering when traveling alone on long, overnight flights, where airline sexual assault is most common...*

• **Book an aisle seat if possible.** You're more visible to flight attendants and fellow passengers on the aisle, making it more difficult for a sexual predator to target you without being seen.

• **React firmly to possibly accidental contact.** Sexual predators sometimes employ "accidental" touching to test how much they can get away with. Firmly say, "Please do not touch me."

• **If you get a bad vibe from a passenger in a neighboring seat**—if, for example, he makes inappropriate remarks—get up and quietly ask a flight attendant if you can change seats.

• **Don't leave your drink unsupervised.** You would be especially vulnerable if someone slipped a "date rape" drug into your drink.

• **React loudly if you are groped.** This typically stops the predator by attracting the attention of nearby passengers. Then tell a flight attendant what you want done—do you want to move to a different seat? Do you want the perpetrator moved to a different seat? Do you want to press charges? Conflicts on aircraft typically are handled by separating the people involved—and the misconduct is reported to law enforcement.

## Working Out? Stay Off the Cell-Phone

Hiram College, news release.

Talking or texting on your cell phone may spell trouble during exercise, researchers say.

In two studies, they found that talking or texting on a cell phone during a workout lowers the intensity of your exercise session. More importantly, the study team noted that cell phone use affects balance, which can increase the risk of injuries.

"If you're talking or texting on your cell phone while you're putting in your daily steps, your attention is divided by the two tasks and that can disrupt your postural stability, and therefore, possibly predispose individuals to other greater inherent risks such as falls and musculoskeletal injuries," study author Michael Rebold, assistant professor of integrative exercise science at Hiram College in Ohio, said in a school news release.

Specifically, texting on a cell phone reduced postural stability by 45%. Even talking on a cell phone reduced postural stability by 19%.

But, if you want to pump up your workout with some tunes, go right ahead. Listening to music on a cell phone had no significant effect on postural stability during a workout, according to the study of 45 college students.

The studies about the effects of cell phone use during workouts were published in the journals *Computers in Human Behavior* and *Performance Enhancement & Health.*

## Brain Scan Test Predicts Fall Risk in Elderly

Joe Verghese, MBBS, MS, director, Montefiore Einstein Center for the Aging Brain, New York City.

Paul Wright, MD, chair, neurology, North Shore University Hospital, Manhasset, New York, and Long Island Jewish Medical Center, New Hyde Park, New York.

Gayatri Devi, MD, neurologist, Lenox Hill Hospital, New York City.

*Neurology*, news release.

Falls can prove very disabling for the elderly, and recent research suggests that measurements of healthy older adults' brain activity may help determine their future risk.

"Our findings suggest that changes in brain activity that influence walking may be present long before people exhibit any sign of walking difficulty," said study lead author Joe Verghese, MBBS. He directs the Montefiore Einstein Center for the Aging Brain in New York City.

Verghese believes the research might even help in fall prevention. "We need to find the underlying biological mechanisms or diseases that may be altering brain activity and, if possible, correct them to prevent falls," he explained.

### Research Details

The recent research involved 166 people averaging 75 years of age with no disabilities, dementia or difficulty walking at the beginning of the study.

All of them underwent brain scans to assess activity in the prefrontal cortex of the brain while they performed specific tests—walking, reciting alternate letters of the alphabet and then doing both at the same time.

Over four years of follow-up, 71 of the participants (43%) reported a total of 116 falls, and 34 of them fell more than once. Most of the falls were minor, with only 5% resulting in fractures, the researchers said.

Higher levels of brain activity in the combined "walking and talking" test were associated with a higher risk of falls, with each incremental increase in brain activity linked with a 32% higher risk of falling.

This association remained even after the researchers accounted for other fall risk factors, such as slow walking speed, frailty and previous falls.

However, there was no link between fall risk and brain activity levels while either just walking or talking (but not both at once), Verghese's group found.

### Expert Comment

Two experts in brain health who reviewed the study said it gives insight into why falls are more common with age.

"The human brain is an incredibly efficient organ, that when healthy, uses precise activation of focal circuits for different activities," said Gayatri Devi, MD, a neurologist at Lenox Hill Hospital in New York City. "The loss of such precision with associated widespread recruitment may be a sign of impending brain illness."

The recent study showed that "those who activated more areas of their brain while walking—in other words expended more brain effort—were more likely to fall in the subsequent four years," she said.

Verghese said: "These findings suggest that there may be changes in brain activity before physical symptoms like unusual gait appear in people who are more prone to falls later."

Paul Wright, MD, is chair of neurology at North Shore University Hospital in Manhasset, New York. He believes that a brain scan test like the one used in the study might someday be used to help predict and prevent falls in the elderly.

Using the results of the test, "physicians may then be able to use this information to educate and counsel their patients with behavior-modification techniques" to reduce fall risk, Dr. Wright said.

The study was published online in the journal *Neurology.*

Visit the U.S. National Institute on Aging at NIHseniorhealth.gov for more information about falls and older adults.

# The Best Yoga for Your Bones

Loren Fishman, MD, assistant clinical professor at Columbia University College of Physicians and Surgeons, and physical and rehabilitative specialist in private practice in New York City. He is coauthor with Ellen Saltonstall, MA, of *Yoga for Osteoporosis*.

Caitlin McArthur, MScPT, physical therapist and doctoral candidate, department of kinesiology, University of Waterloo, Ontario, Canada.

Study titled "Twelve-Minute Daily Yoga Regimen Reverses Osteoporotic Bone Loss," by Loren Fishman, MD, and colleagues, published in *Topics in Geriatric Rehabilitation*.

Study titled "Suggestions for Adapting Yoga to the Needs of Older Adults with Osteoporosis" by Caitlin McArthur, MScPT, Judi Laprade, PhD and Lora M. Giangregoria, PhD, published in *The Journal of Alternative and Complementary Medicine*.

You know that weight-bearing exercise such as walking strengthens your bones. But there's growing evidence that yoga—already pretty popular for making muscles stronger and more flexible, reducing stress and improving brain health—may also be an effective way to prevent osteoporosis. It even can strengthen bones if you already have osteoporosis.

But not all yoga shores up skeletal health. The wrong kind of yoga moves may actually put your bones at risk.

To learn the best way to use yoga to strengthen bones safely, we talked to Loren Fishman, MD, a physiatrist at Columbia University in New York City who has practiced yoga for more than 30 years, regularly prescribes it for his patients, and is coauthor (with Ellen Saltonstall, MA) of *Yoga for Osteoporosis*.

## Stronger Bones in 12 Minutes a Day?

"Yoga actually puts more stress on bones than weight-bearing exercise," Dr. Fishman explains. "The poses require opposing one group of muscles against another, which generates more force on bones than other types of activity."

He recently put the practice to the test in a study of 227 participants, 202 of them women. Their average age was 68, and 83% had lower-than-normal bone density, based on lab tests. Following an instructional DVD, they practiced 12 poses specifically designed to strengthen bone at least every other day for two years.

***Results:*** The program significantly improved bone density in the spines and femurs (thighbones)—by about 9%. Hip-bone density showed improvement, too, but it was not statistically significant. "What's particularly encouraging about these results is that in the two years preceding the study, there was a decrease in bone mineral density at all three sites—spine, hip and femur," says Dr. Fishman. It's a pilot study and the first of its kind. In addition to bone density, notes Dr. Fishman, the study showed improvements in bone quality—the internal structure of bone. "That inner structure provides between 30% and 70% of the bone's resistance to fracture," he says.

There's another, perhaps even more important, way that yoga can help, Dr. Fishman emphasizes—by improving balance and thus preventing falls that lead to fractures. It is falls and fractures, after all, that lead to disability—and often loss of independence. "Most fractures are the result of poor posture or a fall," he says. "Not only does yoga improve posture, it also improves balance, range of motion, coordination—all factors that contribute to the risk of falling." Pills and injections can't provide these types of benefits.

## The Best Kind of Yoga for Bones

For skeletal health, Dr. Fishman recommends Iyengar yoga, which focuses on proper alignment of the body—rather than Vinyasa-type yoga, which moves quickly through a series of asanas, or poses...or working up a sweat with Bikram or hot yoga. Iyengar yoga is a particularly good choice if you already have osteoporosis, because it's safe. But it's a great practice for anyone who wants to improve posture, strength, balance—and bone strength. (You can find a practitioner in your area on the Iyengar website.) If you want to practice the 12 bone-building poses designed by Dr. Fishman, you can order the DVD for $25 from Sciatica.org.

If you do have low bone density or actual osteoporosis, it's particularly important to choose the right kind of class—and practitioner. Caitlin McArthur, MScPT, a physical therapist and doctoral candidate in the department of kinesiology at University of Waterloo in Ontario, has been researching how yoga can be adapted for people with osteoporosis. "People with osteoporosis should focus on alignment and control in poses—rather than pushing themselves beyond what their bodies can do," she says.

She recommends sticking with yoga poses that focus on slow, controlled movement and on balance, proper muscle use, body alignment and sensory awareness rather than pose intensity. "You want to focus on keeping the spine aligned rather than bent forward," she explains. These include poses you do while lying on your back (Bridge, Corpse), on your stomach (Crocodile, Sphinx, Locust) or while standing (Warrior, Mountain, Chair). She advises against poses that require complete flexion, extension or rotation of the spine (Child's Pose, Spinal Twists, Ragdoll, Saw and Plow) and those that involve pushing your hip outward in an extreme way (Thread The Needle, Pigeon). These kinds of moves can put excess stress on the vertebrae, and there have been cases in which patients doing these kinds of poses have actually experienced spine fractures.

With a properly trained instructor, however, even some of the "avoid" poses can be made safe, notes McArthur. That's especially true if you use props such as blocks, blankets and bolsters. "For example, rather than let your forehead touch the floor in Child's Pose, which flexes the vertebrae in the neck, you can use a block to prop up your head and keep it in line with your spine."

One option is to seek out a class that is designed for older people—and run by an instructor who has training in how to adapt yoga exercises for people with osteoporosis. McArthur explains that these skills aren't taught in most entry-level yoga teacher education. You want an instructor who will work one-on-one with you to tailor poses to your abilities. (On Dr. Fishman's Sciatica.org website, you can also find a list of practitioners who are trained in yoga for people with osteoporosis.)

***Another route:*** Work with a physical therapist who has experience with osteoporosis and a knowledge of yoga. You can start by looking for a physical therapist with a specialty in geriatric or orthopedics on the website of the American Physical Therapist Association. When you find one, ask if he/she has yoga training, too.

Finally—and importantly—go slowly and gently. Don't be tempted to compete with your human pretzel classmates. But don't be afraid either. Over the past 10 years, Saltonstall and Dr. Fishman have worked with many people, mostly over age 65, almost all of whom had significant osteoporosis—helping them put in more than 100,000 hours of yoga—without a single case of fracture or, indeed, serious injury of any kind. Says Dr. Fishman, "My colleagues and I are amazed and encouraged to learn that yoga can help those with bone loss take charge—and significantly lower their risk for dangerous fractures."

# Chapter 7

# DIABETES BREAKTHROUGHS

## 4 Hidden Causes of Diabetes

High blood sugar (glucose) is an obvious sign of diabetes. It's worrisome because elevated blood glucose can, over time, lead to serious diabetes-related complications, such as stroke, heart disease and eye damage.

***We've long known how diabetes develops:*** Cells gradually become less responsive ("resistant") to the glucose-regulating hormone insulin...the ability of the pancreas to produce insulin flags...and glucose readings creep upward.

However, it has not been clear, until recently, why people become insulin-resistant in the first place—and what they can do to stop it. Now that's changing.

### New Thinking

The conventional wisdom is that carbohydrates—particularly foods that are high in "simple" carbs, such as soft drinks, white bread and desserts—are a main driver of insulin resistance and diabetes. *But other factors, some of which are largely hidden, are also important...*

***RISK FACTOR #1:*** **Ectopic fat.** It's clear that being overweight increases risk for diabetes. But we're learning that a specific type of fat that accumulates in the liver and muscles is especially harmful. This ectopic fat impairs the ability of insulin to metabolize glucose and can lead to insulin resistance. Certain people—including some who aren't overweight—have a genetic tendency to develop ectopic fat.

***RISK FACTOR #2:*** **Inflammation.** Persistent, low-grade inflammation—caused by air pollution, obesity, a poor diet, gum disease, etc.—causes cells to produce inflammatory molecules that increase insulin resistance.

***RISK FACTOR #3:*** **Mitochondrial dysfunction.** Mitochondria, the "batteries" that fuel the body's cells, naturally produce free radicals and other by-products. The harmful molecules are kept in check by endogenous (produced by the body) and dietary antioxidants. A shortage of either type of antioxidant can cause mitochondria to work less

George L. King, MD, a professor of medicine at Harvard Medical School. He is also research director, head of the vascular cell biology research section and chief scientific officer of Harvard's Joslin Diabetes Center, the world's largest diabetes research center and clinic, and the author, with Royce Flippin, of *The Diabetes Reset.*

efficiently, resulting in less insulin production—and more insulin resistance.

***RISK FACTOR #4:*** **Psychological stress.** A Dutch study found that people who had suffered at least one major stressful event (such as the death of a loved one or serious financial troubles, etc.) within the past five years were 1.2 times more likely to have diabetes.

Why is stress linked to diabetes? Stressed people are more likely to be overweight, eat poor diets and avoid exercise. Also, stress raises levels of cortisol, a hormone that increases insulin resistance and can cause the liver to manufacture excess glucose.

## What Can You Do?

Fortunately, the factors described earlier can be managed—and sometimes reversed—with diet, exercise and other changes. *Here's how...*

• **Double the fiber, halve the fat.** The Joslin Diabetes Center recommends an eating plan that's low in fat (15% of total calories) and high in high-fiber veggies, fruits and grains.

• **Forget what you've heard about carbs being bad.** Processed carbs (sugar, high-fructose corn syrup, etc.) are obviously a problem. But healthy complex carbohydrates (such as whole grains, veggies and legumes) are absorbed slowly...do not cause blood sugar spikes...and many are high in inflammation-fighting antioxidants.

***Best:*** An eating plan with a lot of complex carbohydrates—70% of total calories.

We've found that people who follow this diet for eight weeks show significant drops in insulin resistance...have improved blood glucose levels—and lose about 3% of their weight...and have a decrease in abdominal and overall body fat.

• **Be aware of hidden fat.** Excess body fat is one of the main causes of insulin resistance and diabetes—even when the fat isn't readily visible. People with a fatty liver, for example, are five times more likely to develop diabetes. Fat that accumulates in muscle cells might be completely invisible, but it increases inflammation levels and disrupts the action of insulin.

Fat that is visible—on the hips, buttocks and particularly around the waist—is especially troublesome. Most belly fat is visceral fat, which secretes higher levels of inflammatory chemicals than other types of fat. It also increases levels of "hidden" muscle fat. One large study found that obese men (with a BMI of 30 or higher) were seven times more likely to get diabetes than those with a BMI below 25. For obese women, the risk was 12 times higher than that for normal-weight women.

• **Boost natural antioxidants.** Millions of Americans supplement their diets with large doses of vitamin C, vitamin E and other antioxidants. But research has shown that these supplements are unlikely to improve insulin resistance/diabetes—and may be harmful because they can inhibit the action of the body's natural antioxidants.

***What helps:*** Broccoli, blueberries, green tea and other plant foods that are high in phase 2 antioxidants—beneficial plant compounds that activate a protein called Nrf2, which triggers genes that produce antioxidant molecules. People who eat a lot of plant foods have less inflammation, less mitochondrial dysfunction and less insulin resistance.

• **Get off your duff!** Exercise is great for weight loss, but that's not the only reason to do it. People who are sedentary tend to accumulate more fat deposits in muscle cells. These fats inhibit insulin's ability to transport glucose into muscle cells, and insulin-resistant muscle cells are now thought to be a leading cause of diabetes.

It doesn't take hard-core exercise to get the benefits. If you walk three miles a day (about 6,000 steps)—all at once or in five- or 10-minute increments—you'll reduce your diabetes risk by more than 25%.

• **De-stress.** Take up an enjoyable hobby...go for leisurely walks...spend time with loved ones...and try stress-reducing habits, like yoga or meditation. For severe stress (or depression), consider seeing a professional. Any form of stress relief will help manage diabetes—and reduce your risk of getting it.

## Diabetes and Dense Breasts

Women with diabetes who take insulin may have an increased risk for dense breasts—a risk factor for breast cancer.

***Small, preliminary study:*** Postmenopausal diabetic women who take insulin are about twice as likely to have dense breasts as women without diabetes. In contrast, those who do not take insulin—they control their diabetes with diet or drugs, such as *metformin*—are at decreased risk. Women who take insulin may benefit from more rigorous breast cancer screening.

Gerald Bernstein, MD, coordinator of the diabetes program at Friedman Diabetes Institute at Lenox Hill Hospital, New York City.

## Diabetes: 5 Mistakes to Avoid

Gretchen Becker, a Halifax, Vermont–based science and medical writer who was diagnosed with type 2 diabetes in 1996. She is author of *The First Year: Type 2 Diabetes.* GretchenBecker.com

One of every four American adults age 65 or older has diabetes—and many don't know it. Even so, every 19 seconds, an American is diagnosed with type 2 diabetes.

***My story:*** After I was diagnosed with type 2 diabetes 20 years ago, I vowed to help people avoid some of the missteps that are commonly made when navigating the trickier aspects of this complex disease. *Mistakes you can avoid...*

***MISTAKE #1:* Assuming that you'll have obvious symptoms.** You may be able to name a few of the classic diabetes symptoms, such as excessive thirst, frequent urination and blurred vision. But maybe you don't have any of these red flags.

Perhaps you do feel a little more tired than usual or have numbness or tingling in your hands or feet that you can't explain. These could be subtle signs that your blood glucose levels are out of whack. The symptoms that I initially dismissed were frequent bathroom breaks, increasing nearsightedness and scratches on my arms that wouldn't heal for more than a month.

Surprisingly, you could even be losing weight. Even though diabetes is commonly associated with being overweight, sometimes people drop a few pounds because they're losing water weight when they are urinating frequently and/or their metabolism is not allowing them to properly absorb calories.

***What you should know:*** If you notice any changes—even if they seem minor—write them down and be sure to discuss them at your next doctor visit.

***Important:*** If your doctor doesn't routinely test your blood glucose levels, ask him/her to do so at least every three years if you're past age 45. If you have any risk factors, such as a family history (in a parent, sibling or child) or being overweight, you may need more frequent testing...and perhaps starting at an earlier age.

***Also:*** Be sure that you're not fighting a cold or some other infection when you're tested—such illnesses can elevate blood glucose levels.

***MISTAKE #2:* Worrying only about sugar.** Lots of people assume that individuals with diabetes simply need to avoid sugar. The truth is, it's much more complicated than that. In fact, virtually everything you eat affects your blood glucose in one way or another.

Carbohydrates (which include starchy foods, such as bread, rice and potatoes, that turn into sugar when they are digested) as well as sugar itself actually have the greatest effect on your blood glucose. Fiber (both soluble fiber, the type that slows down digestion and is found in oat bran, barley, nuts, seeds and beans...and insoluble fiber, the type that adds bulk to your stool and is found in wheat bran and whole grains) also plays a role. It's soluble fiber that can be used to improve your blood glucose levels.

***What you should know:*** Food labels are confusing. Because fiber is a healthy carbohydrate, food labels in the US include it in the total carbohydrate count—for example, a product with 34 g of carbohydrates and 14 g of fiber, has an actual carbohydrate content of 20 g. In other countries, such as those in Europe, the food label would list this same product as having 20 g of carbohydrates and 14 g of fiber. Understanding such quirks in food labeling will help ensure that you're not getting more or less carbs than you think.

***MISTAKE #3:*** **Not keeping close tabs on your numbers.** If you are diagnosed with diabetes, your doctor will no doubt explain that the condition is largely a numbers game—with the prime target being your blood glucose level. Whatever advice your doctor gives you in terms of testing, take it seriously.

Especially in the first year, it's important for most people with diabetes to monitor these levels three to five times throughout the day. Don't try to cut corners. It's true that the test strips you use can be expensive if your insurance limits the number you receive, but the cost of diabetes complications is much greater. If you must economize on test strips, ask your doctor for advice on the best times to test during the day.

Frequent testing will help you understand what causes your blood glucose levels to become elevated. You can then develop strategies to keep them in the normal range—this is the single best way to prevent serious complications, such as kidney failure, diabetic neuropathy and amputation of lower limbs.

In addition to diet, there are other factors that affect blood glucose. Managing stress and increasing physical activity are also important. Aim for 30 minutes of aerobic exercise (such as brisk walking) at least five days a week, but be sure to add some weight lifting a few times a week—it also helps with blood glucose control.

***What you should know:*** Even when your blood glucose levels improve, you can't revert back to old behavior. The improvement simply means that you're doing what you need to do to control your disease and now have the flexibility to make small modifications, such as adding a few more carbs to your diet if you've lost some extra weight. Be sure to keep testing to make sure you don't overdo it. And never stop taking your diabetes medication without consulting your doctor!

***MISTAKE #4:*** **Settling for daily blood glucose testing alone.** Even though your daily blood glucose levels are the main number you need to focus on, other tests are helpful. For example, your doctor should also order (usually quarterly) a hemoglobin A1c test, which measures your average blood glucose for the past two to three months. This will tell you how well your overall diabetes treatment is working. Closely tracking your blood pressure and lipid levels (including cholesterol and triglycerides) is also important.

***What you should know:*** No matter what test you are receiving, always insist on knowing the normal range for the lab. Just asking for the result (without knowing the lab's range) can be very misleading.

***MISTAKE #5:*** **Going it alone.** Other diabetes patients can often provide crucial tips, insights and lifestyle advice that you won't hear from a physician who doesn't live with diabetes on a daily basis.

***What you should know:*** You'll save yourself time and trouble by going online for practical tips. In addition to support groups such as DLife.com and the American Diabetes Association's online community at Diabetes.org, there's an excellent resource that was founded by David Mendosa, a fellow diabetes patient—Mendosa.com/advice.htm. His site is especially useful because he reviews other websites so you can go directly to the ones that offer the best information.

# Do You Have Diabetes? What Your Skin Says...

Yellow-red bumps on your arms and legs may signal problems with blood sugar control. Known as eruptive xanthomas, these bumps can pop up anywhere on the body but are especially common on the buttocks, shoulders, arms and legs. They're caused by very high levels of triglycerides, a type of fat in the bloodstream that is common with insulin resistance, a condition that causes excess blood sugar and can result in prediabetes and diabetes. Once diabetes is treated, triglyceride levels often normalize and skin lesions resolve.

Jeffrey P. Callen, MD, a professor of medicine and chief of the division of dermatology at the University of Louisville School of Medicine in Kentucky.

# How to Fight Diabetes with Your Mind

Kyle W. Murdock, PhD, a postdoctoral research fellow in psychology at Rice University and coauthor of the study "Executive functioning and diabetes: The role of anxious arousal and inflammation," published in September 2016 in *Psychoneuroendocrinology*.

The ability to tune out distractions and negative feelings—a cognitive trait psychologists call "inhibition"—can mean less anxiety in your everyday life. And now recent research shows us that it may also protect you from developing diabetes—or help you manage diabetes if you have it.

***The good news:*** This is one psychological trait that you can change. That's right—you can fight diabetes with your mind.

## Stress and Anxiety

The recent research isn't the first to show that stress and anxiety can increase the risk of developing type 2 diabetes. But it does show precisely how it can happen...and points to effective mind-body treatments.

The key cognitive trait linked to increased diabetes risk in the recent study is low "inhibition." It's a necessary coping skill—the ability to control your attention and behavior and ignore distracting thoughts and emotions...especially negative emotions.

People with poor inhibition tend to respond impulsively and are easily distracted by anxious thoughts. They also tend to have poor coping skills, including less ability to respond to new challenges with flexible problem-solving. Poor coping, in turn, can increase anxiety, so it can be a vicious cycle.

Researchers at several American universities hypothesized that this inhibition/anxiety connection might affect diabetes risk. So they enlisted 835 midlife men and women (average age 57) who had already taken a battery of psychological tests to also take blood tests that measure inflammation (a key driver of diabetes) and blood sugar.

When individuals are stressed, anxious or depressed, inflammation goes up. The inflammation marker interleukin-6 (IL-6) is also a marker for stress—and it's linked to higher insulin levels, which can set the stage for insulin resistance and, eventually, diabetes. The blood sugar marker was hemoglobin A1c, a measure of blood sugar over the past two or three months.

***Results:*** After adjusting for other variables, people with low inhibition, compared with those with high inhibition, had more anxiety symptoms...higher levels of IL-6...higher levels of hemoglobin A1c...and greater incidence of type 2 diabetes.

People with poor inhibition are also less likely to eat healthy foods, exercise, stick with diets and get enough sleep. So tackling this psychological trait can be a key to unlocking a bounty of health benefits.

## Strengthening Inhibition

Low inhibition is a psychological trait that can have its origins in childhood, so it's not something you can change in a snap. But it can change—and the benefits for your health and your well-being are tremendous. *The first step is to check yourself for common red flags...*

- **Thinking excessively about something stressful.**
- **Restricting yourself to only certain activities because of fear or anxiety.**
- **Acting impulsively.**
- **Engaging in high-risk activities.**

What helps...

- **Mindfulness-based stress reduction therapy (MBSR).** With this therapy, you're taught to keep your attention on the present. Training teaches you to detect and reduce distracting and stressful thoughts. You can try to learn MBSR on your own—there are many books, websites and CDs that teach it. (But seeing a professional will be much better for some people, especially those who tend to need structure imposed from the outside.)
- **Cognitive behavioral therapy (CBT).** This type of talk therapy has been shown to be an effective treatment for many anxiety disorders—and it's also been shown specifically to strengthen inhibition. The goal of CBT is to learn how to change some negative thought patterns and to modify how you cope with stressful situations. By reducing stress and your body's response to it, you can more easily avoid behaviors (such as impulsive eating) that increase your risk for diabetes.

Anything you can do to reduce your overall stress levels may reduce your risk for diabetes, too. For example, the ancient Chinese mind-body practice of Qigong, which gently exercises the body as it calms the mind, has been shown to reduce stress and reduce blood sugar. The key is to look for a stress fighter that feels right to you!

## Common Virus May Be Linked to Diabetes and Heart Disease in Some Women

University of California, San Francisco, news release.

A common virus may make some women more susceptible to both type 2 diabetes and heart disease, a recent study suggests.

Scientists at the University of California, San Francisco found normal-weight women under age 50 who were infected with cytomegalovirus (CMV) were more likely to have metabolic syndrome than their peers.

Metabolic syndrome is a collection of risk factors for heart disease and diabetes that includes excess belly fat, unhealthy cholesterol levels, high blood pressure and high blood sugar levels.

CMV, a herpes virus, is believed to infect roughly half of the US population over the age of 40. Typically there are no symptoms unless the person's immune system is weakened.

Ironically, obese women infected with CMV were less likely to have metabolic syndrome than obese women not infected with the virus, the researchers found. However, obese women were still far more likely to have metabolic syndrome than their normal-weight peers.

"The likelihood that women infected with CMV will have metabolic syndrome varies dramatically, depending on the presence, absence and severity of obesity," study first author Shannon Fleck-Derderian said in a university news release. She's with UCSF's department of pediatrics.

Research has suggested that metabolic syndrome may be triggered by long-acting, low-intensity inflammation. The study authors pointed out that CMV infection has been linked with other inflammatory conditions, such as inflammatory bowel disease and blood vessel diseases.

## Study Details

For the study, the researchers examined data on more than 2,500 individuals nationwide between the ages of 20 and 49, from 1999 to 2004. Associations were compared between CMV and signs of metabolic syndrome in participants divided into one of four categories—normal weight, overweight, obese and extremely obese.

After taking into account other contributing factors such as age, ethnicity and poverty, the researchers found that nearly 5% of normal-weight women infected with CMV had at least three risk factors for metabolic syndrome. But, the same was true for less than 1% of normal-weight women who were not infected.

More than 27% of women infected with CMV also had lower levels of HDL "good" cholesterol, compared with 19% of the normal-weight women who didn't have the virus.

Curiously, 56% of the extremely obese women infected with CMV had three or more risk factors associated with metabolic syndrome. This compared with almost 83% of the extremely obese women who didn't have the virus.

These very obese CMV-infected women also had higher levels of "good" HDL cholesterol and lower levels of triglycerides, a type of blood fat that increases the risk for heart disease.

The researchers concluded that CMV might protect very obese women from metabolic syndrome.

No such association was seen among the men in the study.

Study senior author Janet Wojcicki is an associate professor of pediatrics and epidemiology at UCSF. "Women who have extreme obesity may be metabolically different from others, and CMV infection might confer some kind of protection for them against the harmful effects we generally associate with excess body fat," she said.

More research is needed to understand these associations, the researchers said. And the study did not prove a cause-and-effect link.

The findings were published in the journal *Obesity*.

The U.S. Centers for Disease Control and Prevention has more on CMV infection at CDC.gov/cmv/.

# Check Your Neck

Neck size is a better measure of disease risk than waist size—which can be influenced by time of day, clothing and other factors. In a study of 1,206 people, those with higher-than-average neck circumference had a higher incidence of prediabetes, hypertension and metabolic syndrome. The average neck size of study participants was 14.2 inches for women and 16.5 inches for men.

Study by researchers at University of Puerto Rico, Medical Sciences Campus, San Juan, published in *Journal of Diabetes Research.*

# Diabetes Drug May Help the Heart

The injectable blood sugar–lowering drug *liraglutide* (Victoza) can reduce heart attack and stroke risk in people with type 2 diabetes. Heart disease is the leading cause of death in people with type 2 diabetes. People who took Victoza, one of a newer class of diabetes drugs known as GLP-1 agonists, had 13% lower risk for heart attack and stroke than those who took a placebo...22% lower risk for death from heart disease...and 15% lower risk for death from any cause.

Study of 9,340 adults with type 2 diabetes and at high risk for heart disease by researchers at University of North Carolina, Chapel Hill, published in *The New England Journal of Medicine.*

# Pregnancy-Linked Diabetes Poses Risks for Mom, Baby

Sophie Jacqueminet, MD, Pitie-Salpetriere Hospital, Paris.

Robert Courgi, MD, endocrinologist, Northwell Health's Southside Hospital, Bay Shore, New York.

Gerald Bernstein, MD, endocrinologist and coordinator, Friedman Diabetes Program, Lenox Hill Hospital, New York City.

*Dibatetologia*, news release.

Diabetes that develops during pregnancy—known as gestational diabetes—carries health risks for both the mom-to-be and her baby, recent research confirms.

## Research Details

A team of French researchers analyzed data from more than 700,000 births in France occurring after 28 weeks of pregnancy in 2012.

Compared with other pregnant women, those with gestational diabetes were 30% more likely to experience preterm birth, 40% more likely to require a C-section and 70% more likely to have preeclampsia/eclampsia, a dangerous spike in blood pressure.

Risks weren't confined to the mother, however. Babies born to women with gestational diabetes were 80% more likely to be of significantly larger-than-average size at birth; 10% more likely to suffer respiratory issues; 30% more likely to experience a traumatic birth; and 30% more likely to have heart defects, the study found.

Babies born after 37 weeks to women with gestational diabetes also had an increased risk of death, compared with babies born to women without the condition, the study authors said.

The study clearly shows that gestational diabetes "is a disease related to adverse pregnancy outcomes," concluded a team led by Sophie Jacqueminet, MD, of the Pitie-Salpetriere Hospital in Paris.

The study also found that the risk of death was 30% higher among babies born to women whose gestational diabetes was treated with a special diet. There was no increased risk of death among babies born to women whose gestational diabetes was treated with insulin, however.

This difference in death risk could be because women with diet-treated gestational diabetes tend to give birth later than those who are insulin-treated, the research team said.

Outcomes were worse for mothers with gestational diabetes "who gave birth later because the baby was exposed to higher blood sugar levels for a longer period of time," explained Robert Courgi, MD, an endocrinologist at Northwell Health's Southside Hospital, in Bay Shore, New York.

## Expert Comment

Two experts in diabetes care weren't surprised by the findings, and they noted that while a woman's weight isn't always a factor, the odds for gestational diabetes go up in the obese.

"Gestational diabetes is a dangerous entity, and the child is at risk," said Dr. Courgi.

"As obesity increases, so does [the risk of] diabetes," he added. "We need to do a better job at diagnosing and treating gestational diabetes."

Gerald Bernstein, MD, coordinates the diabetes program at Lenox Hill Hospital in New York City. He stressed that gestational diabetes requires prompt and proper treatment.

"Once diagnosed, treatment is geared to maintain normal blood sugar but without the risk of hypoglycemia [low blood sugar]," Dr. Bernstein explained. "This may range from nutritional and other lifestyle changes to the addition of insulin. The goal is to give the baby a maximum opportunity for growth and development without an unusual early delivery, so that key organs are as mature as possible.

"Most patients are followed by an endocrinologist, a high-risk ob-gyn and diabetes educators in various disciplines," Dr. Bernstein added. "To reduce birth complications, early diagnosis along with aggressive therapy with a full health-care team is essential."

## Gestational Diabetes a Risk Factor for Postpartum Depression

Icahn School of Medicine at Mount Sinai, news release.

Gestational diabetes and a previous bout of depression can increase a first-time mother's risk of postpartum depression, a recent study suggests.

The analysis of data from more than 700,000 women in Sweden showed that gestational diabetes (developing diabetes during pregnancy) alone raised the risk for postpartum depression.

However, that risk rose even more if a woman had previously been diagnosed with depression.

"Most practitioners think of these as two isolated and very different conditions, but we now understand gestational diabetes and postpartum depression should be considered together," said study lead author Michael Silverman, PhD. He's an assistant professor of psychiatry at the Icahn School of Medicine at Mount Sinai in New York City.

"While having diabetes increases [postpartum depression] risk for all women, for those women who have had a past depressive episode, having diabetes during pregnancy makes it 70% more likely that they will develop [postpartum depression]," Dr. Silverman said in a school news release.

The researchers said they also identified other risk factors for postpartum depression.

Among women with a history of depression, diabetes before pregnancy and giving birth prematurely at 32 to 36 weeks (full-term delivery is 39 to 40 weeks) increased the risk, the researchers said.

Also, among women with no history of depression, giving birth at a young age, having an instrument-assisted or cesarean delivery, and giving birth before 32 weeks increased the risk.

The study was published online in the journal *Depression and Anxiety*.

"The reason a doctor asks if you smoke is because they know you are 20 times more likely to get cancer if you do. We believe ob-gyns should now do the same for depression history," Dr. Silverman said. "With this information, we can now intervene early, before the mother gives birth."

## Menopause Can Raise Diabetes Risk

Early—or late—menopause can raise diabetes risk, we hear from Erin LeBlanc, MD, MPH. The average age of menopause is 51, but a recent study found that women who had their last period before age 46 were 25% more likely to develop diabetes. Women who had their last period after age 55 were 12% more likely to develop diabetes.

***If you've had an early or late menopause:*** Ask your doctor whether you should be tested for diabetes.

Erin LeBlanc, MD, MPH, investigator, Kaiser Permanente Center for Health Research, Portland, Oregon.

## Better Time to Walk

Walking for 10 minutes after breakfast, lunch and dinner lowered post-meal blood sugar in people with diabetes about 12% more than taking a half-hour walk at any other time of day.

***Especially helpful:*** A 10-minute walk after dinner, which tends to be the meal with the most carbs, had the biggest impact on blood sugar.

***Theory:*** Blood sugar is needed to fuel muscles during exercise, so walking has the most impact when done after meals, when blood sugar levels are highest.

Andrew Reynolds, PhD, researcher, department of human nutrition, University of Otago, Dunedin, New Zealand.

# Lessons from Diabetes Boot Camp

Michelle Magee, MD, endocrinologist, director, MedStar Diabetes Institute, associate professor of medicine, Georgetown University School of Medicine, both in Washington, DC. Her study, titled "Diabetes Boot Camp Reduces A1c and Health-Care Services Utilization," was presented at the 2016 annual meeting of the American Diabetes Association in New Orleans.

The name makes you think of raw recruits sweating it out on an Army base. "Diabetes Boot Camp" takcs the same mental commitment but is a good bit simpler, kinder and easier than that.

The intensive 12-week professionally monitored program for people with hard-to-manage diabetes is also remarkably effective at helping people with type 2 diabetes bring their blood sugar under control, according to a recent study.

***Even better:*** Even if you're not in a boot camp, you can reproduce its essential elements yourself with a little help from your health-care team. To find out more, we spoke with study leader Michelle Magee, MD, director of the MedStar Diabetes Institute and an associate professor of medicine at Georgetown University School of Medicine in Washington, DC. She didn't invent the diabetes boot camp concept, but she is one of the first to study it.

## When Diabetes Is Out of Control

If you have diabetes, your body responds quickly to what you eat, how active you are and the medications you take. But even if you are checking your finger-stick blood sugars, if you see your doctor only every few months to review your results, it's hard to understand exactly how your daily actions can make a difference.

It is also complicated to live with diabetes if you haven't learned enough to balance all of what you need to know about it. There's a lot to learn about nutrition, not to mention exercise, psychology and medicine. You might have areas of ignorance holding you back.

No wonder millions of Americans have trouble controlling their diabetes. They show up on an urgent basis at their doctor's office. They miss days of work. They get hospitalized or go to the emergency room with episodes of too high or too low blood sugar.

In search of a better way, five primary care practices in and around Washington, DC, enrolled 125 people with hard-to-control diabetes in boot camp. Everyone had had diabetes for at least a year, was taking glucose-lowering medication or insulin, and was asked to regularly monitor their blood sugar.

They all had A1c levels—a measure of average blood sugar over the past two or three months—above 9% and at least one other health concern, such as high blood pressure. (The average A1c level for these patients was even higher—11.4%.) A target A1c for someone with diabetes is usually around 7%, and people with an A1c of 9% or higher are considered to have uncontrolled diabetes.

The great thing is that those out-of-control numbers went down dramatically.

## Boot Camp Curriculum

Here's the program…

In the first week, each participant met twice with a certified diabetes educator (CDE)—a health-care professional who is specially trained to teach people how to manage diabetes. They took a survey to identify knowledge gaps about diabetes—and then were given video clips that addressed the specific diabetes-related information that they didn't know. They were also surveyed on medication adherence and then given tailored support so that they could take their medications as prescribed. Both diet and medications—as well as exercise and other issues—were covered in the two sessions.

That's it for the face-to-face interactions—just two visits. But each participant was also given a "cellular-enabled" blood glucose monitor. As soon as each patient completed a normal finger-stick blood glucose test, the results were displayed in real-time on a "dashboard" visible to their diabetes educator.

Next, participants graduated to "virtual visits," with phone calls, e-mail or text messages instead of face-to-face meetings. Over the course of the next 12 weeks, most patients had eight to 10 interactions with their diabetes educator. "Educators were able to adjust their patients' medications frequently via the virtual visits to help them get to their goal for blood glucose control and to continue to deliver critical 'survival skills' information about lifestyle management," said Dr. Magee.

One of the main benefits was immediate feedback to tie actions taken by the patient to blood glucose results. Say a participant had a big dessert and did a finger-stick test, and the blood glucose dashboard showed a higher-than-desired reading. This would signal a teaching point—the diabetes educator who was monitoring that patient could call or text the patient right away. "Normally, patients wait months in between primary care visits, when their doctors discuss blood sugar levels," says Dr. Magee. "But this almost-immediate response led to a lot of 'eureka moments,' when patients can markedly increase their understanding of how their lifestyle impacts their blood sugar."

## Big Benefits

The results were astounding. Within three months, the average A1c levels declined from 11.4% to 8.3%. "Each 1% reduction in A1C is associated with a roughly 15% decline in risk for major cardiovascular events," explains Dr. Magee. *Within six months, when compared with prior use of health-care services by the same participants...*

- **Urgent visits to primary care practices dropped by 92%.**
- **Missed days of work or other activities declined by 77%.**
- **Hospitalization declined by 66%.**

The study is being prepared for publication, so its results are still preliminary—and we don't yet know how well the participants maintained their A1c levels after the intervention ended. But the results do show just how effective personalized education and counseling combined with timely medication management can be in helping people who are floundering on their own with this complex disease.

## Bringing It All Back Home

While this boot camp program is being further developed, almost anyone with diabetes can incorporate its lessons and take steps to help improve their diabetes-care outcomes by working with their own doctor and a certified diabetes educator. *Here's how...*

- **Ask your primary care doctor to refer you to a certified diabetes educator (CDE).** Many large health-care systems and hospitals have them on staff, but you can also find a certified one online at the National Certification Board for Diabetes Education. Most insurance plans pay for this service with a referral from your doctor.
- **Once you meet with your diabetes educator,** ask him/her if he can work with you if you use a glucose monitor that can relay data wirelessly so that you can look at your sugars together more often. These meters are relatively recent, but new ones are coming on the market now. This will allow you to work with your new "coach" more easily.
- **Your provider or educator may recommend that you also try a smartphone diabetes-coaching app program**—these often-free programs provide nutrition info and help you track your carbs and blood sugar—to help you manage your diabetes. "There is emerging evidence that these apps can help with diabetes control, too, and some people do find them helpful," says Dr. Douglas, "but an app is no substitute for working closely with your doctor and your CDE."
- **If you have worked with the CDE on your lifestyle management** and your sugars still are not where they should be, you also need to work with your own doctor so that your diabetes medications can be adjusted to help get you to your targets for blood glucose control.

• **"The more you know, the better you do" may never be more true than it is for people with diabetes.** Get educated.

Working with a diabetes educator isn't new, of course—the profession has been around for decades. But here's what's changing—now that your blood sugar numbers can be transmitted immediately, you, your educator and your doctor can become a much more powerful team. This Diabetes Boot Camp has shown that just a few face-to-face meetings with a handful of "virtual visits" can get you on the right track and keep you on the right track—managing diabetes much better than you have ever been able to do.

## Bike Away Diabetes

The more you pedal a bicycle, the less likely you are to develop diabetes, according to a recent study of more than 52,000 adults over age 50. Those who cycled more than two-and-a-half hours a week had a 20% lower risk for diabetes than those who didn't cycle at all.

***Tip:*** Ride a bike whenever possible and/or use a stationary bike.

Martin Rasmussen, MSc, research assistant, department of sports science and clinical biomechanics, University of Southern Denmark, Odense.

## Inhaled Insulin Is a Bust

The French drugmaker Sanofi recently canceled its agreement to sell Afrezza in the US due to poor sales. Afrezza was launched in the US in February 2015, but many doctors were put off by the need for spirometry testing before prescribing the drug, and others were concerned about the long-term side effects of inhaled insulin, such as breathing problems in those with chronic obstructive pulmonary disease (COPD) and other lung conditions. The drug was also higher-priced than injectable insulin.

Osama Hamdy, MD, PhD, director, inpatient diabetes program, Joslin Diabetes Center, Boston.

## Insulin and Breast Cancer Risk

Insulin users may be at more risk for breast cancer, reports Zorana Andersen, PhD.

***Recent finding:*** Diabetic women who take insulin are twice as likely to have dense breasts as women without diabetes. Diabetic women who do not take insulin—they control their condition with diet or other drugs, such as *metformin*—are about 60% less likely to have dense breasts.

***Bottom line:*** Women who take insulin may benefit from more rigorous breast-cancer screening.

Zorana Andersen, PhD, associate professor of epidemiology at University of Copenhagen, Denmark.

## Drink Water!

Water beats diet beverages for weight loss. Overweight women with type 2 diabetes who were placed on a supervised weight-control diet and who drank water five times a week after their main meal at lunch lost an average of 14 pounds in 24 weeks. Those who drank diet beverages lost an average of 11.5 pounds. Body mass index fell by 2.49 in the water drinkers, compared with 2.06 in those using diet drinks. Water drinkers also had greater improvements in fasting insulin, postmeal glucose levels and other measures of diabetes severity.

Study of 81 women led by researchers at University of Nottingham, UK, published in *Diabetes, Obesity and Metabolism.*

## Psoriasis-Diabetes Link

If you have psoriasis, you are at increased risk for diabetes and vice versa, warns Ann Sophie Lønnberg, MD.

### Breakthrough Device Now Available for Type I

FDA approves breakthrough device for type I diabetes, says Robert A. Gabbay, MD, PhD. Medtronic MiniMed 670G monitors blood sugar in people with type I diabetes and automatically delivers insulin as needed. Patients still have to count and enter carbs to teach the device how much insulin they need for their intake. Also, the insulin delivery site dressings have to be replaced every three days, so patients must be capable of doing that.

Robert A. Gabbay, MD, PhD, chief medical officer at Joslin Diabetes Center and associate professor of medicine at Harvard Medical School, both in Boston.

***Recent finding:*** People with the chronic skin condition are 53% more likely to have type 2 diabetes than other people.

***Probable connections:*** Both diseases involve inflammation and have dietary and lifestyle factors in common.

***To decrease risk for both:*** Keep your weight and blood sugar under control. If you have psoriasis, ask your physician to screen you for diabetes.

Ann Sophie Lønnberg, MD, a psoriasis researcher at Gentofte Hospital, University of Copenhagen, Hellerup, Denmark.

# Do Eggs Promote Diabetes? Only in America

Katherine Zeratsky, RD, LD, a registered dietician and nutrition educator at the Mayo Clinic, Rochester, Minnesota.

Eggs are funny. If you eat eggs in the US, they increase your risk for diabetes. But if you eat them in Spain or France or Japan, you're fine. No increased diabetes risk. Buen provecho! Bon appetit! Itadakimasu!

So, does living in America somehow make eggs dangerous? Of course that's ridiculous. Here's the real story.

## A Scrambled Tale

Eggs, once beloved by all, then shunned because they're high in cholesterol, now are back in nutritionists'—and home cooks'—good graces. After all, dietary cholesterol is no longer a "nutrient of concern" according to the latest Dietary Guidelines.

The only potential spoiler has been diabetes risk. Truth be told, the research has been totally confusing. While a few studies have suggested that dietary cholesterol might increase the risk for diabetes, others show that eating eggs actually improves sensitivity to insulin, which protects against diabetes.

To shed light on the issue, researchers looked at 12 studies from the US, Europe and Japan (nearly 220,000 people).

Taken as a whole, the studies showed no increase in risk for people who ate more eggs compared with those who ate fewer or none.

But when the researchers looked just at the US studies, they found that people who ate three eggs or more a week were 39% more likely to develop diabetes than people who ate fewer eggs or none. Even here, it was dicey—some American studies found no such link.

Some non-US studies even found that eggs were protective. In one Finnish study, for example, men aged 42 to 60 who ate the most eggs on a weekly basis over 19 years were 38% less likely to develop diabetes. A Japanese study also found less diabetes in egg eaters, but only in women.

To put these findings in perspective, we spoke with Katherine Zeratsky, RD, LD, a registered dietician and nutrition educator at the Mayo Clinic in Rochester, Minnesota.

## Cracking the Egg Mystery

First, let's acknowledge that these are primarily observational studies that can't prove cause and effect, explained Zeratsky. *But the studies do hold key clues...*

• **Who's eating lots of eggs?** In the US, people who eat the most eggs tend to also be less physically active, eat more meat and smoke. Egg consumers tend to have a higher body mass index (BMI) than those who don't eat eggs, too. These findings aren't observed outside our borders.

• **What else are they eating?** In the US, people who eat the most eggs tend to also eat more processed meat, such as sausage and bacon.

Since avoiding eggs, especially egg yolks, had long been a health recommendation in the US, it's not surprising that healthier people have been eating fewer eggs—or that people with less healthy lifestyles eat more eggs. That may change now that healthier people are likely to be eating more eggs. We also tend to serve our eggs with bacon, sausage, home fries and lots of toast with butter, not to mention orange juice, which is high in sugar and low in fiber—not the healthiest breakfast pattern.

## A Healthier Way to Eat Eggs

A single large egg has only 78 calories, a substantial 6 or 7 grams of protein (more than 10% of the Daily Value) and good amounts of iron and zinc, B-12, B-6 and choline, an amino acid key for brain health.

***Another egg bonus:*** They're satiating. In one weight-loss study of people who already had diabetes, those who ate two eggs a day, six days a week, reported feeling less hungry than those who took in the same number of calories but only two eggs a week. Nor was there any difference in blood cholesterol levels between the two groups.

"In the context of an overall healthy diet, eggs are a great, economical source of protein," says Zeratsky. However, she cautions, eggs do contain a moderate amount of saturated fat, which can increase blood cholesterol levels, so moderation is still the best guide. Her recommendation? "Eating up to one egg a day is reasonable." That jibes with earlier research that eating an average of one egg a day has no effect on risk for heart disease or stroke. Like a two-egg omelet? That's fine to have three times a week or so. No need to avoid yolks.

Just make the rest of your plate healthy, too. A poached egg or two, with some fruit on the side, is a lovely breakfast, suggests Zeratksy. So is a scramble with red peppers and kale, which add their own nutrients. For lunch, a sliced hard-boiled egg adds protein to any salad—and helps you absorb more vitamins from the greens. When making dinner, try sliding a sunny-side-up egg on top of, say, sautéed chopped Brussels sprouts, for a little extra nutritional punch.

***Bottom line:*** Eggs are once again what they've always been—a versatile, inexpensive, good-tasting, nutritious, low-cal, high-protein staple. For everyone.

# Got Diabetes? Don't Let Exercise Mess with Your Blood Sugar

Richard Cotton, MA, ACSM-CEP, exercise physiologist and national director of certification, American College of Sports Medicine, Indianapolis.

If you've been diagnosed with type 2 diabetes, you know that exercise is key for long-term blood sugar control. But it also can affect your blood sugar levels in the short term—and not always in good ways. Exercise too enthusiastically, and you could find your blood sugar level dropping too low—or even spiking.

Here's how people with type 2 diabetes can handle (and even better, avoid) the two most common exercise/blood sugar problems...

## Problem #1: Blood Sugar Drops During Exercise

When you exercise, your body gets energy first by using blood sugar (glucose) and then by depleting glycogen, the storage form of glucose, from your muscles and liver. (You may also start burning fat for energy.)

The short-term effect is that blood sugar levels fall—and can stay reduced for as long as 24 hours. That's the benefit. But if levels fall too low (hypoglycemia)—below 70 mg/dL if your meter measures whole blood, or below 80 mg/dL if it measures plasma glucose—you may feel symptoms, including shakiness, clammy skin, blurred vision and confusion. A severe drop can be scary or even dangerous.

The good news is that it's rare—and easily prevented. Exercise-induced hypoglycemia is most common in people who take insulin—that is, everyone with type 1 diabetes and some people with type 2. It can also happen if you are taking certain medications that promote insulin secretion, including sulfonylureas and glinides. If low blood sugar during or after exercise happens to you regularly, talk to your doctor about possible solutions such as eating a small snack before (and maybe during) exercise, adjusting your medication dose—or both.

Fortunately, exercise-induced hypoglycemia is quite rare in people who manage their diabetes with lifestyle alone or with a medication such as *metformin*, which instead of promoting insulin secretion makes your body more sensitive to the insulin it already makes. Still, it's possible for a mild drop in blood sugar to happen, especially if you train really hard or for more than an hour. Even a mild blood sugar drop might make you feel tired afterward.

The best advice for everyone with diabetes, especially at the beginning of a new exercise program, is to test your blood sugar three times—before, during and after your workout. Once you get a sense of how your exercise routine is affecting your blood sugar, you can cut back on the testing. Just make sure that you have access to a quick energy source such as an energy bar or fruit juice in case your blood sugar drops.

***Tip:*** To reduce your risk for hypoglycemia, do resistance exercise before aerobic exercise.

## Problem #2: Blood Sugar Is Too High Before or During Exercise

Sometimes, blood sugar levels get too high—250 mg/dL or 300 mg/dL or even higher—which can cause you to feel symptoms such as thirst, headache, blurred vision and fatigue. It's called hyperglycemia. It's an indication that you need to adjust your eating pattern, your medications or both so that you can bring blood sugar to more acceptable levels, such as the mid-100s.

Is it safe to exercise if your blood sugar is already somewhat elevated? The answer is yes as long as you're feeling good. Exercise can bring high blood sugar levels down quickly. Indeed, with exercise your muscles can burn up glucose at almost 20 times their normal rate. That's a key reason that regular exercise is so effective in controlling diabetes. Exercising, even a nice brisk walk, is one good way to bring levels down. Make sure you're staying well-hydrated, too, since high blood sugar can lead to frequent urination and thus dehydration.

***Exception:*** Sometimes, if you start exercising when your blood sugar is already running high, rising adrenalin or other exercise-stimulated hormones can stimulate your body to release even more sugar into the blood—temporarily overwhelming the sugar-burning effect of exercise. If that hap-

### Be Sure to Get Your Flu Shot

Flu shots may prevent stroke and heart failure in people with type 2 diabetes. Diabetics who received the flu vaccine had a 30% lower risk for stroke, 22% reduced risk for heart failure and 24% lower risk for death from all causes than those who did not get flu shots. The flu is known to be particularly dangerous for people with diabetes.

Study of more than 124,000 people with type 2 diabetes led by researchers at Imperial College London, UK, published in *CMAJ* (*Canadian Medical Association Journal*).

pens, don't sweat it. Just cool down as you would any time you exercise aerobically and then sit quietly to allow your body to rest. After 30 minutes, when you test your blood sugar again, you should find that your blood sugar has gone down to more normal levels. In some cases, it might take an hour.

## Tailoring Your Exercise Program to Your Blood Sugar Pattern

The good news is that for most people with diabetes, exercise won't cause any short-term blood sugar problems—and it's one of the best things you can do to control your diabetes.

Check with your doctor before starting a new routine to see if you have any exercise limitations. If you're planning exercise more intense than walking and you have certain risk factors or conditions (such as high blood pressure, high cholesterol, heart disease, kidney problems), your doctor may also recommend that you undergo exercise stress testing, which involves walking fast on a treadmill while your heart is monitored. But most people with diabetes don't need this test.

If you have health issues such as foot problems, eyesight issues, arthritis or other limitations, your doctor can help you tailor an exercise plan that works for you or can refer you to a diabetes educator or an exercise physiologist who can help. It's a good thing that exercise is so safe, because it's so beneficial for people with diabetes.

# Chapter 8

# FIGHT INFLUENZA, PNEUMONIA AND OTHER INFECTIOUS DISEASES

## The Germ Hot Spots You've Never Thought About

Whether it's Zika virus, Ebola or MERS (Middle East Respiratory Syndrome), there is a long list of infectious diseases that get our attention when they dominate the news. Even though these are frightening illnesses, this intense level of scrutiny of exotic diseases minimizes the real threat.

The microbes that pose the biggest threat—in terms of annual sickness rates and death—are the potentially fatal ones that we are exposed to every day, such as influenza and hospital-acquired infections known as superbugs.

***Why it matters to me:*** My research on the transmission of infectious disease is fueled, in part, by personal tragedy. Following heart bypass surgery at a highly regarded American hospital, my mother died after contracting a type of virulent hospital-acquired bacterial infection. Hospital-acquired infections kill about 75,000 patients in the US each year. But hospitals aren't the only place where pathogens hang out.

Most people think that they have a good idea where these germs reside. Doorknobs, elevator buttons and handrails in public places are among the best-known hot spots. But hardly anyone thinks about the numerous other places that harbor pesky pathogens.

What you need to know...

### Hidden Germs

Effective handwashing removes the germs that can make you sick. But sometimes we fail to recognize hidden sources of microbial contamination, which so often do not get cleaned properly (or at all).

Many of the germs we encounter are not harmful, and a healthy immune system can often handle most of the rest. In fact, some exposure to germs helps strengthen the immune system. However, with the smart hygiene practices described below, you will greatly reduce the odds of putting yourself, your colleagues and your loved ones at risk for a variety of illnesses, ranging from the

Miryam Z. Wahrman, PhD, professor of biology at William Paterson University in Wayne, New Jersey, where she specializes in microbiology, hand hygiene and the interactions between bacteria and environmental surfaces. Dr. Wahrman also is author of *The Hand Book: Surviving in a Germ-Filled World.*

common cold to the flu and pneumonia. *Germ hot spots that will surprise you...*

• **Neckties.** Some doctors have stopped wearing ties in order to protect their patients. A study at a New York hospital found that nearly half of the ties tested were contaminated with Staph, K. pneumoniae and other disease-causing organisms.

I advise all men (not just doctors) to keep in mind that ties pick up and transmit germs, since they are rarely cleaned, dangle and sweep across surfaces, and are handled frequently. Men who are not working in health-care settings are less likely to pick up drug-resistant superbugs on their ties, but risks still abound, so it's a good idea to clean your ties now and then.

***My advice:*** Buy ties made from microfiber—these textiles tend to resist bacterial contamination more than silk, cotton or polyester. Some ties made of cotton, linen, polyester and/or microfiber can be hand-washed with detergent, air-dried and ironed, but silk and wool usually must be dry-cleaned, which isn't foolproof in killing germs.

***Note to women:*** Handbags have been found to harbor deadly germs, but a sanitizing alcohol wipe can be used to clean straps and the exterior of bags. Vinyl may be easier to clean than cloth or other material.

• **Cell phones.** Have you ever washed your smartphone? It is certainly not recommended to immerse any cell phone in water, but most people don't even wipe off the surface of their phones.

***Important finding:*** A 2011 British study reported that 92% of cell phones had bacteria, with 16% carrying E. coli, bacteria typically found in feces.

***My advice:*** Clean your phone every day by wiping it down with a microfiber cloth (the kind used to clean eyeglasses) that's been moistened with 70% ethyl or isopropyl alcohol (commonly found in drugstores). Or try other products, such as Wireless Wipes, that are made specifically for cell phones.

***Another option:*** An ultraviolet (UV) cellphone sanitizer, such as PhoneSoap Charger or Cellblaster, which uses exposure to UV radiation to kill most bacteria. These products are available online for about $50 to $110.

• **Rings and other jewelry.** Whether you're wearing a plain band or a ring with elaborate settings, bacteria can thrive underneath it—an area that's usually missed by handwashing.

***My advice:*** When possible, remove rings before washing your hands. You should also clean your jewelry, including wristwatches. To avoid water damage, swab the surfaces with 70% ethyl alcohol or use a UV sanitizer device (described earlier).

• **Paper money.** On average, paper currency stays in circulation for about six years. During that time, it comes in contact with wallets, purses, sweaty palms and filthy fingertips. When we tested dollar bills that we collected as change from New York food vendors, we found that about two-thirds were contaminated with different strains of bacteria...and two-thirds of those harbored coliform (fecal) bacteria.

If you use credit cards, you can largely avoid touching money, although sometimes you must hand your credit card to the cashier, which exposes it to someone else's germs. You also have to touch the scanner and stylus, which have been touched by many customers.

***My advice:*** Try to cleanse your hands after handling money, especially before you eat or touch your eyes, nose or mouth. And do not lick your fingers when counting out bills. Coins aren't germ-free, but the metal alloys in the coins tend to inhibit bacterial growth. So it's mainly paper currency that you have to worry about.

• **Airports.** People who travel a lot encounter germs from other travelers. In airplanes, the tray tables, armrests and seat-back pockets can be teeming with pathogens. But there are other hot spots as well.

***My advice:*** At the airport, for example, it's a good idea to put your cell phone, keys and other personal possessions in a Ziploc bag before putting them in a security bin, which has held innumerable shoes, phones...and who knows what.

• **Rental cars.** Even though most rental car agencies vacuum and quickly wipe down surfaces between rentals, studies show the steering wheel may harbor nasty bacteria. Who knows where the previous drivers' hands have been?

***My advice:*** When you rent a car, consider wiping down the steering wheel and door handles with sanitizing alcohol wipes.

# Herbs That Boost Your Immunity

Kathy Abascal, RH, a registered herbalist who practices in Vashon, Washington. A member of the American Herbalists Guild, she is coauthor of *Clinical Botanical Medicine.*

Within the last century, three influenza pandemics—in 1918, 1957 and 1968—killed millions of people worldwide. Medical science has changed dramatically since the outbreaks, but a little-known yet highly effective approach to treating the flu of 1918 may prevent people from contracting the illness during a future outbreak—or help aid in recovery if they do become sick.

## New Lessons from Old Research

In 1918 and 1919, a strain of influenza dubbed "the Spanish flu" (in part because it received the most press coverage in Spain, which was not preoccupied with World War I) circled the globe and resulted in not just one, but two (and in some places three) waves of deadly illness. The Spanish flu and its associated complications, including pneumonia and pleurisy (inflammation of the covering of the lungs), killed as many as 50 million people worldwide.

Some people received what were then believed to be the most progressive and scientific conventional treatments available—mercury, strong laxatives, aspirin, arsenic, quinine and a mixture of ipecac and opium called Dover's powder. According to the Centers for Disease Control and Prevention, more than 2.5%, or 25 out of every 1,000 people treated conventionally, died.

Surveys from the period show that patients given herbal remedies used by a nationwide group of physicians who called themselves the "Eclectics"—because they practiced "eclectic" medicine (what we today might call herbal or alternative medicine)—died at a rate of 0.6%, meaning that six out of every 1,000 who received these botanical treatments died.

Who documented this huge disparity? At the onset of the Spanish flu outbreak, John Lloyd was a respected pharmacist, plant extract researcher, past president of the American Pharmaceutical Association, and owner, with his brothers, of Lloyd Brothers, a Cincinnati, Ohio–based distributor of pharmaceutical botanicals.

In 1919—when the Spanish flu pandemic was on the wane—Lloyd conducted a survey of 222 physicians who had purchased his company's herbal products, asking which ones they had used to treat influenza and pneumonia, how the products were administered and which of the treatments they considered to be the most effective.

Respondents listed more than 40 botanical treatments, including gelsemium (the dried root and rhizome of the yellow jasmine plant native to the Southeastern US), echinacea (purple coneflowers that are native to Midwestern North America), aconite (a bluish flowered herb of the buttercup family) and boneset (a white-flowered plant native to Eastern North America).

Most of the Eclectics practiced "specific medication," treating the flu by addressing each individual patient's specific symptoms—respiratory illness, fever, coughs, vomiting, fatigue, etc. This approach differed from that of conventional doctors, who treated every influenza patient basically the same with purgatives, quinine, aspirin and Dover's powder, regardless of the individual's symptoms.

## Increase Your Immunity

A number of herbal medicines can be used to strengthen the immune system.

The herbs listed below are generally safe and are widely available at health-food stores.* Good manufacturers that offer these herbs include Herbalist & Alchemist (Herb alist-Alchemist.com) and HerbPharm (Herb-Pharm.com).

Adaptogens are herbs used to balance the immune system. They work slowly, so they should be started six to eight weeks before the flu season (typically November to April) and continued throughout that period. Also, adaptogens can be used as needed for general immunity strengthening to help fight colds and other respiratory ailments.

Take one of the following...

• **Ginseng.** Chinese or Asian ginseng (*Panax ginseng*) and American ginseng (*Panax quinquefolium*) have been used for centuries to fight fatigue and increase immunity. Siberian ginseng, or eleuthero (*Eleutherococcus senticosus*), has similar properties but is not a member of the ginseng family.

***Immune-boosting dosage:*** *Chinese or Asian ginseng*: 5 ml to 10 ml of tincture daily ...*American ginseng*: 3 ml to 5 ml of tincture three times daily...*Siberian ginseng*: 3 ml of tincture three times daily.

• **Ashwagandha** (*Withania somnifera*). Ashwagandha has been used for more than 4,000 years in India to treat and fight infectious diseases and immune system disorders.

***Immune-boosting dosage:*** 3 ml of tincture three times daily.

• **Astragalus** (*Astragalus membranaceus* and related plants). Though little research has been conducted on this herb in the West, it has been used here since the 1800s to strengthen the immune and respiratory systems.

***Immune-boosting dosage:*** 4 ml to 8 ml of tincture three times daily.

*Check with your health-care provider before using these herbs, especially if you are taking prescription medications, such as blood thinners or drugs to treat high blood pressure or diabetes. Pregnant and nursing women, in particular, should be especially careful to consult a professional before using herbs.

## The Eclectics' Flu Treatment

Herbs used by the Eclectics to treat influenza included echinacea (*Echinacea purpurea*, *Echinacea angustifolia* and *Echinacea pallida*) and boneset (*Eupatorium perfoliatum*). Echinacea traditionally is used to boost immune functioning at the onset of a cold or flu, while boneset is used to reduce fever and relieve aches and pains caused by the flu.

***Dosage:*** For echinacea, mix one ounce of tincture in four ounces of water and take one teaspoon every waking half hour for up to 14 days. For boneset, mix 1 ml to 2 ml in one ounce of warm water and take every one to two waking hours.

## Using Herbs Safely

The American Herbalists Guild (617-520-4372, AmericanHerbalistsGuild.com) and the American Association of Naturopathic Physicians (866-538-2267, Naturopathic.org) can help you find a qualified practitioner of herbal medicine in your area. Like all medicines, some herbs can be harmful if taken in the wrong quantities or combinations.

# Flu Shots Are Worth It

University of Alabama at Birmingham, news release.

The flu can be a serious threat to your health, but you can protect yourself by getting a flu shot, health experts say.

"The flu shot can reduce the risk of hospitalization and severe disease due to the influenza virus in addition to reducing the incidence or severity," said Kevin Harrod. He's a professor in the department of anesthesiology and perioperative medicine at the University of Alabama at Birmingham.

The flu vaccine is especially beneficial to children, the elderly, people with underlying chronic disease, such as heart disease, and women during and after pregnancy, he added.

About 970,000 Americans were hospitalized due to the flu in 2014, and more than 40 million were affected by flu-related illnesses, according to the U.S. Centers for Disease Control and Prevention.

During recent flu seasons, up to 90% of flu-related deaths have occurred in people 65 and older.

During the 2016-2017 season, the flu shot protected against two influenza A viruses (H1N1 and H3N2) and select influenza B viruses, Harrod said.

"While getting the flu shot may not keep you from getting the flu, it will limit the severity and duration of the illness, and provide you with some protection against future infections in subsequent seasons," Harrod said in a university news release.

Even when the vaccine is a "bad match" for the flu strains that develop, it offers partial protection, he added.

"One's immune system can make antibodies that still recognize and bind to the influenza virus even when new strains emerge unexpectedly," Harrod explained.

The U.S. Centers for Disease Control and Prevention has more on CDC.gov/flu/protect/keyfacts.htm.

---

# Flu or Flu Shot During Pregnancy Won't Raise Autism Risk in Child

Jennifer Wu, MD, obstetrician-gynecologist, Lenox Hill Hospital, New York City.

Lisa Croen, PhD, director, Kaiser Permanente's Autism Research Program, Oakland, California.

Andrew Adesman, MD, chief, developmental and behavioral pediatrics, Cohen Children's Medical Center, New Hyde Park, New York.

*JAMA Pediatrics*, news release.

---

Women who catch the flu or receive a flu shot during their pregnancy may rest easy knowing that neither event seems to raise their child's risk for autism.

That's the finding from a recent study of nearly 200,000 children born in California between 2000 and 2012.

"This large study is reassuring for expectant mothers. The results of this study confirm that neither getting influenza during pregnancy or getting a flu vaccine in the second or third trimester is associated with risk of autism in the child," said study author Lisa Croen, PhD. She directs Kaiser Permanente's Autism Research Program in Oakland.

## Study Details

The study, published in the journal *JAMA Pediatrics*, involved nearly 197,000 children born over a 10-year span. According to the researchers, 1,400 (about 0.7%) of the children's mothers were diagnosed with the flu during their pregnancies, and around 45,000 of the moms-to-be got a flu shot.

About 3,100 of the children went on to develop an autism spectrum disorder. However, there was no link seen between autism and maternal influenza or the mom receiving a flu shot during the last two trimesters of pregnancy, Dr. Croen and her colleagues said.

There was a "suggestion" of increased risk for autism in the child if the mom got a flu shot during her first trimester, but this statistic disappeared after the researchers further refined their analysis.

They stressed that this study was a retrospective look at data, so it can't prove or disprove any cause-and-effect relationships, but only point to associations.

Based on the findings, Dr. Croen said that "we are not recommending changes in our vaccination policy, which currently is to encourage all women to be vaccinated against the flu during their pregnancy."

## Expert Comment

Jennifer Wu, MD, an obstetrician-gynecologist at Lenox Hill Hospital in New York City, reviewed the recent findings. She said that "despite lack of evidence, many pregnant patients still worry about a link between vaccinations and autism."

On the other hand, she said, "the flu vaccine is very important for pregnant patients as they have higher risks of hospitalization and needing ventilation with flu infection. This study helps doctors to reassure their patients that flu vaccination in the second and third trimesters is safe.

"There should be some caution about giving the flu vaccination in the first trimester," Dr. Wu said, "as there was an increase in autism spectrum disorders—which was not found to be significant."

Her advice? Women who are "planning a pregnancy may want to get the [flu] vaccine before conceiving," Dr. Wu said.

One pediatrician said more research is needed to settle the first trimester finding.

"Additional studies are needed to clarify whether or not there is an association between first trimester influenza vaccinations and later autism spectrum disorders, so that more informed recommendations can be made to pregnant women," said Andrew Adesman, MD. He's chief of developmental and behavioral pediatrics at Cohen Children's Medical Center in New Hyde Park, New York.

For more on the flu and pregnancy, head to the U.S. Centers for Disease Control and Prevention at CDC.gov/flu/protect/vaccine/pregnant.htm.

## When Does Flu Testing Help?

William Schaffner, MD, professor of preventive medicine, Vanderbilt University Medical Center, Nashville.

Flu tests are sometimes given to rule out other infections with similar symptoms that may require different treatment. The test is most accurate when given within three days of the onset of symptoms.

However, the antiviral medication *oseltamivir* (Tamiflu) can be given within 48 hours after symptoms begin—even without a flu test. It will help shorten symptoms such as fever, chills, cough and muscle aches. Prompt treatment is especially important for older people and anyone whose immune system is compromised, such as cancer patients or those with chronic kidney or lung conditions. They are more likely to get complications from the flu, such as pneumonia, which can be deadly.

Treated or not, the flu generally goes away within a week or two in healthy people, although some may have a lingering cough or fatigue. Rest, drink plenty of fluids and wash your hands often to keep from spreading the flu to others.

## Women's Estrogen Stops the Flu

Women fight the flu better than men. The female sex hormone estrogen makes it harder for flu cells to replicate, so flu-infected women tend to have less severe symptoms and are less likely to spread the disease.

Study led by researchers at Johns Hopkins Bloomberg School of Public Health, Baltimore, published in *American Journal of Physiology—Lung Cellular and Molecular Physiology.*

## Flu Shot Fights Other Serious Conditions

Adults with diabetes who got the seasonal flu vaccine were 24% less likely to die from any cause than those who were unvaccinated, a recent seven-year study of nearly 125,000 adults with diabetes found. They were also less likely to be hospitalized for such conditions as heart failure, stroke or pneumonia.

***Why:*** Flu may lead to other serious conditions, such as heart attack or stroke, in people with chronic conditions, such as diabetes, and the elderly. The CDC recommends flu shots for children and adults, especially those with most chronic health conditions.

Eszter Vamos, MD, PhD, research fellow, Imperial College London, UK.

## How Long the Flu Shot Protects

Flu vaccines protect for six months—enough to get most people through the annual flu season. Vaccination reduces the chance of a doctor's visit for flu by 50% to 70%.

Study of more than 1,700 Americans by researchers at US Naval Health Research Center, San Diego, presented at the 2015 International Conference on Emerging Infectious Diseases, Atlanta.

## Don't Wear Dentures While You Sleep

Wearing dentures while sleeping raises pneumonia risk.

***Probable reason:*** Bacteria that breed easily in the mouth when dentures are left in can be inhaled into the lungs and cause pneumonia. People who leave their dentures in overnight likely have other poor oral-health habits as well—a study found that they visited the dentist less often than people who removed and cleaned their dentures nightly. Always take out your dentures at night, and clean them thoroughly.

Study of 524 denture wearers, ages 85 and older, by researchers at Nihon University School of Dentistry and Keio University School of Medicine, both in Tokyo, Japan, published in *Journal of Dental Research.*

### Be Careful at That Super Bowl Party!

Flu deaths are tied to the Super Bowl. People whose home team is in the Super Bowl have a significantly higher rate of death from the flu.

***Theory:*** The game takes place during flu season—and fans of the home team are more likely to attend Super Bowl parties, where the flu virus can spread.

Analysis of mortality data from 1974 to 2009 led by researchers at Tulane University, New Orleans, and College of William and Mary, Williamsburg, Virginia, published in *American Journal of Economics*.

## Another Reason to See Your Dentist

Regular dental cleanings lower pneumonia risk. In a study of the records of more than 26,000 people, those who never saw a dentist were 86% more likely to get bacterial pneumonia than those who had dental checkups twice a year. Regular dental cleanings reduce levels of bacteria that cause the lung infection.

Michelle E. Doll, MD, MPH, assistant professor and associate hospital epidemiologist in the department of internal medicine, division of infectious diseases, Virginia Commonwealth University School of Medicine, Richmond.

## My Winter Wellness Secrets

Jamison Starbuck, ND, a naturopathic physician in family practice and a guest lecturer at the University of Montana, both in Missoula. She is a past president of the American Association of Naturopathic Physicians and a contributing editor to *The Alternative Advisor: The Complete Guide to Natural Therapies and Alternative Treatments.* DrJamisonStarbuck.com

Cold weather is tough on our bodies. So it's not surprising that, as a family doctor, I spend a good part of my days peering down throats and otherwise examining patients who have been stricken by wintertime ailments such as colds and flu. To keep myself well, I've developed my own "winter protection program," which includes several simple immune-boosting steps in addition to frequent handwashing. *My winter-survival secrets...*

• **Humidify and hydrate.** Most heating sources lower humidity, drying and inflaming the mucous membranes of our eyes, nose, throat and lungs. This makes us more vulnerable to cold- and flu-causing germs.

***My advice:*** Purchase a small device known as a hygrometer (available at hardware stores for $30 or less) to keep an eye on the humidity of your home. Research varies on optimal humidity levels, but I strive for about 40%. I also use a warm-mist humidifier for a few hours in the bedroom each evening to keep the humidity levels stable. Other humidifiers are available, but whatever type you choose, be sure to keep it clean to avoid releasing mold and allergens into the air. Rinse it out with a 50/50 vinegar/water solution about three times a week. Also, without summer heat to remind us, some people forget to drink enough water. Doing so in winter is just as important as it is in the summer!

• **Eat the right fruits and veggies.** Antioxidants, including vitamins A, C and E, help keep us well during winter months.

***My advice:*** To get the biggest antioxidant boost from your food, make powerhouse veggies, such as squash (acorn, butternut and pumpkin), carrots and leafy greens, as well as "super" fruits, including berries and citrus, a routine part of your winter diet. Frozen berries and fruit are good alternatives if fresh produce looks a bit peaked.

• **Get outdoors.** Cold fresh air is invigorating. Our bodies respond to it by bringing blood to our skin and lungs to keep us warm and our blood oxygenated. This gives our entire circulatory system a boost.

***My advice:*** Spend 15 to 30 minutes outside each day. If you are unable to do so, open a couple of windows for about 15 minutes each morning. You'll feel some coldness, but the real payoff comes from breathing the fresh, oxygen-rich air.

• **Take an immune-boosting herbal.** As extra protection against colds and flu, I use elderberry, an immune-boosting herb, throughout the winter.

***My advice:*** Take one tablespoon of elderberry syrup or fresh juice...or one-quarter teaspoon of tincture daily, mixed with water if desired. Sambucol is my favorite brand of elderberry syrup.

• **Try vitamin D (2,000 international units daily).** It can also help prevent colds and flu, but check with your doctor first, since it may interact with certain medications.

• **Get extra sleep.** Years ago, a landmark study found that people who slept eight to nine hours a night in the winter months had fewer colds and flu than those who got less sleep.

***My advice:*** Get at least eight hours of sleep per night November through February.

# Xanax, Valium May Boost Pneumonia Risk in Alzheimer's Patients

*CMAJ (Canadian Medical Association Journal)*, news release.

Alzheimer's patients given sedatives such as Valium or Xanax may have an increased risk for pneumonia, a recent study warns.

People with Alzheimer's disease are often given these drugs, called benzodiazepines, over the long term, the researchers said.

Examples of benzodiazepines include *alprazolam* (Xanax), *clonazepam* (Klonopin), *diazepam* (Valium) and *lorazepam* (Ativan).

"An increased risk of pneumonia is an important finding to consider in treatment of patients with Alzheimer's disease. Pneumonia often leads to admission to hospital, and patients with dementia are at increased risk of death related to pneumonia," Heidi Taipale, PhD, of Kuopio Research Center of Geriatric Care at the University of Eastern Finland, and coauthors wrote.

### Study Details

For the study, the researchers reviewed data from nearly 50,000 Alzheimer's patients in Finland. The patients' average age was 80 and about two-thirds were women.

The study found that people with Alzheimer's who took benzodiazepines were 30% more likely to develop pneumonia than those who weren't given the sedatives.

The risk of pneumonia was highest in the first 30 days after starting the drugs, the findings showed.

The researchers said their findings are consistent with previous studies.

Because benzodiazepines are sedating, it's possible that people taking them may breathe saliva or food into the lungs, increasing the risk of pneumonia, the study authors suggested.

Dr. Taipale's team said the benefits and risks of these drugs—including pneumonia—need to be carefully considered before giving them to someone with Alzheimer's disease.

The study was published in the *CMAJ (Canadian Medical Association Journal)*.

### Expert Comment

The study is "a good reminder to clinicians to 'first do no harm' when prescribing these drugs for frail older women and men with dementia," Paula Rochon, MD, and her coauthors wrote in an accompanying editorial in the journal. Dr. Rochon is from Women's College Hospital and the University of Toronto.

Non-drug "approaches should be the starting point when managing neuropsychiatric symptoms in this patient population, which should help to limit inappropriate use of these drugs," the editorial authors said.

## Better Abscess Healing

Patients with an abscess recover better when an antibiotic is added to the usual treatment of surgical draining. Giving patients a seven-day course of *trimethoprim-sulfamethoxazole* (also known as Bactrim) led to a 93% cure rate, compared with an 86% rate for those who had drainage plus a placebo... and it limits the spread of methicillin-resistant Staphylococcus aureus (MRSA). MRSA is the most common cause of skin infections in the US and many other parts of the world.

Study of more than 1,200 patients at five hospital emergency departments by researchers at David Geffen School of Medicine at UCLA and Olive View–UCLA Medical Center, Sylmar, California, published in *The New England Journal of Medicine.*

## Antibiotics and Delirium

More than 50 of the most commonly prescribed antibiotics, including sulfonamides (such as Bactrim) and fluoroquinolones (such as Cipro), were linked to temporary mental confusion (delirium) in a review of nearly 400 patients (hospitalized and outpatient).

***Self-defense:*** If you're taking an antibiotic and experience symptoms of delirium, such as disorientation, agitation or social withdrawal, a loved one should talk to your doctor about your medication.

Shamik Bhattacharyya, MD, instructor in neurology, Harvard Medical School, Boston.

## Watch Out for Your Nurse

Nurses' uniforms pick up dangerous bacteria, including the antibiotic-resistant superbug MRSA. In a study of 40 hospital nurses, there were 22 instances in which at least one of five germs was spread from a patient or a room to a nurse's uniform. *Editor's note*: After a nurse or doctor visits, patients or family members can use antiseptic wipes on bed rails and other surfaces.

Deverick J. Anderson, MD, MPH, an associate professor of medicine at Duke University School of Medicine, Durham, North Carolina, and leader of a study presented at IDWeek, the annual meeting of several infectious disease associations.

# Valley Fever Is Often Misdiagnosed

Valley fever often is misdiagnosed, with deadly consequences. The disease, caused by fungi that live in desert soil, is clinically indistinguishable from many other diseases with severe respiratory symptoms. If you live in or have visited the West or Southwest—especially Arizona or central California—and have pneumonia or flu symptoms, ask for a blood test for valley fever.

John Galgiani, MD, is professor of medicine at University of Arizona College of Medicine and director of the university's Valley Fever Center for Excellence, both in Tucson.

# Zika Can Attack Adult Brains, Too

Nikos Vasilakis, PhD, assistant professor, department of pathology, and a member of the Center for Biodefense and Emerging Infectious Diseases at the University of Texas Medical Branch, Galveston.

Zika has become a disease to fear for pregnant women and women who may become pregnant—because babies who are infected with the Zika virus while in the womb can come into the world with devastating birth defects including the "tiny head" condition called microcephaly that can lead to severe developmental problems, seizures, blindness and more.

But there is new evidence that this mosquito-borne and sexually transmitted virus also damages adults—especially *older* adults. If so, it's dangerous to *all* of us.

## A Paralyzing Disease

Since Zika hit the headlines in the fall of 2015, there's been a *suspected* association between the virus and the autoimmune disorder Guillain-Barré syndrome (GBS) in adults.

In GBS, the body attacks its own nerves, especially in the legs and arms. GBS can lead to muscle weakness, temporary paralysis and, if untreated, death. There's no cure, although treatment can minimize complications. Recovery can take years. The elderly are more prone to GBS than younger people, and GBS symptoms last longer in older people as well.

Now there's stronger evidence that Zika really can cause GBS. A recent study published in *The New England Journal of Medicine* evaluated 164,237 cases of Zika infection and 1,474 cases of GBS in seven South American and Central American countries in one year, from April 2015 to April 2016.

***Findings:*** During Zika outbreaks, GBS cases increased anywhere from 100% to nearly 900%.

***Perspective:*** On average, the risk of developing GBS is still very small even if you become infected with Zika, says Nikos Vasilakis, PhD, assistant professor in the department of pathology and member of the Center for Biodefense and Emerging Infectious Diseases at the University of Texas Medical Branch. He's an expert on mosquito-borne diseases. In the study (Dr. Vasilakis was not associated with the study), about one in 300 people infected with Zika developed GBS. The real-world risk is likely much less, however, according to Dr. Vasilakis.

***Here's why:*** The study covered people who had *hospital-confirmed* cases of Zika, but most people with Zika never even get symptoms. GBS, on the other hand, is almost always reported because the symptoms are so severe. In the US, there are only about 3,000 to 6,000 cases of GBS a year from all causes. Says Dr. Vasilakis, "Guillain-Barré is a very rare disease."

Guillain-Barré isn't the only neurological disease that Zika can cause in adults. It is associated with acute myelitis, an autoimmune condition. It may also lead to peripheral neuropathy—damage to the nerves in the arms and legs, leading to tingling or numbness in the hands and feet. The likely cause is inflammation as a result of the Zika viral infection. But this effect has been shown only in a case study, so it's not known how common it is.

## Zika and Adult Brains

The new GBS findings confirm a link that's been suspected. Recent animal research also opens up the possibility that Zika may affect adults in ways we *haven't* suspected before—it focused on adult brains.

In the fetus, Zika attacks *neural progenitor cells*—stem cells that form more specialized brain cells as a baby develops. Damage to these cells interferes with normal development, leading to birth defects.

In healthy adults, these stem cells have already become fully formed neurons. But our brains hang onto some of these stem cells, it turns out. They cluster in the *hippocampus*—the part of the brain involved in memory and learning—helping to develop new neurons as we learn new things. Having these stem cells as we age may help prevent dementia and depression.

Researchers at The Rockefeller University in New York and the La Jolla Institute for Allergy and Immunology in California wanted to see whether Zika also attacked these progenitor cells in adult brains. Using biomarkers in adult mice infected with the Zika virus, they tracked where the virus went in the brain.

***Result:*** The virus clustered around the progenitor cells, especially those in the hippocampus, attacking them—so that there were fewer new neurons. "It was very clear that the virus wasn't affecting the whole brain evenly, like people are seeing in the fetus," said Joseph Gleeson, MD, one of the study authors and head of the Laboratory of Pediatric Brain Disease at The Rockefeller University in New York City. "These cells are special and somehow very susceptible to the infection." By attacking these adult stem cells, the authors suggest, Zika may affect the brain's "neuroplasticity"—its ability to change. Over time, that could lead to cognitive decline.

***Perspective:*** It's a preliminary study in mice. Although human studies often show similar results to mouse studies, we can't draw conclusions about Zika in people, who may be able to mount an effective immune response that prevents the virus from attacking the brain. However, a warning flag has now been raised—Zika could be much worse for adults than we thought.

## How to Avoid It

Zika is an unusual virus. It's spread not just by mosquito bites but also through sexual transmission (as well as blood transfusions). So far there is no evidence that it can be transmitted by deep kissing. It's horrifically scary for women who are or want to become pregnant and for their partners. There is risk for adults getting GBS...and there may be risk to the adult brain as well.

***One reassuring point:*** A Zika epidemic in the continental US is unlikely. Indeed, even in and around Miami, where there has been some local transmission—not just from travelers coming back from Zika-infected countries—it's now coming under control. In the Wynwood section of Miami, which recently had a Zika outbreak, for example, transmission of the virus has been halted. Says Dr. Vasilakis, "We have air conditioning, window screens and mosquito-prevention strategies such as aerial spraying. They are very effective."

If you're traveling to another country that has Zika, though, check the Centers for Disease Control and Prevention (CDC) website for the latest guidance. *Some tips...*

- **If you're pregnant, avoid any Zika area.** These include much of Central and South America, parts of Southeast Asia and, in the US, the island of Puerto Rico and certain areas around Miami. If you may become pregnant, or are a man whose partner may become pregnant, avoid nonessential travel to these areas. Because Zika is sexually transmitted—and the virus can be found in a man's semen for up to six months after initial symptoms—it is recommended that if a man has symptoms of Zika infection, he should use condoms for six months after the start of his symptoms. If he has been in a Zika-infected area, even if he doesn't have symptoms, he should use condoms for six months after his travel. (Symptoms may include fever, rash, joint pain, conjunctivitis [red eyes], muscle pain and headache. Flu, in contrast, doesn't include red eyes or a rash.)

• **If you do travel to a Zika-infected area, try hard to avoid mosquito bites.** The Aedes mosquito, which carries Zika, is active night and day, inside houses as well as outside. Wear insect-repellent clothing, and spray yourself with a repellent containing DEET or other effective mosquito repellents.

• **If you have a chronic condition that may affect your susceptibility to viral infections**—and especially if you are immunocompromised—you may want to consider staying away from Zika areas entirely. This isn't official CDC advice, but the same Aedes mosquito that carries Zika also carries other potentially debilitating diseases, including chikungunya and yellow fever. At the least, if you are considering such travel, talk with your own doctor before planning a trip.

## Surprising Cause of Constipation

Chronic constipation might be caused by a viral disease, according to Yale researchers. In people infected with the herpes simplex virus, the infection can spread from the genitals and damage nerves in the colon, inhibiting normal digestion.

*Cell Host & Microbe.*

## Don't Get Bitten by Mosquito Myths

Jonathan F. Day, PhD, professor of medical entomology at the University of Florida, Vero Beach. He has published more than 100 peer-reviewed scientific articles about mosquitoes and the diseases they transmit.

Somewhere out there—likely very near you—mosquito eggs are waiting to hatch.

While some people consider mosquitoes to be little more than a minor, itchy annoyance, these pesky insects can put you at risk for a number of mosquito-borne diseases.

One of the most common diseases transmitted by mosquitoes to humans in North America is West Nile Virus (WNV), which can cause flulike symptoms and, in rare cases, inflammation of the brain (encephalitis). The illness has been reported in every state in the continental US except Maine.

The most recent mosquito-borne disease to cause alarm in the US is Zika virus. If a pregnant woman is infected with Zika virus, her child may be born with a serious birth defect called microcephaly, which is associated with incomplete brain development. *Here are additional "truths" behind some commonly held myths about what makes the little buzzers bite—and what we can do to stop them…*

***MYTH #1:* Mosquitoes bite only at dusk and dawn.**

***Truth:*** While most common types of mosquitoes feed mainly at dusk and dawn, some species feed during the day while other species feed at night. In fact, the Aedes aegypti mosquito that transmits Zika virus is most active during the day.

***MYTH #2:* Mosquitoes are attracted to people who have type O blood.**

***Truth:*** You may have heard that mosquitoes prefer to bite people with type O blood. Not true. Aside from the fact that type O is the most common blood type in the US, mosquitoes do not choose a host based on blood type.

***What does attract mosquitoes:*** Carbon dioxide. People with high metabolic rates produce more carbon dioxide than do people with low metabolisms—those producing high levels of CO2 (as may occur, for example, during vigorous exercise such as running or biking) attract more mosquitoes.

Another mosquito draw is lactic acid, a compound found in sweat. This means that you'll be more likely to get an armload of bites if you sit outside after a run.

***MYTH #3:* You don't need to worry about mosquitoes if you live in a dry climate.**

***Truth:*** While mosquitoes are not as abundant in dry climates as they are in tropical rain forests, you will find them ready to bite in dry habitats, including the desert Southwest and the High Plains east of the Rocky Mountains.

Research shows that mosquito populations increase with higher spring soil moisture levels—heavy snowpack, snowmelt and spring rain all provide sufficient standing water to allow the development of immature mosquitoes, even in typically "dry" areas.

***For up-to-date forecasts on mosquito activity:*** Go to the website AccuWeather.com. Add your location to the search box, then look for "mosquito" in the drop-down menu under "Personalized Forecasts."

For mosquito prevention, keep standing water away from your home. And don't just look for the obvious places like empty flowerpots or kiddie pools. Be sure to check for water that collects in rain gutters and buckets, too. Empty and refresh water in birdbaths and fountains at least once a week to keep mosquitoes from maturing. Small ponds can be treated with Bti Briquets, a sustained-release larvicide that floats on the water's surface. Vegetation around larger ponds should be controlled, especially cattails and water hyacinth.

***MYTH #4:* DEET is toxic to humans.**

***Truth:*** Developed by the US Army in 1946, DEET (short for N,N-diethyl-meta-toluamide) is one of the few products that is effective against mosquitoes and biting flies. It was registered for human use in 1957 and has been found to be safe even for pregnant and nursing women when applied according to label instructions.

Concerns about DEET come primarily from the toxic effects seen when it is ingested, inhaled or used in other ways inconsistent with label instructions. Do not apply DEET products more often than recommended...and do not apply over cuts, wounds or irritated skin. For more information on DEET, consult the EPA website, EPA.gov/insect-repellents/deet.

***MYTH #5:* Non-DEET repellents don't work.**

***Truth:*** Research published by the Centers for Disease Control and Prevention (CDC) demonstrated that products containing oil of lemon eucalyptus, whose active ingredient para-menthane-diol is derived from the eucalyptus tree, can be as effective as low-concentration DEET. But most botanical formulations require frequent reapplication—usually every 10 to 20 minutes.

Another option is Avon Skin-So-Soft. Its current formula contains picaridin (a synthetic compound that resembles the natural compound found in the plants used to produce black pepper) and IR3535 (structurally similar to the naturally occurring amino acid B-alanine). Both ingredients are registered with the EPA as effective and safe.

***MYTH #6:* Sprays are more effective than creams.**

***Truth:*** When it comes to efficacy, what really matters is the concentration of the active ingredient—for example, the CDC recommends DEET, oil of lemon eucalyptus and picaridin-based repellents. This means that a 3% DEET spray and a 3% DEET lotion are equally effective. The downside of an aerosol is the risk for inhalation.

But there are ways to apply a DEET spray without inhaling it. For instance, when using an aerosol, spray the product onto the palm of your hand and apply the liquid to areas you want to treat—your arms, neck and forehead.

***Note:*** Sunscreen/repellent combinations are not recommended—the effectiveness is less than if you used two separate products. When both are needed, apply sunscreen first...then bug repellent.

***Also:*** For unknown reasons, mosquitoes are attracted to dark colors, so wear tightly woven, light-colored apparel. And if you must wear sandals, apply a CDC-recommended insect repellent. Some mosquitoes reportedly love the smell of feet!

## Zika Can Be Sexually Transmitted

Did you know that the Zika virus can be sexually transmitted from a woman to a man? The first case of female-to-male sexual transmission was reported in New York City. Prior to this case, sexual transmission of the Zika virus had been reported only from male to female. The virus is most commonly spread through mosquitoes and poses the greatest risk to pregnant women because it can cause microcephaly, a condition in which babies are born with abnormally small heads and neurological issues.

*Morbidity and Mortality Weekly Report*, Centers for Disease Control and Prevention, Atlanta.

## DEET Repellents Safe in Pregnancy to Prevent Zika, Researchers Say

Blair Wylie, MD, MPH, associate professor, Harvard Medical School, division of maternal-fetal medicine, and department of obstetrics and gynecology, Massachusetts General Hospital, Boston.

R. Phillips Heine, MD, professor of obstetrics and gynecology, Duke University, Durham, North Carolina.

*Obstetrics & Gynecology.*

DEET insect repellents won't harm a pregnant woman or her fetus when used as instructed to prevent infection with the Zika virus, a recent research analysis suggests.

Exposure to the mosquito-transmitted virus during pregnancy can cause devastating birth defects, including microcephaly, which results in abnormally small heads and brains.

Because of this, recommendations to mothers-to-be include protecting themselves from mosquito bites by using products containing DEET in areas where Zika is circulating.

But some women worry that the repellents themselves might pose a toxic threat to an unborn child. Not so, say the authors of the recent research review.

"Given what we know about both Zika and DEET, the evidence overwhelmingly favors use of DEET-containing products," said Blair Wylie, MD, MPH, an associate professor at Harvard Medical School's division of maternal-fetal medicine.

### About Zika Virus

While the Zika epidemic is concentrated in South America and the Caribbean, 105 cases of "local transmission" have occurred in Florida. However, the vast majority of Zika infections in the US have been linked to patient exposure during travel outside the mainland 48 states.

Some cases of Zika have been transmitted sexually.

Symptoms of Zika can last several weeks, and include a fever, rash, joint pain, red eyes (conjunctivitis), muscle pain and/or headaches.

But most healthy adults will experience only a mild reaction, or none at all.

### Using DEET Effectively

Dr. Wylie's team noted that a 1998 Environmental Protection Agency review determined that DEET posed no health risk to users. The EPA reaffirmed that finding in 2014.

"An infection during pregnancy with Zika can put babies at risk for death, birth defects including brain problems, poor growth and hearing or eyesight loss," Dr. Wylie said. "Insect repellents are key to prevention."

Typically, that means repellents containing DEET (N,N-diethyl-meta-toluamide). The insecticide has been used since the 1950s and is available in more than 200 products.

These repellents are "considered safe with few side effects if used properly," added Dr. Wylie, lead author of the recent study published *Obstetrics & Gynecology*.

"Proper" use, Dr. Wylie added, means avoiding the eyes, mouth, cuts and irritated skin when applying to the face. Also, apply DEET after sunscreen (don't use combination products), wash your hands after application and don't apply it under clothing.

Another ob-gyn agreed with the study's conclusion that DEET is safe for pregnant women.

"The available data suggests that DEET is safe in pregnancy," said R. Phillips Heine, MD, a professor of obstetrics and gynecology at Duke University Medical Center in Durham, North Carolina.

"There is little that is absorbed systemically, so the fetus will be exposed to very low amounts. I would recommend DEET, as well as other mosquito-avoidance measures," Dr. Heine said.

These measures generally include covering arms and legs, using window screens and avoiding geographic areas where Zika is prevalent.

DEET products are available in concentrations ranging from 5% to nearly 100%, Dr. Wylie said, adding she would never recommend using anything above 30%.

Why? "Because their effectiveness at repelling insects plateaus around there," she said. "The added concentration would not increase benefit."

This advice, Dr. Wylie added, applies to any user, male or female.

For more information on Zika and pregnancy, visit the website of the U.S. Centers for Disease Control and Prevention (CDC), cdc.gov, and search "Zika and pregnancy."

To see the CDC list of sites where Zika virus is active and may pose a threat to pregnant women, go to its website, CDC.gov, and search "Zika travel information."

## What Spreads Mosquito-Borne Viruses...

The itchiness of mosquito bites could be what allows mosquito-borne viruses to spread.

***Recent discovery:*** The immune cells that rush to bitten areas can themselves become infected with these viruses and allow them to move to other parts of the body.

*Immunity.*

## Bacterial or Viral?

An inexpensive blood test that identifies gene activity that's unique to viral and bacterial infections is now in development.

***Possible benefit:*** A cutback in unnecessary antibiotic use—a current problem since viral and bacterial infections often cause similar symptoms.

Stanford University School of Medicine.

## OK to Refreeze?

Is it OK to refreeze food that has thawed?

Yes. You can refreeze food that has been thawed as long as the food was thawed safely in a refrigerator. If you put it in cold water or the microwave to thaw, you must cook the food before refreezing. As perishable foods begin to thaw at temperatures above 40°F, bacteria begin to multiply. Ground meat, poultry and seafood should remain safe in the refrigerator for one to three days after removing it from the freezer. Pork or beef roasts, chops and steaks are OK generally for three to five days.

Julie Garden-Robinson, PhD, RD, professor of nutrition and food safety, North Dakota State University, Fargo.

# Food-Safety Secrets Restaurants Don't Want You to Know

Darron Cardosa, who has more than 25 years of experience waiting tables in the New York City area.

Eating out means trusting strangers to prepare and handle your food. Usually that trust is well-placed—but at times, the hectic pace and financial pressures facing restaurants result in corners being cut in ways that could jeopardize jeopardize your health. *A veteran waiter shared what restaurants don't want you to know...*

## Food Quality and Safety

• **Seafood stew, soup and pasta "specials" often feature fish that's too old to serve any other way.** Restaurants do not like to throw away expensive ingredients. When seafood is no longer fresh enough to serve on its own, it might be chopped up and served in a stew, soup or pasta dish, where sauces and other bold flavors can be used to hide its age. This can happen with meat and poultry, too, but it's most common with seafood, which has an especially short shelf life.

***Tip from the waiter:*** It's generally OK to order a seafood stew, soup or pasta dish if it is on the regular menu. But when these are listed as specials, the odds are high that the restaurant is trying to sell past-its-prime seafood.

• **Restaurant menus rarely are cleaned.** Responsible restaurants take cleanliness very seriously. Almost everything in the kitchen and dining room is cleaned regularly—except the menus. At most restaurants, menus are rarely, if ever, wiped down, even though they are handled by many people and occasionally dropped on the floor.

***Tip from the waiter:*** Wash your hands after you've ordered and handed your menu back to the waiter.

• **Complimentary bread or chips might have been served to other tables before yours.** A Mexican restaurant in Michigan recently received negative press when it was caught taking chips and salsa that were not consumed at one table and serving them to a second table. That restaurant is far from alone—it is not uncommon for uneaten slices of complimentary bread to find their way onto multiple tables rather than get thrown away. And even restaurants that hold themselves to a very high standard usually send out the butter packages that accompany bread to table after table until they are used.

***Tip from the waiter:*** It might be worth skipping complimentary premeal items such as bread and chips unless the restaurant has an open area where you can watch these items being prepared specifically for you.

• **The week following an extended power failure might be the wrong time to eat out.** Cash-strapped restaurants often cannot afford to throw away everything that was in their fridges and freezers after power outages, so ingredients may no longer be as fresh as they should be.

***Tip from the waiter:*** If you want to eat out following a long power failure, choose a restaurant in a neighboring area that did not lose its power.

• **You might not want to eat your leftovers if you saw how they were put into to-go containers.** This task might be delegated to a busboy who has little training in hygienic food handling...or it might be done by a harried server who uses the same spoon to transfer multiple customers' partially eaten meals.

***Tip from the waiter:*** Ask your server to bring to-go containers to your table, and then transfer your leftovers yourself.

• **Your water might not be as pure as you are told.** Some restaurants serve only filtered water...and some patrons pay extra for bottled water. But if there is ice in the water, that ice is almost certainly made from unfiltered tap water. Restaurant ice makers rarely have filters.

***Tip from the waiter:*** If water purity is important to you, skip the ice.

• **Drink garnishes sometimes are germy or old.** That lemon or lime slice in your drink might have been cut hours earlier and then left to sit in an open, unrefrigerated container where numerous restaurant employees pick out pieces with their bare hands. Restaurants may have policies requiring the use of tongs for grabbing these garnishes, but rushed servers and bartenders frequently skip that.

***Tip from the waiter:*** Tell your server to "hold the lemon" when you order a drink.

# Bagged-Salad Warning

Prepackaged salad could contain harmful salmonella bacteria on leaves that are wilted or damaged, recent research has found.

***What happens:*** Juices that form when lettuce leaves break down can cause a biofilm to form, prompting the growth of salmonella.

***If you purchase bagged salads:*** Choose leaves with minimal damage...rinse salad before eating...and consume by the "best by" date on the package.

Primrose Freestone, PhD, associate professor in clinical microbiology, University of Leicester, UK.

# Parasites: Your Body May Be Hosting These "Stealth Germs"

Erno Daniel, MD, PhD, an internist and geriatrician at the Sansum Clinic in Santa Barbara, California, and a former clinical assistant professor of medicine at the University of Southern California in Los Angeles. He is author of *Stealth Germs in Your Body.*

Most people think that parasitic infections are a problem only in less-developed countries. Not true. Up to 40% of US adults harbor Toxoplasma gondii, the parasite that causes toxoplasmosis, an infection marked by flulike symptoms. Meanwhile, the Centers for Disease Control and Prevention estimates that more than 100,000 cases of giardiasis, a parasitic infection that causes watery diarrhea, occur annually in the US.

Many parasitic infections cause only mild symptoms or no symptoms at all. But some organisms can cause brain and nervous system damage or long-lasting symptoms such as chronic fatigue or muscle aches. Some of these infections can turn deadly, especially in people whose immune systems are suppressed by illness or chemotherapy.

***Good news:*** Once you're diagnosed (usually with a stool sample), most parasites can be eliminated with medication. Virtually all can be prevented with good hygiene and the safe handling of food and water.

Common parasites in the US...

## Toxoplasma gondii

Healthy adults with this potentially dangerous single-celled organism typically have no symptoms. Occasionally, however, a scar can form on the retina. During a routine eye exam, the scar can be noted and serve as a clue to previous exposure. In people with impaired immunity, such as those undergoing chemotherapy or AIDS patients, untreated toxoplasmosis can suddenly reemerge and cause brain or nervous system damage and even can be fatal.

Although medications are usually recommended for those with compromised immunity, symptoms usually go away without treatment in people who are otherwise healthy. However, the dormant organism may reemerge.

T. gondii is often present in the feces of otherwise healthy-appearing cats. People may get infected while cleaning a cat's litter box or working in the yard and touching soil where a cat has defecated.

Be sure to wash your hands thoroughly after contact with a cat or its feces and after yard work or gardening. The disease also can be contracted by eating any type of undercooked contaminated meat, which can harbor the organism.

***Symptoms:*** Swollen lymph nodes, headache, fever, body aches and sometimes a sore throat.

***Treatment:*** *Pyrimethamine* (Daraprim), an antimalaria drug that also kills T. gondii. It's combined with an antibiotic to increase the effectiveness of the treatment. Treatment usually lasts several weeks, but those with compromised immunity may need to continue for the rest of their lives.

***Important:*** Pyrimethamine inhibits the absorption of folate (folic acid). Patients who take high doses for extended periods are usually advised to supplement with 400 micrograms (mcg) of folic acid daily.

Toxoplasmosis can cause problems with pregnancy, including miscarriage. Pregnant women should speak to their doctors for precautions to take.

## Cryptosporidium parvum

This one-celled parasite—and its close relative Cyclospora cayetanensis—infects the small intestine. People with this infection, known as cryptosporidiosis, release enormous quantities of the parasite in their stools. People may get infected if they drink (or swim in) contaminated water, eat uncooked foods that were prepared by someone with the infection, or touch their mouths after touching a contaminated surface or object.

***Note:*** Chlorination of water will not kill this organism.

***Symptom:*** Watery diarrhea. This may continue for one to two weeks—or even up to a month—in people who are otherwise healthy. The infection is potentially deadly for those with weak immune systems.

***Treatment:*** Patients who are generally healthy don't require treatment and usually recover within two weeks. In those with compromised immunity, in addition to treating the underlying illness if possible, fluid/electrolyte replacement may be required as well as antidiarrheal medications and/or antiparasitic medications to reduce symptoms.

## Tapeworms and Larvae

The largest intestinal parasite is the tapeworm. It can survive in the intestine for more than a decade and can potentially reach up to 50 feet in length. Infection is usually caused by eating infected raw or undercooked pork, beef or fish.

***Symptoms:*** Most people have no or only mild gastrointestinal symptoms, such as occasional diarrhea. Equally important, tapeworm larvae can migrate to parts of the body outside the intestine and cause seemingly unrelated symptoms, such as seizures (if they enter the brain).

Depending on the species and the nature of the infection (worm or larval), some patients may suffer damage to the central nervous system.

***Treatment:*** *Praziquantel* (Biltricide) kills adult tapeworms. A stool sample is usually taken one to three months after the initial treatment. If the parasite is still present, the drug is repeated.

It also may be useful to take probiotics to ease severe diarrhea—speak to your doctor.

## Parasite Self-Defense

Food and water sanitation, as well as good hygiene, are the best ways to prevent parasitic infections. *Recommended...*

- **Use a countertop or under-the-sink activated carbon water filter to trap cryptosporidium, giardia and other parasites.**
- **Wash your hands not only after using the bathroom,** but also after working in the yard or handling laundry—particularly when the laundry includes underwear or bedsheets. You would be surprised at how many people don't follow these simple guidelines.
- **Always rinse fresh fruits and vegetables.** This will remove most organisms. In high-risk areas (such as tropical or underdeveloped countries), soak these foods in water disinfected with iodine. Add five to 10 drops per quart of water. Let the food soak for about 20 minutes.

- **Wash knives, cutting boards and other kitchen equipment**—as well as your hands—with warm, soapy water before and after handling raw meats.
- **Wear gloves when cleaning a litter box, and wash your hands afterward.**
- **Don't walk barefoot in the yard/garden,** particularly if you have cats (or livestock).

## Can You Eat Around Mold on Food?

Mold spreads deep beneath the surface rather quickly in soft foods such as breads and strawberries but does not penetrate as deeply in hard foods. You can safely eat firm vegetables and fruits, such as apples and carrots, or hard cheeses if you can cut away at least one inch around the mold and discard it. Any other foods, such as sliced bread, soft fruits and vegetables and meat, that are moldy should be thrown out. Some molds make toxins that can cause severe illness.

Stephanie Smith, PhD, food safety specialist, Washington State University, Pullman.

## Better Tick Protection

Most ticks are very sensitive to dryness. The first thing you should do once you're in the house after taking a hike or working in the yard is to strip your clothing off and throw it in the dryer—not in the washing machine. Run it on high heat for about 10 minutes to kill deer ticks as well as Lone Star ticks and other species. Gas dryers tend to get hotter than electric dryers, so you might want to add five minutes if you're using an electric dryer.

Ticks are not killed by washing, even in hot water. Clothing just left in the hamper or on the floor may put the next person who touches it at risk. Dry clothes first, then wash. You can also keep ticks off your clothing with insect repellents, such as Insect Shield or Sawyer, that contain long-lasting permethrin.

Thomas Mather, PhD, director, TickEncounter Resource Center, The University of Rhode Island, Kingston. TickEncounter.org

## Rodent Danger

Any activity that puts you in contact with droppings, urine, saliva or nesting materials from mice or rats can put you at risk for hantavirus pulmonary syndrome (HPS)—which can be fatal—and other diseases. HPS occurs when people breathe in air that contains the virus, so it's important to avoid actions that raise dust, such as sweeping or vacuuming.

The CDC website has specific instructions for safely cleaning up after rodents (go to CDC.gov/rodents/cleaning/index.html).

***Key steps:*** Air out the area that contains urine, droppings or nesting material. Then, while wearing gloves, spray the area with a disinfectant or a bleach-water mixture (one-and-a-half cups of bleach in one gallon of water). Let soak for five minutes before gently removing the droppings/urine with a paper towel. Wash hands thoroughly after you are done.

Elizabeth Ervin, MPH, health scientist, Centers for Disease Control and Prevention (CDC), Atlanta.

## Cancer Drug Fights Sepsis

A minuscule dose of a topoisomerase inhibitor, a cancer drug, attacks the "inflammatory storm" caused by sepsis, a "top 10" leading cause of death in the US.

Icahn School of Medicine at Mount Sinai.

## Turmeric for Tuberculosis

Drug-resistant tuberculosis (TB) may respond to turmeric, a popular anti-inflammatory, recent research has found.

***Why it helps:*** The curcumin in turmeric stimulates the immune cells that fight TB.

*Respirology.*

## Infection-Free Hip Surgery

If you're considering hip replacement, you may want to put it off for a few months if you've just received a steroid shot in your hip.

***Recent study:*** Infection rates jumped 40% in hip replacement patients who received a steroid injection in the three months prior to surgery...but those who received an injection earlier showed no increased risk. Steroids may weaken the immune system, which could account for the higher infection rate. Although rare, an infection in the hip joint could require additional surgery, intravenous antibiotics and a prolonged recovery.

William Schairer, MD, orthopedic surgeon, Hospital for Special Surgery, New York City.

### Sleep Away Your Risk of Illness

People who sleep less than six hours a night are 400% more likely to get a cold than people who sleep seven hours or more.

Prevention.com

## Sunlight Boosts Immunity

Sunlight boosts immunity by energizing infection-fighting T cells. The blue light found in the rays of the sun makes T cells move faster, so they get to the site of an infection and begin their protective activity more quickly. Thus, short sun exposure can be beneficial.

Gerard Ahern, PhD, associate professor in the department of pharmacology and physiology at Georgetown University, Washington, DC.

## Whooping Cough Still a Threat

Whooping cough is a threat to teenagers. Children get five vaccinations against the disease (pertussis) starting before kindergarten and continuing until age 10. Children 11 to 12 years old should receive a Tdap booster. The shot protects 69% of 11- and 12-year-olds in the first year, but within one year after the booster, only 9% have sufficient protection.

***Recommendations:*** Give another booster shot at 15 years and 18 years. Adults who should have the booster include all people living with or caring for a newborn or infant...pregnant women...all health-care workers...and people age 65 and older.

Analysis of 175,000 adolescents by researchers at Kaiser Permanente's Vaccine Study Center, Oakland, California, published in *Pediatrics.*

# Chapter 9

# KIDNEY, LIVER AND BLADDER HEALTH

## Kidney Stones... Never Again!

If you've ever endured the searing pain of a kidney stone—it's often described as worse than childbirth—then you probably felt like celebrating once the pain was gone and now consider yourself home free. But that's a mistake.

***What most people don't realize:*** Once you've suffered a kidney stone, which can be as small as a grain of sand or as large as a golf ball, you have a chronic condition that must be managed over a lifetime to prevent a repeat performance.

Here's what you need to know to control this condition over the long haul—and prevent it in the first place if kidney stones run in your family...

### A Growing Problem

Even if you've never had a kidney stone, that doesn't mean you're in the clear. About one in every 10 Americans will have a kidney stone during his/her lifetime.

***Eye-opening recent finding:*** For unknown reasons, the prevalence of kidney stone disease has doubled in the past 15 years, especially in women—more than three million Americans receive medical care for the condition each year.

### Best Treatment Options

Treatment for a kidney stone mainly depends on its size. If you develop a small stone (less than 4 mm—or about one-sixth of an inch), count yourself lucky. You may be able to simply drink lots of water (about three liters per day)...take an over-the-counter nonsteroidal anti-inflammatory drug, such as *ibuprofen* (Motrin)...and wait for it to pass on its own within a few days, though it sometimes takes a week or longer. A prescription medication, such as *tamsulosin* (Flomax), may also be used to help pass the stone.

***Important:*** It's crucial that a urologist monitor the patient (for example, with an abdominal X-ray or ultrasound), since the stone may cause an obstruction that damages the kidney—even if the pain has subsided.

A larger stone (4 mm or more) usually needs more extensive medical intervention. While doctors once relied on external sound waves (shock wave lithotripsy), which

Fredric L. Coe, MD, a nephrologist and professor of medicine at The University of Chicago Pritzker School of Medicine. Dr. Coe has published more than 250 peer-reviewed medical journal research articles and an additional 200 reviews, chapters and books.

was only moderately successful at breaking apart a kidney stone in the body, there's now a more effective method. An ultra-thin lighted tube (ureteroscope) can be threaded into the urethra, into the bladder, then up to the ureter. A laser at the tip of the scope pulverizes the stone, turning it into dust that is urinated out.

When a kidney stone exceeds 2 cm (or about three-quarters of an inch), surgery is usually required. With percutaneous nephrolithotomy, the surgeon creates a small incision in your back to remove the stone.

## Know Your Stone

To avoid a recurrence, the key is to know the composition of your kidney stone. *Main types of stones...*

- **Calcium oxalate.** These small, black or dark brown stones account for about 80% of all kidney stones.
- **Calcium phosphate.** These stones, which are usually tan to beige, form when urine is more alkaline.
- **Uric acid.** These red or orange stones form when urine is too acidic due to heredity, obesity or kidney disease.
- **Cystine.** These lemon yellow stones are associated with the hereditary disorder cystinuria, which causes high urine concentrations of the amino acid cystine.
- **Struvite.** These brownish-white stones are produced when bacteria get introduced into the urinary tract—due, for example, to the use of a urinary catheter.

## Prevention Secrets

To prevent a kidney stone recurrence, your goal is to stop the stone-forming process by changing the composition of your urine.

Here's how to do that...

***STEP 1:* Get your kidney stone analyzed.** If you pass a stone at home, save it so that your doctor can have its composition analyzed. Urine analysis shows what stone-causing compounds are in your urine so that you can take appropriate preventive steps.

***What to do:*** Strain your urine through gauze in a funnel and then put the stone into a small plastic bag.

***Important:*** It's best to have all stones analyzed, since your kidneys can produce stones of varying crystals at different times in your life, which may require a change in treatment. Anyone who has ever suffered a kidney stone should also see a doctor at least once a year for urine analysis.

***STEP 2:* Provide two 24-hour urine samples after the stone has passed.** This requires catching and saving all your urine for 24 hours after you've resumed your normal diet and lifestyle habits. Getting two samples provides a more accurate view than a single sample.

***STEP 3:* Raise your urine volume.** The more dilute your urine becomes, the less likely that stones will form. The goal is to produce about 2.5 liters daily in urine volume. This will require drinking three liters or more of fluid daily (spaced out during waking hours). People who sweat a lot due to heat or physical activity may need to drink four to six liters of water per day.

***Note:*** High water intake can sometimes be harmful for people with heart, kidney or liver disease...the elderly...and people taking certain medications (such as diuretics). Consult your physician for advice on how much water you should drink.

***STEP 4:* Change your diet.** This should start immediately when you have a kidney stone and continue for a lifetime. A kidney stone prevention diet is...*

- **Low sodium and high calcium.** If your daily sodium intake is below 1,500 mg, you can eat 1,000 mg to 1,200 mg of calcium daily (mainly from dairy foods and leafy green vegetables, except for spinach), and urine calcium losses will be as low as possible. Why do you need calcium? High calcium intake

*If you have chronic kidney disease, your dietary and treatment needs may differ—consult your doctor.

will reduce oxalate absorption—oxalate is a component of most kidney stones.

***Helpful:*** After following a low-sodium/high-calcium diet for about a month, repeat the 24-hour urine test to see if additional dietary restrictions are required.

***Important:*** If urine oxalate remains high (over 30 mg per day) despite a high calcium intake, then you need to go low oxalate. To reduce your risk for calcium oxalate stones, avoid high-oxalate foods (such as spinach, rhubarb, beets, cocoa, raspberries and soy products).

***Note:*** Even though many of these foods are healthful, there are safer substitutes—for example, instead of spinach, you can try arugula or kale. For a full list of high-oxalate foods and good substitutes, go to KidneyStones.UChicago.edu/how-to-eat-a-low-oxalate-diet.

- **High potassium.** When food sources of potassium—all fruits and most vegetables—are consumed, they are converted to bicarbonate. This process reduces the risk for calcium and uric acid stones.

***Recommended daily potassium intake:*** 4,700 mg.

- **Low protein and refined sugar.** These foods can promote uric acid stones. Ideally, intake of refined sugar should be less than 10% of total caloric intake, and protein intake should be about 0.8 g to 1 g of protein per 2.2 pounds of body weight.

***STEP 5:*** **Ask your physician about medication.** A variety of medications can help prevent a kidney stone recurrence. These include potassium citrate tablets for people who have had uric acid stones or calcium stones...thiazide diuretics, which help prevent calcium stones...and antibiotics for struvite stones that are triggered by, say, a urinary tract infection.

For more on kidney stones, go to KidneyStones.UChicago.edu.

### Kidney Stone Basics

When a stone forms in the kidney, it typically moves through the urinary tract to exit the body in urine. At various points along that journey, the stone may become lodged, leading to extreme pain (usually in one's side or back near the bottom of the rib cage, though it may spread to the lower abdomen and groin).

***Important:*** Kidney stones may also cause blood in the urine, an inability to pass urine, nausea and vomiting and/or fever and chills. Get to an emergency room if you suffer from any of these symptoms—they may signal an infection that requires immediate medical care.

## Healing Roller Coaster

In a quirky experiment, researchers created a silicone kidney model (containing urine and stones) and took it on 60 roller-coaster rides.

***Result:*** The passage rate of stones rose by 64% in some tests.

*The Journal of the American Osteopathic Association.*

## Diet Supplement May Help Prevent Kidney Stones

University of Houston, news release.

A dietary supplement may hold the power to dissolve a key component of kidney stones, potentially offering a new prevention tool against this painful condition, researchers say.

It's too early to be sure if the compound hydroxycitrate will become a preventive treatment for kidney stones, since extensive research in people hasn't begun. Still, it could offer an alternative to potassium citrate, which treats kidney stones but has side effects, the study authors explained.

***At issue:*** The calcium oxalate crystals that are the most common component of kidney stones, mineral deposits that form inside the kidneys. They may get stuck in the urinary tract, blocking urination and causing great pain.

Kidney stones affect an estimated 12% of men and 7% of women, but is on the rise in women and teens. High blood pressure, diabetes and obesity can increase the risk.

Physicians often urge people who are at risk to drink a lot of water and avoid foods high in oxalate, such as spinach, almonds, okra and rhubarb. Doctors may also recommend potassium citrate, a dietary supplement that can slow the growth of crystals.

In the recent study, researchers looked at a similar compound known as hydroxycitrate. It is a natural fruit extract available as a dietary supplement.

The investigators found that hydroxycitrate did a better job of slowing the growth of calcium oxalate crystals. Hydroxycitrate appears to form a stronger bond with the crystals, helping to break them up.

The study authors briefly tested the supplement in people, but more in-depth research is needed. There's no information now about long-term safety and dosages.

The study's lead author, Jeffrey Rimer, called the findings promising. He is an associate professor of chemical and biomolecular engineering at the University of Houston.

If it works in people, "similar to our trials in the laboratory, hydroxycitrate has the potential to reduce the incidence rate of people with chronic kidney stone disease," he said in a university news release.

The study was published online in the journal *Nature*.

For more about kidney stones, try the U.S. National Institute of Diabetes and Digestive and Kidney Diseases.

# Thirsty? Dehydrated? Don't Drink THIS!

An article titled "Rehydration with soft drink–like beverages exacerbates dehydration and worsens dehydration-associated renal injury" researchers at Instituto Nacional de Cardiología-Ignacio Chávez, Mexico, University of Colorado, Aurora, and INSERM and Centre de Recherche des Cordeliers, both in France, published in *American Journal of Physiology—Regulatory, Integrative and Comparative Physiology.*

When it's really hot and you're super-thirsty, it might be tempting to reach for a soda pop. But that's one of the worst ways to hydrate—and might not be doing your kidneys any good either.

In a recent four-week animal study, mildly dehydrated rats that drank water with glucose and fructose—the types of sugars in soda—became more dehydrated and showed signs of kidney damage. Rats that drank plain water or water sweetened with stevia (a noncaloric plant-based sugar substitute) were fine. The glucose-fructose water, it turns out, stimulated oxidative and inflammatory processes and increased vasopressin, a hormone secreted by the pituitary gland that, in excess, harms kidneys.

## Symptom of Kidney Disease

Frequent constipation is linked to kidney disease. People with constipation had an average 13% higher risk of developing kidney disease and 9% higher risk for kidney failure than people who were not constipated. Kidney function declined faster in people with more severe constipation.

***Possible reason:*** Constipation may indicate changes in the mix of microorganisms in the gut, and those changes may lead to kidney disease. Further research is needed.

Study of the medical records of 3.5 million US military veterans by researchers at University of Tennessee Health Science Center, Memphis, and Memphis VA Medical Center, published in *Journal of the American Society of Nephrology.*

It's an animal study, to be sure, but the researchers believe that it has meaning for us humans. "Our studies raise serious concerns for the common practice…to drink soft drinks as a means to quench thirst following an episode of dehydration," they write.

You already know what's best for hydration—water. If you like soda, one that's sweetened with stevia might be a good second choice.

# Marathon Running May Cause Short-Term Kidney Injury

Chirag Parikh, MD, PhD, professor of medicine, and director of applied translational research, Yale University, New Haven, Connecticut.

Cathy Fieseler, MD, primary care sports medicine physician, Christus Trinity Mother Frances Health System, Tyler, Texas.

Peter McCullough, MD, vice chief of medicine, Baylor University Medical Center, Dallas.

*American Journal of Kidney Diseases.*

Any marathoner will tell you that the grueling 26-mile races can do a number on the hips, knees, ankles and feet.

Now, a small study suggests that these tests of endurance are also tough on the kidneys.

"Marathon runners demonstrate transient or reverse short-term kidney injury," said Chirag Parikh, MD, PhD, professor of medicine at Yale University.

In his study of 22 participants in the 2015 Hartford, Connecticut Marathon, Dr. Parikh found that 82% showed acute kidney injury after the race. In this condition, the kidneys fail to filter waste from the blood.

The good news is that the kidney injury seems to clear up within two days of the race, he said.

"On day two, they are all fine," Dr. Parikh said.

Runners likely don't even know they've had this transient injury, Dr. Parikh said. "For the short term, I don't think they would notice anything," he said.

Dr. Parikh isn't certain why the strenuous event is linked with kidney injury. But some potential causes include the sustained rise in core body temperature, dehydration or the decreased blood flow to the kidneys that occurs during a marathon, he explained.

When the blood is pumped to the skin and muscles while running, he said, the kidneys may not get as much blood as they normally do.

Nor can Dr. Parikh say whether the effect might be cumulative, getting worse with more marathons run. It may be that the kidney adapts over time instead, he noted.

## Study Details

To evaluate this type of kidney injury, his team looked at blood and urine samples collected before and after the marathon. These tests included measuring blood creatinine levels and proteins in the urine, along with looking at kidney cells on a microscope. Creatinine is a waste product excreted by the kidneys; measuring it in the blood helps assess kidney health.

In a previous study, published in 2011, Peter McCullough, MD, vice chief of medicine at Baylor University Medical Center in Dallas, and colleagues evaluated 25 men and women marathoners. They found 40% of the runners met the definition of acute kidney injury based on their blood creatinine levels.

In the recent study, Dr. Parikh's team also "performed an in-depth evaluation of the urine and found evidence of injury," Dr. McCullough said.

"The larger question looming is whether these repeated bouts of injury in endurance athletes lead to chronic kidney disease years later. Can anything be done about the injury at the time including hydration strategy?" Dr. McCullough said. More study is crucial, he added.

Dr. Parikh said additional research is also needed to assess whether certain people may not recover as quickly. For now, those with a family history of kidney disease should let their physician know they run marathons, he suggested.

## Additional Expert Advice

Cathy Fieseler, MD, said marathoners who want to reduce their risk of kidney injury should avoid anti-inflammatory drugs before the race. Those drugs include over-the-counter *ibuprofen* (Advil, Motrin IB) and *naproxen* (Aleve), Dr. Fieseler said. *Acetaminophen* (Tylenol) is cleared through the liver.

Dr. Fieseler is a primary care sports medicine doctor at Christus Trinity Mother Frances Health System in Tyler, Texas. She's also medical director of the American Running Association.

The study was published in the *American Journal of Kidney Diseases.*

# Past Kidney Damage Linked to Pregnancy Problems

*Journal of the American Society of Nephrology*, news release.

Women with prior kidney damage may have an increased risk for pregnancy complications, a recent study suggests.

"We believe that this study highlights an important finding that will be useful for medical providers caring for reproductive-age women," said study author Jessica Sheehan Tangren, MD, a nephrologist from Massachusetts General Hospital in Boston.

The researchers reviewed data from almost 25,000 women who gave birth at Massachusetts General Hospital between 1998 and 2007. Just over 100 of the women had previously experienced acute kidney injury. This is a sudden decrease in kidney function.

All of the women had recovered normal kidney function before they were pregnant.

Women in the kidney damage group had much higher rates of a condition called preeclampsia that causes high blood pressure and other problems during pregnancy—23% compared with 4% in the non-injury group.

Women who had kidney damage were also more likely to have small-for-gestational-age babies (15% versus 8%), and to give birth earlier (average 37.6 weeks compared with 39.2 weeks), the study showed.

Dr. Tangren and her colleagues adjusted the findings to account for other factors that could contribute to the risk.

Although the study wasn't designed to prove a cause-and-effect link, the researchers found prior kidney damage was tied to a nearly six times higher risk for preeclampsia.

Women with previous kidney damage also had more than twice the risk for poor infant outcomes.

The study was published online in the *Journal of the American Society of Nephrology.*

"Our goal in future studies is to address why women with a history of acute kidney injury are at higher risk for pregnancy complications and to identify strategies to lower their risk," Dr. Tangren said in a journal news release.

She also said that the varying rates of preeclampsia seen worldwide may be partly explained by the findings.

# Women Don't Like Male Kidneys

*Clinical Journal of the American Society of Nephrology*, news release.

Weight and gender differences between donors and recipients can affect the success of kidney transplants, a recent study says.

Researchers reviewed data from more than 115,000 people in the United States who received a kidney from a deceased donor. The transplants took place between 2000 and 2014.

The average follow-up time was about four years. During that time, more than 21,000 patients developed transplant failure.

After accounting for other possible causes, the researchers concluded that weight was a factor in transplant failure. Specifically, if a kidney transplant recipient was more than 66 pounds heavier than the donor, there was a 28% higher risk of transplant failure, compared with recipients who weighed about the same as donors.

The researchers also noted a difference if the donor and recipient's genders were mismatched. The risk of transplant failure was 35% higher for a male receiving a kidney from a female donor. In women receiving a man's kidney, the odds of transplant failure were 50% higher.

That level of risk is similar to that faced by a recipient who receives a kidney from a donor who has diabetes, the study authors said.

The findings were published in the *Clinical Journal of the American Society of Nephrology*.

A kidney donor's weight and sex are not typically considered when choosing a recipient. These findings suggest that such factors may need to be considered, the researchers said.

"This study is extremely important because we have shown that when all else is considered, something as simple as the combination of a kidney donor's weight and sex is associated with a marked increase in kidney transplant failure," study coleader Amanda Miller, MD, said in a journal news release. Dr. Miller is from Dalhousie University and the Nova Scotia Health Authority, Canada.

She said more research is needed before taking weight and gender into consideration when matching donors and recipients. But the findings suggest that current matching strategies may need to take other factors into account, she added.

However, matching donors and patients by weight and gender would be complex and could leave some potential recipients at a disadvantage, Bethany Foster, MD, and Indra Gupta, MD, of McGill University in Montreal, said in an accompanying editorial.

"Restricting transplant options by prioritizing sex matching may also lead to longer waiting times," they wrote. "Females with a large body size would be particularly disadvantaged by an approach that favored allocation of sex- and body size-matched kidneys."

The U.S. National Institute of Diabetes and Digestive and Kidney Diseases has more on kidney transplant.

## Coming Soon: A Wearable Artificial Kidney?

Maria DeVita, MD, associate director, nephrology, Lenox Hill Hospital, New York City.

Robert Courgi, MD, hospitalist and endocrinologist, Northwell Health's Southside Hospital, Bay Shore, New York.

Victor Gura, MD, internist and nephrologist, Cedars-Sinai Medical Center, Los Angeles.

University of Washington, news release.

Someday, dialysis patients might free themselves of clunky machines, moving about with a "wearable artificial kidney" instead.

That's the promise of a new clinical trial that suggests this type of technology is finally within reach.

"This would be a game changer," said one kidney specialist, Maria DeVita, MD. "The fact that clinical trials are beginning gives us all hope that we will have a significant improvement in the care of those patients requiring ongoing hemodialysis."

Dr. DeVita is associate director of nephrology at Lenox Hill Hospital in New York City.

### Background

People with advanced kidney disease must often resort to spending hours a day several times a week at dialysis centers, with special machines cleansing their blood as their kidneys once did.

The dream has long been a small portable device that could perform dialysis as patients went about their usual day.

## New Study

***That dream may be getting nearer:*** A prototype of such a device was recently tested on seven patients at the University of Washington Medical Center in Seattle. The study was led by the device's inventor, Victor Gura, MD, of Cedars-Sinai Medical Center in Los Angeles and chief medical officer of Blood Purifications Technologies in California.

The trial was designed to see how well the wearable kidney might work to safely take over some of the functions of failed kidneys. Patients used the device for up to 24 hours.

***It did seem to work:*** The device successfully cleared the blood of urea, creatinine and phosphorus—all waste products, the resarchers said. It also helped rid the blood of excess water and salt.

Patients seemed to tolerate the therapy well, with no effect on circulation and no serious adverse effects, Dr. Gura's team found.

And there was another bonus. During standard dialysis, patients have to adhere to a strict diet to keep blood electrolytes stable. But the participants in the trial had no such problems, even when they ate what they wanted, the researchers said.

## Implications

Overall, the research team believes that a wearable artificial kidney is feasible. However, the researchers said some redesigns are needed to correct device-related technical problems that occurred during testing.

For example, there was excessive formation of carbon dioxide gas bubbles in the dialysis solution, and intermittent variations in solution and blood flow, Dr. Gura's team explained.

The device redesigns will also focus on ease of use and reliability during use, because the objective is to enable patients to undergo dialysis at home.

The study was published in the journal *JCI Insights.*

## Expert Commentary

"The wearable artificial kidney is a concept that has been discussed for years," said Robert Courgi, MD, an endocrinologist at Northwell Health's Southside Hospital in Bay Shore, New York.

"It is exciting to see this technological breakthrough come to reality in clinical trials," he said.

"Unfortunately there were some shortcomings, in the form of technical problems, and traditional hemodialysis remains the standard of care for the moment," Dr. Courgi said. However, "the wearable artificial kidney may become a reality in the very near future," he added.

The National Kidney Foundation website has more information about dialysis at Kid ney.org. Search "hemodialysis."

# Kidney Failure Linked to Some Forms of Cancer

Kidney and thyroid cancers are more common in people who are on dialysis for kidney failure, possibly because of their severely impaired kidney function. Kidney transplant patients also have higher cancer risk—specifically for non-Hodgkin's lymphoma, lung cancer, melanoma and other skin cancers. The increased risk may be related to drugs that suppress the immune system after the transplant.

***Self-defense:*** Discuss your cancer risk with your doctor.

Analysis of data on 202,195 people by researchers at U.S. National Cancer Institute, Bethesda, Maryland, published in *Journal of the American Society of Nephrology.*

## Beware of Hidden Liver Disease

Jamison Starbuck, ND, a naturopathic physician in family practice and a guest lecturer at the University of Montana, both in Missoula. She is a past president of the American Association of Naturopathic Physicians and a contributing editor to *The Alternative Advisor: The Complete Guide to Natural Therapies and Alternative Treatments.* DrJamisonStarbuck.com

If you think of liver disease, chances are alcoholics and heavy drinkers come to mind. While it's true that these individuals are at increased risk for cirrhosis and certain other liver disorders, there's another condition that can affect this vital organ even in people who drink little (if any) alcohol. Fatty liver is a condition in which fat accumulates in the liver. This disease is very common in people who consume a lot of alcohol, but it's also reaching almost epidemic proportions in the US in nonalcoholics. Among those who aren't drinking heavily, obesity is the main risk factor. Individuals who have high triglycerides or diabetes (or even borderline diabetes) are also at increased risk for fatty liver.

What's most concerning is the insidious way that this condition progresses. As fat continues to accumulate in the liver, the organ becomes inflamed. Months or years of liver inflammation leads to scarring within the liver—and eventually to cirrhosis, possible liver failure (unless the person has a liver transplant) and death. In its early stages, fatty liver causes few symptoms. Your doctor might be able to palpate an enlarged liver, and you may have some indigestion and/or a swollen abdomen. But there is no specific testing for fatty liver, other than a liver biopsy, which involves surgically removing and analyzing a tissue sample from the organ. For this reason, fatty liver disease is usually diagnosed by a doctor based on a physical exam, lifestyle evaluation (red flags include a poor diet and lack of physical activity), excessive body weight and lab tests that show elevated lipids, such as triglycerides, and high blood glucose.

When it comes to treating fatty liver, conventional medical doctors recommend weight loss and perhaps medication for a related condition such as high cholesterol or diabetes. Naturopathic medicine, on the other hand, offers several effective treatment options. *My protocol for fatty liver disease...*

- **Diet.** I agree with medical doctors—if you have fatty liver and are overweight, you must lose weight. But do so slowly. Losing more than three pounds a week is hard on your liver. When planning meals, go low-carb—stay away from pasta, bread and sweets. Limit whole grains to two servings a day. Eat vegetables, fresh fruit, nuts, seeds, legumes and no more than one daily serving each of low-fat dairy, lean meat and fish.

- **Get the right nutrients.** Vitamin C is a powerful antioxidant that can help repair damaged liver cells. And a multivitamin offers other minerals and vitamins necessary for healthy liver function. In addition, I prescribe choline and methionine—these nutrients are essential for the breakdown of fats that can promote fatty liver.

***Typical dose:*** 400 mg each of choline and methionine.

- **Try herbs.** Research shows that artichoke, dandelion and beet can reduce blood fats that promote fatty liver and support the health of liver cells. You can eat these as vegetables...or take them in powdered form in capsules. You can also find general formulas that contain lipotropic botanical compounds, which help protect the liver by breaking down fats in the blood. Follow the manufacturer's recommended dose for each of these supplements.

By taking these steps, under the supervision of your doctor, you may be able to actually reverse fatty liver disease—and in the process improve your digestion...boost your energy levels...and perhaps even increase your life span!

## Yogurt for Liver Health

In animal studies, the probiotics found in yogurt and other foods reduced the size of liver tumors by 40%.

***Theory:*** Probiotics help block angiogenesis, the growth of tumor blood vessels.

Proceedings of the National Academy of Sciences.

## What Your Skin Says About Your Liver Health

Jeffrey P. Callen, MD, a professor of medicine and chief of the division of dermatology at the University of Louisville School of Medicine in Kentucky.

A red, itchy rash...little yellow bumps...extremely dry skin. The list of skin problems can go on and on. But did you know that a skin issue isn't always just about your skin? It might be alerting you to an internal problem, such as hepatits C, that your doctor needs to know about and treat.

Hepatitis C is a liver infection caused by the blood-borne hepatitis C virus. It increases the risk for cirrhosis and liver cancer. New medications can cure the disease, but it's symptomless in three out of four cases. *However, the skin can sometimes provide an early clue...*

- **Blistered, fragile skin on the backs of the hands.** This condition can be a sign of hepatitis C. Called porphyria cutanea tarda, it's characterized by sensitivity to sunlight and is also seen in alcoholics and can occur as a drug side effect, particularly with nonsteroidal anti-inflammatory drugs (NSAIDs) such as aspirin and *ibuprofen* (Motrin, Advil). When the hepatitis C is effectively treated, the skin issue goes away.

- **Red, tender spots on the lower legs.** This can be caused by inflammation of blood vessels, which occurs in some people who have hepatitis C. Like porphyria, it resolves when hepatitis C is treated.

## Liver Disease Is Rampant

Rich Snyder, DO, nephrologist, osteopathic physician and clinical professor at Philadelphia College of Osteopathic Medicine. He is author of *What You Must Know About Liver Disease: A Practical Guide to Using Conventional and Complementary Treatments.*

Alarming fact—about 30 million Americans have some form of liver disease. That's one-tenth of the population. Yet it's normal for people to go undiagnosed for years or even decades.

Unless liver disease is detected and treated early, it can cause severe inflammation that can lead to scarring (cirrhosis), organ failure and/or cancer—and it even may require a transplant. It is a leading cause of death in the US.

***Important:*** I advise patients who have risk factors for liver disease to get their livers checked—the inexpensive group of blood tests can be done during routine checkups. Risk factors include obesity, metabolic syndrome, hepatitis and a history of alcohol or drug abuse.

If you have liver disease, medications may be required, but herbs and supplements can help reduce inflammation, improve liver function and slow ongoing damage. Always speak with your doctor before taking any natural supplements.

I usually advise patients to start with just one remedy at a time. After six to eight weeks, we reassess to see if there's improvement and if an additional supplement is required. Any of the herbs below can be started first, but milk thistle and turmeric are among the more common options.

### Milk Thistle

Milk thistle has been used for thousands of years for liver health. It's among the most studied herbs for treating hepatitis and other liver diseases.

Milk thistle (a member of the plant family that includes daisies and sunflowers) contains a flavonoid called silymarin. It's an antioxidant that reduces inflammation, blocks the movement of toxins into liver cells and increases the output of enzymes that prevent toxin-related damage.

Research suggests that milk thistle can improve liver function and improve survival in patients with chronic hepatitis and/or cirrhosis. One study found that it reduced the viral load (the amount of viral particles in the blood) in hepatitis C patients who hadn't responded to drug treatments.

***Typical dosage:*** If you have risk factors for liver disease or if you've been diagnosed with liver disease, talk to your doctor about taking 100 mg twice a day, to start—your doctor might recommend a higher dose (between 200 mg and 600 mg) if lab tests aren't improving. Milk thistle is unlikely to cause side effects, although it should be avoided if you're allergic to ragweed or one of its relatives, such as sunflower seeds or chamomile.

## Turmeric

The active ingredient in this spice, curcumin, is an exceptionally potent antioxidant that has been shown to reduce jaundice (the dark urine and/or yellowing of the skin or eyes that often occurs in liver patients).

There's also some evidence that it reduces liver scarring. A study published in *Gut* found that turmeric helped prevent a hepatitis-causing virus from moving from one cell to another.

***Typical dosage:*** Between 500 mg and 1,500 mg of a turmeric supplement daily, divided into two or three doses. (Exact dose will depend on your weight, symptoms and other factors.)

***Caution:*** Turmeric has blood-thinning properties, so it may not be best if you are on a blood thinner such as *warfarin* or if your liver disease is advanced and clotting of the blood is a problem.

## N-acetylcysteine (NAC)

Doctors who specialize in natural health recommend this supplement for liver patients. It reduces inflammation and increases intracellular levels of glutathione, the "master antioxidant" that is mainly produced and stored in the liver and that is depleted by liver disease.

Doctors give it to improve the viability of transplanted livers. It also is used in patients with liver damage caused by *acetaminophen* overdose (acetaminophen rapidly depletes glutathione).

***Typical dosage:*** 600 mg, twice daily.

## Glutathione

You don't have to take this supplement if you already are using NAC (which is converted to glutathione in the body), but I often advise my patients to take glutathione because it helps rebuild body tissues, including liver cells.

Glutathione is particularly helpful if you regularly use acetaminophen for treating arthritis or another painful condition because acetaminophen, as mentioned before, can deplete glutathione levels. Oral glutathione usually needs to be taken with cysteine, which helps glutathione get into the cells.

Follow dosing directions on the label.

## Coffee

Coffee isn't a cure for liver disease, but there's good evidence that it reduces liver inflammation and may reduce liver-related health risks, including cirrhosis and cancer.

One study found that hepatitis B patients who drank more than four cups of coffee a week were only about half as likely to develop hepatocellular carcinoma (a form of liver cancer) as those who did not drink coffee.

Another study—one that looked at 430,000 people—found that people who drank an extra two cups of coffee a day could potentially reduce their risk for cirrhosis by 44%.

## Weight Loss Is Crucial for Your Liver

Non-alcoholic fatty liver disease (NAFLD) is the leading type of liver disease in the US. It affects up to 25% of all adults and is linked to obesity and metabolic syndrome (a constellation of problems that includes high blood pressure, high blood sugar and elevated triglycerides, along with obesity).

A liver is considered "fat" if more than 5% to 10% of its weight comes from fatty tissue. This serious disease can lead to severe inflammation, cirrhosis or liver failure.

You have to lose weight if you've been diagnosed with NAFLD. Studies have shown that it may be possible to eliminate the condition altogether by losing as little as 10% of your total weight.

***Also helpful:*** Alpha lipoic acid. It's a well-researched supplement that can decrease insulin resistance and improve metabolic syndrome. I advise patients with NAFLD to take 200 mg daily, increasing the dose by 100 mg weekly until they reach a maximum dose of 400 mg to 600 mg.

If you have diabetes or are at risk for diabetes, you may need to check your blood glucose levels because alpha lipoic acid has the potential to decrease glucose levels in some individuals.

# Even One High-Fat Meal Can Harm Your Liver, Study Finds

Michael Roden, MD, scientific director, German Diabetes Center, Leibniz Center for Diabetes Research, Heinrich Heine University Dusseldorf, Germany.

Hannele Yki-Jarvinen, MD, professor, medicine, University of Helsinki, Finland.

*Journal of Clinical Investigation.*

Eating a high-fat meal—say, a cheeseburger and fries or a pepperoni pizza—disrupts liver function, a recent, small study reveals.

Researchers found that the high levels of saturated fat found in such rich foods immediately alter the work of the liver, possibly setting the body up for serious disease down the line.

"The effects mimic the abnormalities seen in people with severe metabolic disease," said study coauthor Michael Roden, MD, referring to conditions like fatty liver disease and cirrhosis.

"Our findings paint the picture of the earliest changes in liver metabolism leading to fatty liver diseases and liver cirrhosis in the context of obesity and type 2 diabetes," said Dr. Roden. He's scientific director of the German Diabetes Center at Heinrich Heine University in Dusseldorf.

How long these metabolic alterations last after people indulge in a rich meal isn't clear.

The liver plays a crucial role in processing the fats and carbohydrates people eat.

In some cases when fatty foods are repeatedly eaten to excess, fats accumulate and cause a condition known as nonalcoholic fatty liver.

This condition has ballooned along with the US obesity epidemic, and is thought to affect as many as 25% of people in the United States. It can lead to cirrhosis, a serious condition characterized by scarring of the liver.

Hannele Yki-Jarvinen, MD, is professor of medicine at the University of Helsinki in Finland. "We know diets high in saturated fat make the liver fatty," she said.

"Saturated fats such as in butter, fatty cheeses and coconut oil are thus the worst thing to eat from the liver perspective," said Dr. Yki-Jarvinen, coauthor of a commentary accompanying the recent study.

## Study Details

For the study, the researchers assigned 14 healthy, lean young men to consume a placebo or a dose of palm oil that varied according to their weight. The palm oil provided levels of saturated fat equivalent to that from an eight-slice pepperoni pizza or a cheeseburger with large fries, the report said.

This "fat loading" caused the liver to produce 70% more glucose, which could boost blood sugar levels over time, Dr. Roden said. Potentially, this could contribute to insulin sensitivity—a precursor to type 2 diabetes.

Fat loading also caused liver cells to work harder, which could stress them and contribute to liver disease, he noted.

In addition, the saturated fat lowered the liver's ability to store glucose compared with fat, "which over time might favor fatty liver disease," Dr. Roden said.

It's possible that healthy people could easily overcome these effects while those who repeatedly eat fat-laden foods might be less fortunate, Dr. Roden added.

Dr. Yki-Jarvinen said that while cirrhosis is difficult to reverse, most people can boost their liver health.

"If you change your diet to a more healthy one containing healthy fats, such as found in olive oil, your liver fat decreases in a few days," she said.

In addition to their work with humans, the researchers also launched a similar analysis of fat intake in mice. This provided insight into how fat affects the workings of genes, the study authors said.

Next, Dr. Roden said he hopes to learn how long the effects of one high-fat meal last and how that compares with those of other nutrients, such as proteins and carbohydrates.

The study was published in the *Journal of Clinical Investigation.*

## Trace Blood in Urine

Hematuria (blood in the urine) can range in amount from "trace" (invisible to the naked eye) to large, noticeable amounts. There are many reasons for hematuria, including bladder or kidney infections, an inflamed prostate, and certain medications such as aspirin, penicillin and chemotherapy drugs. Strenuous exercise can even cause blood to leak into the urinary tract.

But because blood in the urine is one symptom of urinary tract cancer, it should be monitored. If you had trace amounts of blood and no other symptoms (such as pain and/or frequent urination, which are common with infection), you will need follow-up urine tests in three to six months. If the blood remains, see a urologist, who may recommend imaging tests such as ultrasound or cystoscopy (a bladder exam done with a thin tube equipped with a camera on the end).

Mildred Lam, MD, professor of medicine, Case Western Reserve University School of Medicine, Cleveland.

## Beat Urinary Incontinence with a Stronger Pelvic Floor

Lesli Lo, DPT, a women's health physical therapist (WHPT) at Northwestern Medical Group and an instructor of obstetrics and gynecology at Northwestern University Feinberg School of Medicine, both in Chicago.

If you're a woman who urinates when you laugh or cough, or sometimes feels overcome by a sudden, nearly uncontrollable urge to urinate—that is, if you have urinary incontinence—you've undoubtedly heard of Kegel exercises...and maybe even tried them. The do-anywhere pelvic exercises are often recommended for this condition—and a wide variety of other pelvic problems, including fecal (bowel) incontinence and pelvic organ prolapse, in which the bladder or uterus bulges into the vagina.

But doing Kegels may be making your problem worse. Eventually, Kegels can be part of the solution, but you need to take these steps first.

### A Pelvic Floor Primer

The pelvic floor is a network of muscles, ligaments and tissue that acts like a sling to support a woman's pelvic organs—the uterus, vagina, bladder/urethra and rectum. You control your bowel and bladder by contracting and relaxing these muscles and tissues. About 25% of women ages 40 to 59 will suffer pelvic floor dysfunction (PFD) in their lifetime. Risk factors for PFD include menopause, age, obesity, repeated heavy lifting and traumatic injury—as may happen during childbirth, for example, or from a hip or back injury. Over time, the likelihood of a pelvic floor disorder increases.

## Myths About Kegels

Women with PFD often think their internal muscles are too weak and do Kegels to strengthen them. That's often true, but it isn't the biggest problem. For 99% of my patients, those muscles are too tight, so they often get stuck in a contracted position, unable to control the flow of urine or to fully relax and contract in a pleasurable way during intercourse. Kegels can worsen the situation by strengthening already too-tight muscles. What these patients really need is to relax these muscles.

***The first step:*** Bring up your symptoms with your internist, ob/gyn, urogynecologist or urologist, who can rule out issues that aren't musculoskeletal. If physical therapy is the next best course of treatment, he/she can refer you to a women's health physical therapist (WHPT). WHPTs treat not just the pelvic floor but the body as a whole. Three to six months of weekly manual therapy sessions, combined with homework, usually ease symptoms of urinary incontinence, painful intercourse and/or pelvic pain.

A WHPT will perform an internal exam to assess your areas of strength and weakness and design a plan to retrain your muscles. To find a WHPT in your area, go to WomensHealthAPTA.org for a locator from the American Physical Therapy Association. Insurance typically covers these services.

## Toning the Right Way

A crucial component of treatment is manual therapy—a WHPT uses her hands to gently massage, stretch and release spasms and trigger points within the deep and soft tissues of the vagina. This helps reduce tightness and tension and can even break up scar tissue that's further restricting tissues, allowing the pelvic floor muscles to fully relax and contract. Though it can feel uncomfortable initially, any pain quickly recedes as the muscles and tissues relax.

Manual therapy is a prime opportunity to assess how you do Kegels. During such therapy, I will insert one finger into the vagina and then ask my patient to perform a Kegel by imagining that she is stopping the flow of urine midstream. (Once a woman learns how to do this correctly, she can do it herself.) Two out of three women do this incorrectly, tightening their pelvic floor muscles but not releasing them all the way back down—or not tightening their pelvic floor at all. The goal is to fully relax these muscles. *What helps...*

- **Reverse Kegels.** In a conventional Kegel, you tighten your pelvic floor muscles, hold the contraction for 10 seconds, then fully relax back down. In a reverse Kegel, you begin by relaxing the muscles as you do when you've just sat down on the toilet with a full bladder and are able to urinate. You should feel your anus relax as well. Hold for 10 seconds while you continue to breathe. Then return to normal for 10 seconds. Repeat the reverse Kegel 10 times, two to three times daily.
- **Biofeedback.** This pain-free, nonsurgical technique allows patients to see their pelvic muscles at rest and while contracted—and improves their ability to retrain the pelvic floor. A sensor or small weight is inserted into the vagina, while a nearby computer provides visual feedback.
- **New: Home biofeedback.** The apps Elvie ($199, Apple/Android, Elvie.com) and PeriCoach ($249, Apple/Android, PeriCoach.com) use intravaginal devices to assess the strength and endurance of vaginal contractions, and then send data to your smartphone via Bluetooth. If you've already had a professional pelvic assessment and know how to do Kegels the right way, these products can be helpful.

## A Lifestyle Solution

Shallow breathing also contributes to pelvic floor disorders.

***Why:*** The diaphragm, a sheet of muscle that separates the chest cavity from the abdomen, gets stuck in a contracted position—causing pelvic muscles to contract, too.

***Solution:*** Learn diaphragmatic breathing. Lying down, pretend your belly is a balloon and fill it with air, keeping your chest still. Now exhale, deflating the balloon. Do this once an hour for five breaths...and for five minutes before bed. In two to three weeks, you should notice a change in the way you breathe.

# Staying Trim, Strong May Cut Risk of Urinary Incontinence

Anne Suskind, MD, assistant professor of urology, University of California, San Francisco.

Megan Schimpf, MD, chair, Public Education Committee, American Urogynecologic Society, and associate professor, obstetrics and gynecology, University of Michigan, Ann Arbor.

*Journal of the American Geriatrics Society.*

Urinary incontinence is a widespread complaint among women, but a recent study suggests that older women may find relief from this frustrating problem if they're slimmer and stronger.

The study followed nearly 1,500 women in their 70s for three years. Researchers found that a decrease in body mass index of 5% or more during that time led to a 50% reduction in the risk of new or persistent stress urinary incontinence.

Body mass index (BMI) is a rough estimate of a person's body fat based on height and weight. For example, a woman who's 5 feet 6 inches tall who weighs 175 pounds has a BMI of 28.2. If she lost 5% of her BMI, it would be 26.8, which translates to a weight loss of about nine pounds.

The study also showed that a decrease in grip strength of 5% or more was linked to 60% higher odds of new or persistent stress urinary incontinence. Grip strength is considered an indicator of overall muscle strength, the study authors said.

"Our study found that changes in body composition and grip strength are associated with changes in stress urinary incontinence frequency over time, but not with changes in urgency urinary incontinence frequency over time," said the study's lead author Anne Suskind, MD. She's an assistant professor of urology at the University of California, San Francisco.

## Two Kinds of Urinary Incontinence

Dr. Suskind said that distinguishing between the two types of urinary incontinence is important.

"Stress incontinence is involuntary leakage of urine associated with an increase in abdominal pressure (i.e., coughing, laughing, sneezing)," she explained.

"Urgency urinary incontinence is involuntary leakage of urine accompanied or immediately preceded by a sense of urgency. The underlying mechanisms of each type of incontinence differ and each type of incontinence is treated differently," Dr. Suskind said.

Stress urinary incontinence tends to happen after delivering children, said Megan Schimpf, MD. She's chair of the Public Education Committee for the American Urogynecologic Society.

Urgency incontinence may be caused by neurological issues, Dr. Schimpf said.

## Study Details

At the start of the study, there were 1,475 women aged 70 to 79. Of those, 212 women said they had at least monthly stress urinary incontinence, and 233 said they had at least monthly urgency urinary incontinence.

Women who said they had at least monthly urinary incontinence had an average BMI of about 28. It was slightly lower—27.5—for women who didn't have incontinence. A BMI between 24.9 and 29.9 is considered overweight. A BMI above 30 is considered obese.

After three years of follow-up, 1,137 women were still in the study.

Of those women, 164 women said they had new or persistent stress urinary incontinence, and 320 had new or persistent urgency urinary incontinence.

The study authors suggested that losing weigh—even for a woman in her 70s—may help stress urinary incontinence by relieving some of the pressure on the bladder. Likewise, grip strength may indicate overall strength, and stronger bladder muscles may be able to withstand more pressure.

Neither of these factors was linked to an improvement in urgency urinary incontinence. This may be because urgency urinary incontinence could be the result of years of damage that isn't so easily reversible, the researchers noted.

### Urinary Incontinence Is Treatable

Dr. Schimpf said whatever the cause, women of all ages with urinary incontinence should see their doctor.

"A lot of women are unfortunately under the assumption that incontinence issues are normal, and that's definitely not the case," Dr. Schimpf said.

There are a number of treatments for stress incontinence—from pelvic floor physical therapy to silicone devices called pessaries, to surgery—and these treatments aren't one-size-fits-all, she added.

Dr. Schimpf said caffeine, alcohol, nicotine and artificially sweetened beverages can irritate the bladder and trigger bladder spasms, which can lead to overactive bladder symptoms.

Circling back to the recent study's findings, Dr. Suskind pointed out that weight loss and increased strength can also be effective treatments. "Appropriate diet and exercise would be a good place to start, and may be helpful in decreasing the odds of new or worsening stress of urinary incontinence," she said.

The study was published recently in the *Journal of the American Geriatrics Society*.

There's more on urinary incontinence at ACOG.org/Patients/FAQs/Urinary-Incontinence, the website of the American College of Obstetricians & Gynecologists.

## Drink Cranberry Juice

Urinary tract infections might be prevented with cranberry juice.

***Recent finding:*** Over a 24-week period, drinking an eight-ounce glass of a cranberry beverage once a day cut UTI incidence in women who had had two or more UTIs within the past year by approximately 40%.

***Always best:*** Avoid the sugary versions of cranberry and other fruit drinks.

Tomas L. Griebling, MD, MPH, distinguished professor of urology, University of Kansas School of Medicine, Kansas City.

## PT for Urine Leaks

Physical therapy stops urine leaks.

***Recent study:*** Women with osteoporosis or low bone density who reported more stress incontinence (urine leaks when coughing, laughing or exercising) than women with strong bones had 12 weeks of physical therapy (PT) focusing on pelvic-floor muscles.

***Result:*** The PT group had 75% fewer episodes of urinary leaking than those who did not get PT. The benefit lasted for about a year.

Meena M. Sran, PT, PhD, physiotherapist, BC Women's Hospital & Health Centre, Vancouver, British Columbia, Canada.

Chapter 10

# PAIN RELIEF AND AUTOIMMUNE DISEASE CURES

## Drug-Free Pain Cures You Need to Try

If you're among the estimated 25% of adults in the US who live with moderate-to-severe chronic pain, from conditions such as arthritis, headaches and fibromyalgia, you may be so desperate for relief that you decide to try a powerful opioid—and take your chances with side effects.

It's widely known that people can become dependent on (or addicted to) these drugs—including older standbys such as morphine and codeine...as well as newer heavy hitters such as *hydrocodone* (Vicodin, Norco) and *oxycodone* (OxyContin, Percocet). Yet many doctors are still too quick to prescribe them.

Sadly, these drugs don't stop the root cause of the pain—they simply block the intensity of pain signals that a patient feels. While opioids can be appropriate for acute conditions (including broken bones and postsurgical pain), they rarely are the best choice for chronic pain.

What's more, a recent study published in *JAMA* (*The Journal of the American Medical Association*) found that long-acting opioids, such as OxyContin or *fentanyl* (Duragesic), increase one's risk for death by 65%—due to heart attack and other cardiovascular events.

So what's the best solution for chronic pain?

### The Pain Medicine Paradox

It's an unfortunate paradox that pain medicine can actually worsen pain. In fact, researchers are now finding that patients who are weaned off opioids, using such nondrug therapies as physical therapy and relaxation exercises instead, actually can experience less pain than they did while on opioids, and they have a greater sense of well-being and function better.

***Here's what happens:*** It's relatively easy to develop a tolerance to an opioid, which requires increasingly higher doses for the drug to work. Even when properly prescribed, chronic high doses of these medications can trigger a condition called hyperalgesia, which results in new pain sensitivity either in the primary area of pain or in a new area. For example, a patient who takes an opioid for low-back pain may begin to develop neck pain and headaches.

---

Heather Tick, MD, holds the Gunn-Loke Endowed Professorship for Integrative Pain Medicine at the University of Washington in Seattle and is a clinical associate professor in both the departments of family medicine, and anesthesiology and pain medicine. She is author of *Holistic Pain Relief*.

***The good news:*** Nonopioid therapies that stimulate the parasympathetic nervous system—the branch of the nervous system that helps us feel calm and relaxed—can be highly effective for pain relief.

Chronic pain patients tend to live in the sympathetic nervous system's "fight or flight" mode, which intensifies pain by secreting inflammation-promoting hormones. That's why it's crucial to fire up the parasympathetic system, which tells the body to secrete acetylcholine instead, a neurotransmitter that counteracts inflammation.

There's strong evidence supporting the effectiveness of meditation for fighting pain. It induces the relaxation response—literally altering your body's chemistry. Meditation also lowers stress hormone levels, decreases muscle tension and builds pain tolerance. Other ways to trigger the parasympathetic system's pain-fighting mechanism...*

• **Autogenic training.** Autogenic training (AT) is a relaxation technique based on a set of affirmations (self-directed statements) that are designed to reverse the physical effects of stress. You can buy AT recordings online, in which a person with a soothing voice says the affirmations...or you can repeat them to yourself or make your own recording, using a script like the one below.

***What to do:*** Sit or lie in a comfortable, quiet room. Repeat each of the following statements three times, then dwell on each statement for about 30 seconds afterward. Try to truly feel each sensation in the script. Do this daily.

I am completely calm.

My arms feel heavy and warm.

My legs feel heavy and warm.

My heartbeat is calm and regular.

My abdomen is warm and comfortable.

My forehead is pleasantly cool.

My shoulders are heavy and warm.

*Consult your doctor before trying these methods or the supplement described here—especially if you take blood thinners or have a chronic medical condition such as hypertension.

• **Ujjayi breathing.** Stress causes us to breathe shallowly from the chest instead of deeply from the belly. This leaves stale air trapped in the bottom of the lungs and hinders delivery of healing oxygen to muscles. Any deep-breathing technique can stimulate the parasympathetic system, but Ujjayi (pronounced oo-ja-EE) breathing is particularly effective.

***What to do:*** To get the hang of this technique, inhale deeply through your nose and exhale through your open mouth, gently constricting the muscles at the back of your throat and making a HAAAH sound, as if you were trying to fog up a mirror. Then try to make the same sound on the inhale.

Once you've achieved the correct sound, close your mouth and breathe in and out through your nose, making the HAAAH sound on both the inhale and exhale. Spend equal time (at a pace that's comfortable for you) inhaling and exhaling several times a day. When you first start this technique, try to do it for six  minutes at a time. You can work up to 15 to 20 minutes at a time.

***Important:*** If you have a favorite deep-breathing technique of your own, feel free to use that—just be sure that you keep the flow of air constant, and you don't hold your breath for longer than a beat. Otherwise, you will stimulate the sympathetic nervous system, triggering the pain response.

## Another Nondrug Solution

In addition to the approaches described above, the following supplement can help ease pain by reducing inflammation...

• **Turmeric.** This mildly bitter spice is a powerful analgesic with impressive anti-inflammatory powers. A 2014 study suggested it may be as effective as *ibuprofen* in reducing the pain of knee osteoarthritis.

Capsules are one option to try. But if you like the taste, try making "Golden Milk."

***What to do:*** Combine one-quarter cup of turmeric with one-half cup of water in a pot, and blend to create a thick paste. Heat gently, adding a pinch of ground black pepper and drizzling in water as needed to maintain a thick but stirrable consistency.

Refrigerate the mixture in a glass container, and add one heaping teaspoon to an eight-ounce glass of warm water mixed with a little almond milk every day. You can add some honey to cut the bitterness. Or use warm broth instead of water and a dash of ginger and/or garlic for a tasty soup.

# You May Be Using the Wrong Painkiller

Jianguo Cheng, MD, PhD, professor of anesthesiology and director of the Cleveland Clinic Multidisciplinary Pain Medicine Fellowship Program, and president-elect of the American Academy of Pain Medicine. Recognized by Becker's Review as one of the 70 Best Pain Management Physicians in America, he has published more than 200 research papers, articles and book chapters.

Millions of Americans fight their pain and inflammation with an over-the-counter (OTC) nonsteroidal anti-inflammatory drug (NSAID), such as *ibuprofen* (Motrin, Advil) or *naproxen* (Aleve, Naprosyn)—or a prescription anti-inflammatory, such as *celecoxib* (Celebrex). But if you've got heart disease and/or kidney disease, finding a pain reliever that won't worsen your other condition is tricky.

***What most people don't realize:*** Even in healthy people, NSAIDs—especially when taken for longer or at higher doses than directed by a doctor—increase risk for heart attack and stroke and can potentially harm the kidneys. For those who already have heart disease and/or kidney disease, these risks are even greater.

It's widely known that NSAIDs can cause stomach bleeding as a side effect, but the potential risks to the user's heart and kidneys are not nearly as well recognized.

***Important:*** Short-term use of any NSAID (no longer than 10 days) is always preferable to long-term use. In fact, you may not need drugs at all. *Pain relief options if you have...*

## Heart Disease

***Background:*** NSAIDs raise one's risk for heart attack and stroke by increasing blood clot formation. These medications can also interfere with certain high blood pressure drugs, such as diuretics...angiotensin-converting enzyme (ACE) inhibitors...and beta-blockers, and cause the body to retain fluid—a problem that often plagues people with heart failure.

***If you have known risks for heart disease:*** For people with risk factors such as high blood pressure, diabetes, an enlarged heart or an abnormal EKG reading with no clinical symptoms, NSAIDs may be used, under a doctor's supervision. Celecoxib is generally safer for pain than naproxen or ibuprofen because it is associated with fewer gastrointestinal and/or renal complications.

People treating high blood pressure with an ACE inhibitor drug, such as *captopril* (Capoten) or *benazepril* (Lotensin), should aim for lower doses of celecoxib than typically prescribed (for example, less than 150 mg per day) and use it for no more than 10 days.

***If you have known heart disease:*** NSAIDs increase the risk for new cardiovascular events in people with established heart disease and may lead to heart failure in those with severe heart disease. NSAIDs should be avoided in those with recent heart attack, unstable angina or poorly controlled heart failure. For these individuals, non-NSAID medications, such as *acetaminophen* (Tylenol), may be considered.*

***Note:*** Aspirin is also an NSAID but does not carry the same cardiovascular risks. Low-dose aspirin is widely used for its blood-thinning effects to reduce risk for heart attack or stroke in those who have cardiovascular disease or are at increased risk for it. A doctor should prescribe and monitor such daily aspirin therapy.

*With some cases of heart disease (and/or kidney disease), a topical NSAID, which is absorbed differently from a pill, may also be an option.

## Kidney Disease

***Background:*** NSAIDs can reduce blood flow to the kidneys and/or cause the body to retain fluid, taxing the kidneys.

***If kidney disease is mild:*** It may go unnoticed, except you may have slightly higher blood levels of creatinine (a waste product normally removed by kidneys). Short-term and low-dose NSAIDs, including aspirin, may be used if creatinine levels are not substantially elevated (less than 1.5 mg/dL). Creatinine levels should be monitored if NSAIDs are used in these cases.

***If kidney disease is severe:*** If you have kidney disease and routinely retain extra fluid, it's a severe case. You should avoid all NSAIDs—including daily low-dose aspirin for heart attack prevention. A person with severe kidney disease may use acetaminophen if his/her liver function is normal.

***Important:*** When used as directed, acetaminophen is generally safe but can interfere with liver function when taken in excessive doses (more than 3 g per day) and/or when combined with alcohol.

## Heart and Kidney Disease

What if you have both heart and kidney problems? If your blood work indicates that your liver function is normal, acetaminophen (see above) can often be used for pain, under a doctor's direction.

## Nondrug Pain Relief

Drugs are not the only option—nor should they even be your first choice—especially if you have heart disease and/or kidney disease. *Nondrug therapies that can reduce or replace your use of pain medication...*

- **Noninvasive.** Physical therapy, aqua therapy, exercise, tai chi and yoga are powerful pain-fighters. Acupuncture and massage have also been shown to help, as have behavioral approaches such as cognitive therapy. Most people see results within days to weeks.

- **Minimally invasive.** Nerve blocks—injected anesthetics or nerve ablations (using heat) that are designed to turn off pain signals—are generally given once every few weeks or months and can produce lasting pain relief without resorting to long-term drug use.

***Another option:*** Neuromodulation, in which a small device (electrodes and a pulse generator about the size of a stopwatch) is surgically implanted to deliver electrical stimulation that disrupts pain signals that travel from the spinal cord to the brain. This can be used to treat pain in many locations of the body.

- **Surgery.** This is an option if the cause of your pain is identified and can be surgically corrected.

***Example:*** A herniated disk pressing on a nerve may be surgically removed. Of course, nonsurgical methods should be tried first. Surgeries can cause short-term pain and fail to provide the desired level of pain relief and function. Talk to your doctors so that you understand the risks of surgery and have realistic expectations for your outcome.

# Flirting with Painkillers: Could You Get Hooked?

Michael Weaver, MD, professor of psychiatry and behavioral sciences, and medical director, Center for Neurobehavioral Research on Addiction, The University of Texas Health Science Center at Houston.

If you've heard about the painkiller-addiction epidemic, you're probably scared of these drugs—even wondering if you could become addicted if you ever needed one.

On the one hand, it is very easy to get hooked on painkillers...especially if you're a woman. What tips the balance? Are you at risk? If you started to get hooked, would you recognize the signs? Would you get help—or even know where to start?

## How to Know If You're at Risk

Some factors to consider when facing the risk of painkiller addiction...

• **Gender.** Women are more likely to become dependent on prescription painkillers than men are, and not only because they are more likely to have chronic pain—women tend to weigh less than men, so when they are prescribed standard doses, they are in effect taking higher amounts, which can jump-start them on the path to dependence. Also, while men are more likely to abuse illegal "hard" drugs such as heroin or cocaine, women are more likely to fall prey to prescription addictions, especially to opioids.

• **A family history of addiction to any substance.** There is a scientifically based genetic component to addiction. The closer the family member, such as a parent or sibling, the stronger the genetic risk.

• **Symptoms of anxiety and/or depression.** You may knowingly or unknowingly use opioids to numb these symptoms and not just physical pain.

• **A history of abusing another substance**—whether it's nicotine, alcohol, marijuana, stimulants or sedatives. Substance-use disorders tend to travel in packs. If you have one, you are at higher risk to have another.

## Warning Signs to Watch for

Opioid painkillers often are prescribed for chronic pain even though they aren't very effective for chronic pain and should never be the "first line" prescription, according to recent Centers for Disease Control and Prevention guidelines.

Once they are prescribed, often for a hospital procedure, however, some people get used to the drugs' feel-good effects and keep using them...which is to say abusing them. *Here are some signs that that might be happening...*

• **You're using an opioid painkiller for something other than pain**—to improve a bad mood, relieve stress or help you relax or get to sleep.

• **You feel that you have to take a painkiller just to feel normal**—"or what you think normal should feel like," said Michael Weaver, MD, medical director of the Center for Neurobehavioral Research on Addiction at the University of Texas Health Science Center in Houston.

• **You find yourself taking higher doses to have the same effect**—that means you're building up a tolerance.

• **Family members or friends express concern about your painkiller use.**

• **You spend a significant amount of time trying to get your hands on one or more painkillers,** using them and recovering from their effects.

• **You find yourself trying to cut down on your use of painkillers**—to no avail.

## What to Do If You Think You Might Be Hooked

If any of the above describes you, the first and most important tip is, *Don't go it alone.* Talk to your doctor about your concerns and your pattern of use, and ask for guidance on the best way to wean yourself from dependence.

Unlike with some other drugs, quitting opioids cold turkey can be very difficult because it can lead to opioid-withdrawal syndrome, which is very uncomfortable and often leads to relapse. Symptoms of opioid withdrawal can feel like a bad case of the flu, without a fever but with nausea, diarrhea, muscle cramps and aches, runny nose and watery eyes. These symptoms often are accompanied by considerable anxiety and powerful cravings to use opioids since that will make the symptoms go away immediately.

To prevent withdrawal symptoms and improve someone's chances of overcoming an opioid addiction, medication-assisted therapy is often recommended. This involves substituting a different opioid such as *methadone* or *buprenorphine*, which is much less likely to produce euphoria, for the one that's being abused. It is better to be slowly tapered off over several days or weeks with a longer-acting, less-reinforcing opioid with the help of a qualified physician or treatment program. This is what's often referred to as "detox." Naltrexone, which blocks the effects of other opioids if you do use one, may also be prescribed for long-term maintenance.

Over time, with ongoing counseling or other forms of professional help, people can learn skills to help them quit abusing opioids and avoid relapse for the long haul. There are many effective options available, including individual addiction counseling, group therapy, working with a physician who specializes in addiction medicine or participating in an inpatient or outpatient addiction treatment program.

### How to Avoid Addiction...and When Addiction Is Actually OK

Of course, if you are at risk for opioid dependence—if you're almost addicted, as it were—the best thing to do is to nip it in the bud before it becomes a full-blown addiction that needs treatment. There are lots of nonopioid pain meds available for many different chronic pain conditions, so talk with your doctor about these. Think about whether you need a particular dose of opioid at a particular time, or whether you can try to skip it for now, or wait a while by using nonopioid pain management techniques.

Consider comfort measures such as a heating pad, ice pack, massage or repositioning a painful body part. Other modalities can be useful as alternatives to opioids, such as biofeedback, hypnosis and chiropractic manipulation.

Mind-body approaches can be more effective than opioids for debilitating conditions such as fibromyalgia. Finally, it should be noted that continuing use of opioid painkillers can sometimes have a place in medicine. The CDC's new guidelines, for example, make it clear that they don't apply to people who are actively battling cancer pain or who are being given opioids for palliative care at the end of life. For these patients, opioid painkillers can be perfectly appropriate.

## Better Painkiller Safety

Amidst an epidemic of prescription painkiller addiction and overdose deaths, a recent survey found that 60% of patients prescribed opioids don't take all their pills, with many saving leftover pills for later use or even sharing them with others, raising risk for drug abuse.

***Better:*** Dispose of unused or expired medications on National Prescription Drug Take-Back Day (October 22). To find a drop-off location, go to DEAdiversion.usdoj.gov.

Alene Kennedy-Hendricks, PhD, assistant scientist, Johns Hopkins Bloomberg School of Public Health, Baltimore.

## Do Not Take Opiods for Back Pain

Opioids do not help chronic low-back pain. The slight relief they provide is little better than that of NSAIDs, such as aspirin.

***Self-defense:*** Regular exercise and education about its benefits reduce the risk of developing lower-back pain by as much as 45%.

Analysis of data from 20 trials including 7,295 patients by researchers at University of Sydney, Australia, published in *JAMA Internal Medicine.*

## Expired Meds OK?

Is it OK to take a medication after the expiration date?

In some cases. An FDA review of 122 different drugs found that 88% were still effective a year past their expiration dates. Generally, prescription tablet and capsule medications are good for one year from the date that they are dispensed from the pharmacy...over-the-counter drugs for a year after you open them. However, these medications may have some potency after that. Powders that are mixed with water to make a liquid solution just before being given to the patient are normally good only for 14 to 21 days. Drugs that require refrigeration are also less likely to remain viable past their expiration dates. You may be able to safely take some drugs that are just past their expiration date, such as *acetaminophen* (Tylenol), but never use any critical medicine, such as insulin, that has expired.

Amy Tiemeier, PharmD, associate professor of pharmacy practice, St. Louis College of Pharmacy.

# Link to Hearing Loss

When women ages 48 to 73 used over-the-counter pain relievers such as *ibuprofen* (Motrin) or *acetaminophen* (Tylenol) two or more days a week for more than six years, they were 16% more likely to suffer hearing loss than those who took aspirin or no pain reliever. The exact reason for this link is unknown. Further research is needed to determine whether men could be similarly affected by pain relievers.

Brian M. Lin, MD, resident in otolaryngology, Brigham and Women's Hospital, Boston.

# Stop a Migraine Before It Happens

Mark W. Green, MD, a professor of neurology, anesthesiology and rehabilitation medicine at Icahn School of Medicine at Mount Sinai in New York City, where he directs Headache and Pain Medicine and is the vice chair of Neurology for Professional Development and Alumni Relations. He is coauthor of *Managing Your Headaches* and several medical textbooks.

There are more than 37 million Americans who suffer from migraines, but the odds aren't in their favor when it comes to drug treatment.

***Sobering statistics:*** Preventive drugs work for only about half of the people who have these awful headaches—and even when the medication does help, migraine frequency is reduced by only about 50%.

The drugs that stop migraines once they've started—mainly prescription triptans (such as *sumatriptan*, *rizatriptan* and *almotriptan*) ...as well as OTC nonsteroidal anti-inflammatory drugs, such as *ibuprofen* (Motrin), and Excedrin Migraine, which contains acetaminophen, aspirin and caffeine—are not always effective. They work best when they're taken soon after the pain begins. Some of the drugs also cause side effects, such as fatigue or gastrointestinal bleeding. And taking them too often can lead to more—and more severe—headaches, known as overuse headaches or "rebound" headaches. So preventive drugs may be needed to avoid overuse of these medications.

## A Complex Problem

Why are migraines so hard to manage? Experts once believed that migraines were mainly caused by the dilation (widening) of blood vessels in the brain. That's why drugs usually prescribed for other conditions, such as *propranolol*, a blood pressure drug, have been used to reverse these changes.

But we now believe that migraines have more to do with overstimulation of the trigeminal nerve in the face and head—this can cause blood vessels in the brain to expand and become inflamed. Treatments that affect this nerve (see below) are often very effective.

***Important:*** Everyone who suffers from migraines should pay attention to possible triggers that precipitate attacks. Some people react to strong scents. Others are vulnerable to specific foods (such as bacon, ripened cheeses or alcohol)...food additives such as monosodium glutamate (MSG)...emotional stress... bright lights, etc. Avoiding triggers can be an effective way to prevent some attacks.

## Best Nondrug Options

Preventing a migraine is always better than trying to treat one that's already taken hold. Unfortunately, not all doctors are aware of the more recent effective migraine-prevention approaches. *Among the best...*

• **Cefaly.** Nearly three years ago, the FDA approved the first device for migraine prevention. Cefaly is known as an external trigeminal nerve stimulation unit. It electrically stimulates branches of the trigeminal nerve, which transmits sensations to the face and head.

***How it works:*** The prescription-only device, which blocks pain signals, includes a battery-powered headband with a reusable, self-adhering electrode. Patients position the headband around the forehead, just above the eyes. It may cause a slight tingling, but no pain. It's used for 20 minutes once a day. Anyone who has an implanted device in the head, a pacemaker or an implanted defibrillator should not use Cefaly.

***Scientific evidence:*** One study found that more than half of migraine patients who used Cefaly were satisfied and intended to keep using it. The unit costs about $350 and is usually not covered by insurance. The device manufacturer offers a 60-day guarantee, so people can get their money back if it doesn't seem to help.

• **Biofeedback.** Emotional stress is one of the most common migraine triggers. A biofeedback machine allows people to monitor skin temperature, muscle tension, brain waves and other physical stress responses that affect blood flow in the brain. The idea is that once people feel how they react to stress—with tightened forehead muscles, for example—they can modify their reactions with things like deep breathing, muscle relaxation, etc.

***Scientific evidence:*** There's strong research showing that biofeedback can reduce both the frequency and severity of migraines by 45% to 60%—but only for patients who are willing to practice.

Biofeedback can work about as well as many drugs, but it takes most people a few months before they're good at it. It can also be costly because you have to work with an instructor at first. To find a certified biofeedback practitioner, go to the website of the Biofeedback Certification International Alliance, BCIA.org. Insurance often won't cover it.

• **Supplements.** Some people do well when they combine one or more of these supplements with the previous approaches...*

Riboflavin, a B vitamin, may improve oxygen metabolism in cells. In one study, migraine frequency was reduced by 50% in patients who took riboflavin (400 mg daily).

Feverfew is an herbal headache remedy. Some research shows that 50 mg to 125 mg daily can help prevent and ease migraines, while other studies suggest that it's no more effective than a placebo. For some people, it might be a helpful addition to more mainstream treatments.

Magnesium (500 mg daily) can help reduce the frequency of migraines in people with low levels of the mineral.

## Botox

Known for smoothing facial wrinkles, these injections were FDA-approved for chronic migraines in 2010. Botox is a good treatment option for patients who have 15 or more days of headaches each month.

We still do not know how Botox works to prevent headaches. It probably deactivates pain receptors in the scalp and blocks the transmission of nerve signals between the scalp and the brain.

***How it's done:*** The drug is injected in multiple locations on the head and neck—and the injections are repeated every three months. It sounds terrible, but the injections are only mildly painful. The procedure takes about 15 minutes, and it's usually covered by insurance if drugs or other treatments haven't worked. Botox treatments are given by headache specialists. Side effects may include swallowing problems, blurred vision and speech difficulties.

***Important:*** I advise patients to commit to at least three treatments. If Botox relieves your pain, you and your doctor can decide how frequently you need additional treatments. If you haven't noticed relief after

*Check with your doctor before taking these supplements, since they can interact with certain medications and/or cause side effects such as diarrhea.

three treatments, Botox is unlikely to be a good choice for you.

## No More Neck Pain

Carol Krucoff, a yoga therapist at Duke Integrative Medicine in Durham, North Carolina, and codirector of Integrative Yoga for Seniors teacher training, which helps yoga instructors safely adapt the practice for older adults. She is also author of *Healing Yoga for Neck & Shoulder Pain* and the forthcoming *Relax into Yoga for Seniors*. HealingMoves.com

About 15% of US adults endure the misery of neck pain at some point each year. When neck pain occurs, the sufferer will do almost anything to get relief—whether it's popping strong painkillers, paying for massages or seeing a chiropractor.

While these and other approaches may be appropriate in some cases, one of the most effective—but underutilized—therapies for neck pain is yoga. Almost all causes of neck pain, including arthritis, can benefit from yoga, which is a great adjunct to medical treatment. It is also helpful to relieve neck pain stemming from poor posture.

Why yoga? Key yoga moves not only stretch tight muscles and strengthen weak ones, but also help create proper body alignment and posture—crucial steps in both preventing and treating neck pain.

To alleviate neck pain and keep it from coming back, practice these steps every day—but be sure to see your doctor first if you're experiencing severe pain...*

### Hold Your Head Right

The adult head weighs about 10 pounds—roughly the same as a medium-weight bowling ball. So it is important to correctly balance that weight to avoid strain on the neck.

Many daily activities, including sitting at a desk, working at a computer and talking and texting on the phone, cause our shoulders to round...bodies to lean forward...and heads to protrude in front of the shoulders. This posture puts extreme pressure and tension on the neck and shoulders.

***What to do:*** For correct head posture whether sitting or standing, your ears should be directly over your shoulders and your shoulders directly over your hips. Check yourself several times a day to make sure you're doing it. This posture may feel strange to you when you first try it, but learning to keep your head balanced over your shoulder girdle can make you feel better and will eventually seem natural.

### Check for "Body Armor"

When stressed, many people tighten the muscles in the upper back, shoulders and neck. As this physical response becomes habitual, we develop a "body armor" of tight, overused muscles in the neck and shoulders. The pattern becomes so ingrained that we don't even notice that we hold this tension constantly in our bodies.

To break this cycle, it's important to consciously consider how tension is affecting your neck muscles.

***What to do:*** Set your wristwatch alarm or phone alarm to sound once every waking hour. When you hear the alarm, take a moment to identify any areas of discomfort or tension in your body, including your back, shoulders and neck. Close your eyes, take a deep breath and relax these muscles. With practice and patience, it is often possible to get substantial release of muscle tension.

***Also helpful:*** Repeat a simple mantra, such as "Lips together, teeth apart," throughout the day to avoid clenching the teeth and help relax the jaw, a common site where tension resides. Jaw tightness often radiates downward and exacerbates neck pain.

*Check with your physician before doing any physical activity, including yoga poses, if you have neck pain that is accompanied by numbness, tingling or weakness in your arm or hand...the pain was caused by an injury or accident...you have swollen glands or a lump in your neck...or you have difficulty swallowing or breathing.

## Stretch and Strengthen

Don't worry if you have never done yoga—these are easy poses that will improve your body alignment and gently stretch the shoulders and neck. Practice the following yoga poses throughout the day, while at your desk, a table, while waiting for coffee to brew, etc. The seated mountain pose can be done anytime you're sitting. The other poses can be done once a day. It should take about five minutes to do them all.

- **Seated mountain pose.**

***What to do:*** Sit tall in your chair, with your feet on the floor. Use your hands to gently move the fleshy part of your buttocks aside and allow your "sit bones"—the two rounded knobs at the base of your pelvis—to press down onto the chair seat.

Extend the crown of your head up toward the sky, lengthening your spine. Relax your shoulders down away from your ears, and let your hands rest on your thighs. Be sure your chin is parallel to the ground and neither tilted up nor tucked in.

***What helps:*** Imagine that you have a headlight in the center of your chest at your breastbone—and shine that light forward. Relax your face, and look straight ahead. Linger here for five to 10 slow, easy breaths.

- **Shoulder shrugs.**

***What to do:*** Inhale and lift your shoulders up toward your ears and then exhale as you drop them down. Repeat five to 10 times, moving with the breath—inhale as you lift, then exhale (with a sigh if you like) as you release. Be sure to keep your arms as relaxed as possible.

- **Shoulder circles.**

***What to do:*** Lift your shoulders straight up as high as they will comfortably go. Then bring them behind you as far as is comfortable. Next, release the shoulders down toward your hips, then bring them forward as far as you comfortably can and finish the circle by bringing them up toward your ears.

Continue circling your shoulders, and avoid holding your breath. Let the movement be easy and get as much motion as possible in your shoulders. Circle five times in this direction, then circle five times in the opposite direction. When you've finished, relax your shoulders and take three to five easy breaths.

- **Head turn.**

***What to do:*** Inhale and extend the crown of your head toward the sky. Exhale and turn your head as far to the right as comfortably possible, keeping your shoulders still. Allow your eyes to turn also so you can look toward whatever is behind you. Inhale and turn back to center. Exhale and turn to the left. Repeat the set three to six times, moving with the breath.

- **Ear to shoulder.**

***What to do:*** Sit tall with your hands on your thighs. Inhale and lift the crown of your head toward the sky. Then exhale and drop your right ear down toward your right shoulder, trying not to lift that shoulder toward the ear. Keep your left shoulder down and relax the left side of your neck.

Keep your breath flowing as you take your left hand off your thigh and let your left arm dangle at your side. Stay in this pose for a few breaths while relaxing. Bring your head back to the center and pause. Then repeat on the other side.

# A Simple Fix for Neck Pain

Rebecca Shannonhouse, editor, *Bottom Line Health*, with Shani Soloff, manual orthopedic physical therapist and founder of the Posture People.

If you've got neck pain, you know all too well the misery it causes.

***In your search for relief, don't forget to consider this:*** How much time do you spend on the phone? Even if it's just a few calls a day, using a handheld landline or cell phone causes you to hold your body in ways that nature never intended.

When you're talking, you naturally tip your head toward the phone—and get even more contorted when your hands are busy and you raise a shoulder to prop the phone in place. It's no wonder that these movements were widely cited in a landmark study that found more than 45% of office workers had frequent episodes of neck pain!

You may think that you've solved the problem if you've switched to a speakerphone. But chances are you haven't. A speakerphone may not be a good alternative, because many people tend to move their necks forward—and lean toward the speakerphone.

Fortunately, the solution is often as simple as investing in a good headset. Shani Soloff, a manual orthopedic physical therapist and founder of the Stamford, Connecticut–based ergonomics firm The Posture People, advises everyone who uses a phone to do this. It will help you maintain proper posture—with your body straight and your shoulders square—while talking on the phone.

It doesn't really matter what style you choose, as long as it's comfortable and easy to use. You can start by checking online at such sites as Headsets.com, BestBuy.com or Staples.com. Headsets come in corded and wireless versions...prices range from about $15 to $350. Your neck will thank you!

## Better Way to Ease Low-Back Pain

Adults with chronic low-back pain showed significant improvement after eight weekly two-hour sessions of mindfulness-based stress reduction (MBSR), a program that combines meditation with simple yoga poses, a recent study found. Participants also practiced MBSR at home.

***Details:*** After six months, 60% of those who did MBSR reported less pain and could more easily perform activities such as walking, climbing stairs and standing for long periods—a better result than those who treated their chronic low-back pain with medication and/or physical therapy. To find an online class in MBSR, go to the Center for Mindfulness, UMASSmed.edu/cfm/stress-reduction.

Daniel Cherkin, PhD, senior investigator, Group Health Research Institute, Seattle.

### Meditation Beats Morphine

According to recent research, mindfulness meditation, a technique that focuses on awareness and acceptance of daily thoughts and feelings, activates areas of the brain that reduce pain intensity.

***Details:*** Adults who meditated for 20 minutes a day for four days before being touched with a hot probe reported feeling up to 44% less pain than those who did not meditate—which was twice the benefit provided by opioid drugs such as *morphine*.

Fadel Zeidan, PhD, assistant professor of neurobiology and anatomy, Wake Forest School of Medicine, Winston-Salem, North Carolina.

## How Compassion Relieves Chronic Pain

Emma Seppälä, PhD, science director, Center for Compassion and Altruism Research and Education, Stanford University School of Medicine, California, and author of *The Happiness Track: How to Apply the Science of Happiness to Accelerate Your Success.*

If you suffer from chronic pain, and perhaps the angry emotions that may result, there's a drug-free treatment that takes only 15 minutes a day and can bring real relief.

It's called compassion meditation. It's not like "regular" meditation. Rather than simply calming your mind, you actively direct your thoughts—toward kindness and altruism. Don't believe this could relieve your pain? Rigorous scientific studies have found that it can—and it may even help you live longer.

## The Science of Kindness

At the Center for Compassion and Altruism Research and Education at Stanford University School of Medicine, we study the health effects of compassion and altruistic behavior. *Recent research at our center and other institutions has found that compassion meditation helps...*

• **Chronic pain**—and anger. Among people with chronic pain, a nine-week compassion meditation program at Stanford University led to significantly reduced pain severity and greater pain acceptance by the end of the program.

One benefit was that it reduced levels of anger, based on self-evaluations of the patients. Anger has been shown to be an important predictor of chronic pain symptoms, and cultivating compassion has been shown to positively influence how we process emotions, reducing the tendency toward negativity, including anger.

• **Post-traumatic stress disorder (PTSD) symptoms.** In a study at the Veterans Administration's Puget Sound Health Care System in Seattle, researchers found that when veterans with PTSD practiced loving-kindness meditation (a form of compassion meditation) for 12 weeks, they experienced a reduction in PTSD symptoms and depression. The benefits were still evident three months later.

• **Migraines.** A study from the University of Massachusetts Medical School in Worcester found that migraine sufferers who learned loving-kindness meditation in a single session experienced a 33% decrease in pain and a 43% reduction in emotional tension.

• **Longevity.** While there's certainly no conclusive evidence that learning to be compassionate to yourself and to others will help you live longer, there are intriguing clues that it might.

***The connection:*** Telomeres, which are "caps" on the tips of each strand of DNA on your chromosomes.

A study from Massachusetts General Hospital and Harvard Medical School found that people experienced in practicing loving-kindness meditation had longer telomeres, which are associated with greater longevity.

## How to Practice Compassion Meditation

Compassion meditation aims to strengthen feelings of compassion and empathy toward yourself and other people—to generate feelings of kindness toward yourself and others. It's different from the well-known "mindfulness" meditation, which is mostly focused on calming the mind and increasing awareness. In compassion meditation, rather than letting your thoughts come and go without judgment, you focus your attention in specific ways as you silently repeat benevolent phrases or visualize kind wishes.

The goal is to express your intention to move from judgment or dislike to caring, compassion, acceptance and understanding. Compassion meditation involves bringing to mind people you know and love, feeling their love and spreading caring feelings toward strangers or even people you find challenging.

It isn't hard to do.

***What to do:*** Sit quietly, close your eyes, breathe gently and silently repeat a phrase designed to evoke a feeling of goodwill toward yourself, such as *May I be happy, healthy and strong.* Then, extend the good wishes to someone you feel thankful for, then to someone you're indifferent toward, then to someone you find challenging and finally to the world at large.

Practicing loving-kindness or compassion meditation is a way to stretch the "muscles" of kindness, caring and empathy toward everyone and to remember our common humanity. The key is to give your "compassion muscles" a workout by practicing regularly, just as you might any other skill. Doing so will help you cultivate more loving relationships, greater happiness and better health... and could noticeably reduce your chronic pain.

Ready to do it now? You can use my YouTube video, "A Gift of Loving Kindness Meditation," which runs for less than 15 minutes. Close your eyes and follow the prompts.

Once you know it by heart, you can do it in your own time and voice.

## Arthritis Drug Considered Safe

An arthritis drug is safe despite its similarity to a drug that had to be pulled from the market. *Celecoxib* (brand name Celebrex) is a COX-2 inhibitor, the same type of drug as Vioxx, which was taken off the market in 2004 when long-term use was found to increase risk for heart attack, stroke and death. Logically, celecoxib might seem to pose similar risks—but a decade-long study showed that it does not. In fact, it is at least as effective as the nonsteroidal anti-inflammatory drugs (NSAIDs) *ibuprofen* and *naproxen* and causes fewer gastrointestinal side effects and kidney-related complications.

Steven E. Nissen, MD, MACC, chairman of the department of cardiovascular medicine at the Cleveland Clinic, Ohio, and leader of a study published in *The New England Journal of Medicine.*

## Vitamin D Does Not Help Arthritic Knees

The use of vitamin D to help arthritic knees has been controversial.

***Recent finding:*** It does not ease pain or slow the progression of knee osteoarthritis—even in people who are deficient in the vitamin. There currently is no treatment available to stop the loss of cartilage that eventually leads patients to need knee replacements. Symptoms are treated with painkillers, cortisone injections and anti-inflammatory drugs, but these do not slow the disease's progress.

Study of 413 patients with knee osteoarthritis by researchers at University of Tasmania, Hobart, Australia, published in *JAMA.*

## Beat Knee Pain Without Surgery

Mitchell Yass, DPT, a St. Augustine, Florida–based physical therapist and creator of the Yass Method for treating chronic pain. He is also author of *The Pain Cure Rx: The Yass Method for Diagnosing and Resolving Chronic Pain* and the PBS special *The Pain Prescription.* MitchellYass.com

Do you wince when you walk, kneel, squat or climb stairs? If so, you are definitely not alone. Nearly 20% of all cases of chronic pain are associated with the knee, and it's severe enough to limit the sufferer's mobility and affect quality of life.

Knee surgery, including knee replacement, is a widely used option, but it's rarely the best choice...and should never be the first choice. Knee pain is often caused by weak and/or imbalanced muscles, which surgery or other invasive treatments do not address.

***A much better option:*** For most people with knee pain, exercise is at least as effective as surgery—with none of the risks, according to research. *What you need to know...*

### Muscle Pain

When you see a doctor because of nagging knee pain, you'll probably be advised to have an X-ray or MRI to look for arthritis, torn cartilage or other structural problems that can

### Gut Bacteria

Gut bacteria may fight rheumatoid arthritis. The painful autoimmune disease eventually may be treatable by giving patients specific intestinal bacteria. A study in arthritis-prone mice found that those given Prevotella histicola had fewer and less severe symptoms than those not given the treatment.

Veena Taneja, PhD, immunologist, Center for Individualized Medicine, Mayo Clinic, Rochester, Minnesota, and leader of a study published in *Arthritis and Rheumatology.*

cause joint pain. But the tests, more often than not, point doctors in the wrong direction.

***Eye-opening research:*** A study of nearly 1,000 patients with arthritis-related knee pain found that 63% had a damaged meniscus (cartilage that cushions and stabilizes the knee). But the same study also found that 60% of patients without pain had the same type of damage.

Most patients—and many doctors—fail to realize that there's a poor correlation between structural problems and knee pain. That's why I often advise clients not to have imaging tests—or consider surgery—until they've first tried my program of targeted exercise. In my experience, about 90% of knee patients have a muscle imbalance or weakness that causes all or most of their symptoms.

Here is a 30- to 60-minute workout that helps specific types of knee pain. Do the exercises on the side that is painful until the pain subsides—once the pain is gone, do the exercises on both sides. Stop if the exercise hurts.

A resistance band, ankle weight or machine in the gym can be used for resistance, which is key for strengthening muscles.* Start at a level where you feel you are working hard but not in pain, and gradually increase resistance.

The exercises can be performed by anyone, including those who have had knee surgery, but check first with your doctor. The quad stretch should be done daily. For each of the other exercises below, do three sets of 10 repetitions (resting 45 to 60 seconds between sets) and repeat the workouts three times a week (with a day between workouts).

## Weak Hamstrings

The thigh muscles (quadriceps) tend to be a lot stronger than the opposing muscles (the hamstrings) on the backs of the legs. Why? It's because virtually all of our daily movements—including walking and climbing stairs—are "forward."

*To increase muscle strength, add resistance (with heavier weights or a stronger exercise band) when the exercises become easy.

***The problem:*** Weak hamstrings (they are mainly responsible for knee bending) cannot effectively counteract the force of much stronger quadriceps, causing a muscle imbalance.

***Result:*** The quadriceps shorten and pull up on the kneecap, causing excessive pressure and pain. The majority of people with knee pain will improve when they strengthen the hamstrings and stretch the quads.

***EXERCISE #1:* Hamstring curls.** While sitting in a chair, tie the ends of a resistance band to a doorknob and slip it around the ankle...or try the seated leg curl machine at the gym.

***What to do:*** Begin with the exercising leg pointing straight out, then bend the knee until it reaches 90 degrees. Return to the starting position.

***EXERCISE #2:* Hip extensions.** This exercise works the gluteus maximus muscles in the buttocks.

***What to do:*** While standing, place a resistance band behind one knee. Then attach the ends to a fixed point—such as a doorknob. While standing (you can rest your hand on top of a chair or table for extra support), bring the knee about 10 degrees behind the hip, then return to the starting position.

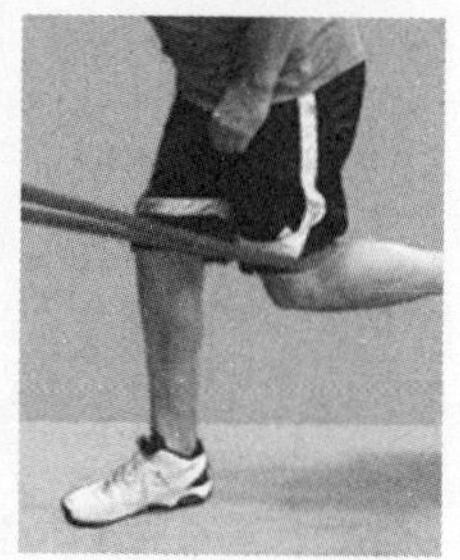

***EXERCISE #3:* Quad stretches.** Tight quadriceps pull the kneecap toward the top of the joint and prevent it from moving smoothly. Tight quads can cause both knee and back pain.

***What to do:*** Stand near a wall (or a dresser, bookcase or other solid support), and use one hand for balance. Reach back with your other hand, and grip the ankle.

Pull the heel upward toward the buttock. The knee should be a few inches behind the hip. Keep pulling until you feel a stretch in the front of the thigh. Hold the stretch for 20 to 30 seconds, and do the stretch twice. Pull gently! If it hurts, you've pulled too far (or too quickly).

## Quad Strain

Another common cause of knee pain is quad strain. What are the telltale signs? You might notice a "pulling" sensation at the top of the knee or in the thigh when you walk or climb stairs. A weak quadricep can cause the kneecap to shift out of place. *Try this...*

***EXERCISE #1:*** **Knee extensions.** They strengthen the quadriceps and help the kneecap stay in a "neutral" position.

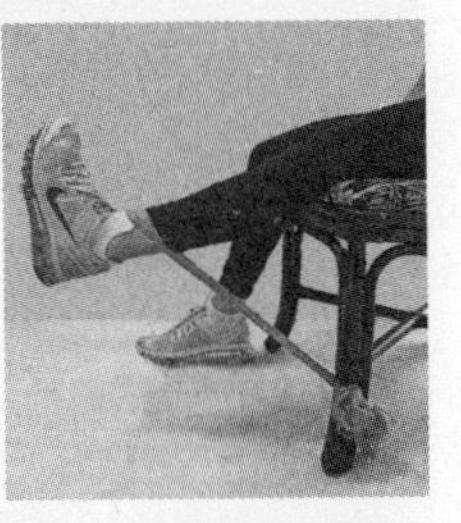

***What to do:*** In a seated position, strap on an ankle weight or tie a resistance band around the front of the ankle and attach the other end to the chair leg. Keep the other foot on the floor. Begin with the knee bent to a 90-degree angle, then straighten it. Return to the starting position.

***Important:*** Make sure that the thigh of the leg being exercised stays on the seat. Raising it will make the exercise less effective.

***EXERCISE #2:*** **Dorsiflexion.** It works the tibialis anterior, a muscle in the front of the shin. Strengthening the muscle can help keep the calf muscle lengthened and allow the knee joint to function properly to prevent knee pain.

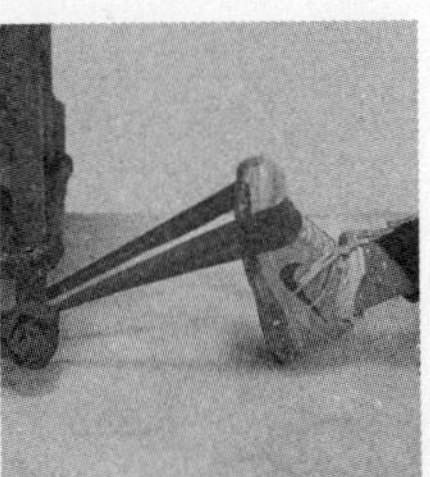

***What to do:*** Sit on the floor with one leg extended. Slip an exercise band over the top of the foot and tie the ends to a sturdy table leg. Start with the ankle angled about 30 degrees forward, then pull the foot toward the upper body until it is 10 degrees past perpendicular. Return to the starting position.

# Beware of This Surgery Risk

Adults recovering from knee surgery were five times more likely to become chronic users of opioids such as *hydrocodone, oxycodone* and *fentanyl* than those who did not have surgery, according to a recent study of more than 650,000 patients. Those who had other types of surgery, including mastectomy and hip replacement, were also at increased risk for opioid abuse.

***If you need surgery:*** Talk to your doctor about alternatives such as other kinds of painkillers and/or physical therapy to manage pain.

Eric Sun, MD, PhD, instructor of anesthesiology, pain and perioperative medicine, Stanford University.

# When Knee-Replacement Patients Can Shower

Knee-replacement patients can shower as soon as two days after surgery if their doctors agree. The usual recommendation is to wait 10 days to two weeks after surgery before showering. But researchers found no difference in bacterial cultures of skin next to incisions in patients who waited and those who were allowed to shower 48 hours after surgery.

Study by researchers at Loyola University Chicago Stritch School of Medicine, published in *Journal of Arthroplasty.*

# Do Compression Braces and Sleeves Work?

Barbara Bergin, MD, orthopedic surgeon, Texas Orthopedics, Sports & Rehabilitation Associates, Austin. She is currently writing a book based on the idea that women should "Sit like a man." DrBarbaraBergin.com

For knee arthritis any kind of sleeve or brace will have a proprioceptive effect, which refers to your brain's ability to sense where your bones, joints and muscles are—even without looking—and take steps to control their function and position.

In other words, the presence of something around the knee—even a piece of duct tape or Kinesio Tape, a type of therapeutic elastic adhesive tape that can be worn for extended periods of time—can actually send more sensory information to the brain, making it more aware of the extremity. Then the brain can send subconscious, corrective impulses down to that extremity—in essence, increasing awareness of the affected part so that your body unconsciously adjusts muscles and joints to accommodate them as you move about.

For example, look at your pinky toe. You might think it is just sitting there limp, resting inside your shoe. But it's not. Your brain is subconsciously putting it there. It's not sticking it up in the air. It's not shoving it down into the sole of your shoe. Now, tell your brain to stick the pinky up in the air. That's not proprioception. That's your conscious brain directing your toe to go there. But let's say you have a blister on your pinky. Now you're not going to walk around all day saying, "Brain! Bend my toe down away from my shoe." Instead, proprioception will eventually take over. The leather on your shoe will act as a messenger to your brain, much as a brace might for your knee, and your wonderful brain will guide that toe away from the abrasive leather.

Proprioception is one reason why a lot of folks with arthritis like the feel of having a sleeve or brace on their knee or anywhere on the body for that matter, such as an ankle sleeve. It's why athletes like to use compression braces and sleeves, tight clothing and Kinesio Tape.

Wearing a compression brace will not directly prevent your knee from twisting in a way that might injure it. But it may help your brain's awareness of your body in space so that you might avoid moves that could cause further injury and pain.

While compression garments and wraps have no potential to cure disorders of bones and joints for those suffering with arthritis or patients with injuries, they just seem to feel better. That's a good enough reason, if you want to try one of these garments or Kinesio Tape—or even an Ace bandage. See if it helps. And yes, you could even try duct tape, a kind of primitive version of Kinesio Tape. It might work quite nicely—although it's going to hurt like hell and give you a waxing when you take it off!

## Exercise Prevents Back Pain Recurrence

Supervised exercise reduced the chance of a repeat episode of back pain by 45% over a one-year period. Shoe orthotics and back belts were almost useless. And the type of exercise did not matter—some programs focused on back muscles, while others combined aerobics with strength and balance training. Patients generally did two to three supervised exercise sessions per week. But the protective effects wore off after a year—probably because many people stopped exercising when they were no longer being closely supervised.

***Troubling:*** About 75% of people who have an episode of debilitating lower-back pain will have another within one year.

Statistical analysis of more than 6,000 studies involving back-pain prevention led by researchers at The George Institute for Global Health, The University of Sydney, Australia, published in *JAMA Internal Medicine.*

## You Can Have Strong, Pain-Free Hands

Mary Formby, OT, CHT, a certified hand therapist at the Curtis National Hand Center at MedStar Union Memorial Hospital in Baltimore. She has practiced hand rehabilitation medicine for more than 25 years and was a contributor to the textbook *Hand and Upper Extremity Rehabilitation.* CurtisHand.com

It's hard to imagine how indispensable your hands are until arthritis limits your ability to use them as you once did. The simplest things, such as turning a doorknob, using a key or opening a jar of pickles, can be intensely painful—or even impossible.

Fortunately, hand exercises can help improve strength and flexibility. Just be sure to do them in moderation—and stop when it hurts!

***What most people don't realize:*** You can make hand exercises more fun by adding a ball, putty and other simple tools to your workouts. You can also do these exercises while you watch TV, so the program can entertain you even if the workout doesn't.

## Who Needs to Exercise?

Osteoarthritis ("wear-and-tear" arthritis) and rheumatoid arthritis (an autoimmune disease) can strike any joint in the body, but when the hands are affected, our day-to-day tasks become difficult.

***Examples:*** An inability to grasp small objects (such as dropped coins or earrings)... or lift or carry more than 10 pounds (such as grocery store purchases). The carpometacarpal (CMC) joint in the thumb is often one of the affected joints, particularly in older women. Stiffness and pain of the CMC joint makes any kind of gripping difficult.

***Self-test:*** Hold up your hand with the palm facing you. Can you touch the tip of your thumb to each fingertip...and bring the thumb to the base of the little finger? Also, can you make a fist and touch each fingertip to your palm? If you can't—or if you struggle with any of the activities described above—you might benefit from hand exercises.

## How to Start

In conventional workouts, people are often advised to do many repetitions for each exercise. This might not be advisable for people with hand pain. High-repetition exercises can strain tendons and cause overuse injuries.

Muscles work and become stronger during both isometric (holding) exercises and repetitive movements, but holding exercises are less stressful to arthritic joints.

***Important:*** The exercises in this article are helpful for a variety of hand symptoms and conditions, but anyone with significant hand limitations should work with an occupational or a physical therapist, preferably with the additional credential of certified hand therapist (CHT). You can find a CHT in your area by going to HTCC.org and clicking on "find a CHT."

***What you will need:*** For the exercises described below, you will need the following items—a hand therapy ball...a small piece of sponge (about the size of a golf ball) or a cotton ball...a rubber band...and hand therapy putty. Sets that include soft, medium and firm balls or putty are available online for about $12 each. Start with soft!

***Stretch first:*** Before using any resistance, start with a few stretches to maximize your flexibility.

***Examples:*** Stretch your thumb gently away from the side of your hand, then toward the bottom of your little finger...make a full fist...then spread your fingers all the way apart. Repeat on the other hand. Do these stretches a few times each.

## Ready, Set...Go!

Do each exercise below for 10 seconds (extend the time to 20, then 30 seconds as your hands get stronger). Relax your hands for a few seconds, then repeat. Continue this cycle for a total of about one minute for each exercise on each hand. You can increase the time gradually to up to three minutes. If you can, do each exercise daily.

- **Ball squeezes.** This exercise can increase overall hand strength, but don't overdo it. Squeezing the ball too often—or too hard—can lead to "trigger finger" (stenosing tenosynovitis), in which a finger gets stuck in a bent position. Stop the exercise if it's painful!

***What to do:*** Hold a ball in your palm... squeeze it with your thumb and fingers... then relax. If your hands are weak or painful, be sure to start with a soft ball. As you improve, you can progress to a harder ball or even a tennis ball. Let your hand be your guide for timing the progression.

- **Scissor squeezes.** This exercise strengthens muscles between the fingers (known as intrinsic muscles). It can help to improve grip strength and is unlikely to cause overuse injuries.

***What to do:*** Simply squeeze a piece of sponge or a cotton ball between two fingers. Hold the item between the index and middle finger, then between the middle and ring finger, then between the ring and small finger. Try to keep the little joints of your fingers straight as you do this.

• **Thumb roll.** This simple exercise can increase thumb mobility and improve your ability to grip things.

***What to do:*** Place a ball in the palm of your hand. Using just your thumb, roll the ball from side to side...and in a circular motion.

• **Finger flicks.** The finger muscles are small, so this easy movement does strengthen them.

***What to do:*** Place a ball on a table in front of your loosely closed fist. Flick the ball away from you with the back of each fingertip (by straightening the fingers), and repeat with your other hand. If you're doing it with a partner, he/she can flick it right back. Stop before you get tired. If you are alone, catch the ball with your other hand.

• **Finger spread.** This exercise improves finger range of motion, which helps with holding large objects, etc.

***What to do:*** With your hand held in front of you, place a rubber band around your thumb and all your fingertips. Spread your fingers out to stretch the rubber band... hold...relax...then repeat.

• **Squeeze, roll, spread and pinch.** This exercise combines flexion, extension and "pinch" movements.

***What to do:*** Mold the putty into a ball. Then roll out the putty with your palm into a cylinder. Next shape the putty into a circle on a table. Place your fingertips inside the circle and stretch it out with your thumb/fingers. You can lift the putty off the table to spread your fingers.

Now mold the putty into a ball again and pinch it using a "three-point pinch"—that is, use the tips of your thumb, index and middle fingers. People with hand arthritis should try to limit their use of a "lateral pinch," in which they pinch with the thumb against the side of the index finger (as though holding a key). This type of pinch pattern can irritate the thumb's CMC joint. When possible, use a three-point pinch—it helps to protect the CMC joint.

---

## Help for Carpal Tunnel

If your doctor says you have carpal tunnel syndrome, you might want to try other forms of therapy before you turn to surgery.

This common condition occurs when tendons within a narrow area of the wrist called the carpal tunnel press on the median nerve, which runs from the forearm to the fingertips, resulting in numbness, pain and sometimes weakness.

Wearing a wrist splint, especially at night, helps decrease tendon swelling and eases symptoms for many people. In some cases, a corticosteroid injection into the carpal tunnel may also provide relief.

A physical or occupational therapist can provide you with hand exercises that can reduce symptoms if done daily. If these techniques do not help relieve pain and stiffness, you may wish to reconsider having surgery, which eliminates pressure on the median nerve, providing permanent relief for most people.

Terry R. Light, MD, professor of orthopaedic surgery and rehabilitation, Loyola University Stritch School of Medicine, Maywood, Illinois.

---

## Foot-tastic! Natural Fixes for Foot Pain

Johanna Youner, DPM, podiatrist and podiatric surgeon. She is founder of Healthy Feet NY, a private practice in New York City. HealthyFeetNY.net and ParkAvenueLaserTreatment.com

Most of us—75% of Americans—will have foot problems at least sometime in our lives. Think about the stresses that your feet endure. They're subjected to significant impact pressure just from walking—and a lot more from running. They're squeezed into tight shoes and stuffed into hot socks.

But you can treat many foot problems at home—without potent drugs or high-priced medical care.

Natural remedies that work...

## Arnica for Injuries

This homeopathic remedy has become the go-to treatment for athletes—including members of the US Men's National Soccer Team—who need to reduce post-injury swelling, inflammation and bruises.

Arnica pellets (taken internally), ointments, creams and gels contain thymol derivatives, compounds that reduce inflammation. A study published in a rheumatology journal found that homeopathic arnica relieved pain as well as *ibuprofen*—without the side effects that often occur with traditional over-the-counter painkillers.

***How to use it:*** Quickly apply arnica gel, ointment or cream (or put five sublingual arnica pellets under your tongue) after you've banged or twisted your foot or ankle. It works best when it's applied or taken within 10 minutes after an injury. Repeat the treatment three times a day until the pain is gone.

For homeopathic products, I recommend Boiron, a leading manufacturer of these remedies. They're available at pharmacies and supermarkets.

## Castor Oil for Arthritic and Chronic Pain

Many doctors advise their patients to apply moist heat for arthritic conditions and other chronic pain. Heat dilates blood vessels, stimulates blood flow and increases the supply of oxygen and nutrients...and it accelerates the removal of fluids that cause swelling.

Castor oil is even better because it's an anti-inflammatory and an antioxidant that is readily absorbed by the skin. It contains the unsaturated omega-3 fatty acid ricinoleic acid, which quickly reduces inflammation and pain. Buy hexane-free castor oil (it will say so on the label). Hexane is a petrochemical that may be hazardous.

***How to use it:*** For foot or ankle pain, soak a piece of flannel (flannels are sold online for this purpose) in castor oil...wrap it around the foot...then wrap a warm towel around that ...and leave it in place for about one hour. It will reduce the inflammation and swelling. (You also can use a heating pad or hot-water bottle to heat the towel.)

***Caution:*** Castor oil stains! Take a shower after you remove the wrapping...and keep the oil away from your good towels. You can store the flannel in the refrigerator in a plastic bag or container for about one month.

## Epsom Salt for Cellulitis

Cellulitis is a common skin infection that often affects the feet, particularly in patients with athlete's foot, fluid retention in the legs (from poor circulation) and/or diabetes. You might notice redness, swelling or warmth in the early stages.

Epsom salt is an osmotic agent. It pulls material (fluids, pus and even splinters) toward the surface of the skin. When your foot is swollen, an Epsom salt soak will reduce swelling right away—it's almost magical. I use it for many nonemergency foot conditions, including cellulitis, painful warts and infected nails.

***How to use it:*** For a foot bath, add one-half cup of Epsom salt to a basin of warm water.

## Tea Tree Oil for Infections and Fungus

Tea tree oil is extracted from the leaves of an Australian tea tree. It has been used for centuries to treat skin infections. Research has shown that it is an effective treatment for athlete's foot as well as nail fungus (onychomycosis).

***How to use it:*** Apply the oil twice a day to new skin infections or toenail infections (don't apply to broken skin). Fungal infections that have gone on for a month or more probably will require a medicated over-the-counter cream such as Tinactin or Lotrimin.

## Coconut Oil to Moisturize

Feet don't have oil glands. Without this natural lubrication, the skin is naturally dry. Too much dryness can cause itching, peeling or even deep cracks that can be painful and sometimes get infected.

Coconut oil is an excellent moisturizer for the feet—one that also has antibacterial and antifungal properties. It is solid at room temperature and is available in jars at supermarkets and pharmacies.

***How to use it:*** Apply it to your feet several times a day. Because it's readily absorbed, it won't look (or feel) greasy.

## Mustard, Pickle Juice or Vinegar for Foot Cramps

It sounds like an old wives' tale, but each of these traditional remedies really can help when you have foot or ankle cramps. In a study published on the website of the American College of Sports Medicine, researchers used electricity to induce toe cramps in young athletes who had just completed a workout. The athletes then drank 2.5 ounces of pickle juice or water—or nothing at all. The pickle juice stopped the cramps about 37% faster than water and 45% faster than drinking nothing.

Researchers speculate that a substance in pickle juice—possibly the vinegar—somehow short-circuits muscle-cramp reflexes. Apple cider vinegar has a similar effect, as does prepared yellow mustard (which contains vinegar).

***How to use them:*** Keep any (or all) of them on hand if your feet are prone to cramps. When you feel a cramp coming on, add pickle juice, vinegar and/or mustard to your food.

***Important:*** For most people, dehydration is the main cause of muscle cramps. You must hydrate after exercise. In addition to the vinegar or pickle juice, drink a few glasses of water, juice or a sports beverage.

## Drug-Free Cures for Plantar Fasciitis

Plantar fasciitis affects about 10% of the US population and is one of the most common causes of heel pain. A thick band of tissue (the plantar fascia) runs across the bottom of the foot. It connects the heel bone to the toes and creates the arch. Small tears in the tissue can cause burning/stabbing pain, particularly in the morning.

- **Apply ice.** Hold an ice pack over the painful area for 15 to 20 minutes, three or four times a day.
- **Replace your shoe insoles.** The Powerstep brand of insoles supports and cushions the plantar fascia and helps it heal more quickly. You can buy insoles at pharmacies, sporting-goods stores and online for $15 to $60. In many cases, they work as well as prescription products (which can cost as much as $550).
- **Use a tennis ball or rolling pin** to gently roll along the bottom of your foot (while sitting).
- **Replace worn-out athletic shoes.** They stop cushioning your feet after about 500 miles of use.

---

# Natural Healing in a Flash

Bill Gottlieb, CHC, a health coach certified by the American Association of Drugless Practitioners. He is author of 16 health books, including *Speed Healing: More Than 2,000 Quick Cures and Fast Fixes to Ease Everything from Arthritis to Wrinkles.* BottomLineStore.com/shl

We all want to feel better faster! *Here are remedies for common pain that take very little time to implement and that often work in a flash...*

- **Arthritis.** Nearly half of Americans age 60 and older suffer with the pain of knee arthritis. Ice is the fastest way to relieve that pain—faster than taking a pain pill, says Jason Theodosakis, MD, coauthor of *The Arthritis Cure* and associate clinical professor at University of Arizona College of Medicine in Tucson. But ice often is used incorrectly, undercutting its pain-relieving power. Many people find the feeling of cold uncomfortable, so they either don't ice often enough or at all.

***Rapid remedy:*** Buy a freezable soft gel ice pack and a compression (ACE-type) bandage. Store the gel pack in the freezer. When your knee hurts, place the pack on your knee over a pant leg or a towel, securing it to your knee with the compression bandage. (Never put the ice pack directly on your skin.) Keep the ice pack on for about 15 minutes—just the right amount of time to provide an hour or two of pain relief. Ice packs can bring relief to other parts of the body, too, including the ankle, shoulder and neck.

- **Back pain.** There are many different causes of back pain. But you can relieve many types by using a simple position that takes weight off your spine while supporting it, says Art Brownstein, MD, director of Princeville Medical Clinic in Hawaii and author of *Healing Back Pain Naturally*.

***Rapid remedy:*** Lie on your back on the floor with your knees bent and your feet resting up on a chair or a bed. Remain in this position for 15 to 20 minutes. Repeat this pose several times a day if needed.

## Fight Joint Pain Without Losing Weight

Study titled "Dietary Intake Mediates the Relationship of Body Fat to Pain," by Charles F. Emery, PhD, Institute for Behavioral Medicine Research, The Ohio State University, Columbus, and colleagues, published in *Pain*.

Is your weight really responsible for your joint pain? When people gain weight, especially around the middle, they are more likely to experience painful joint-related conditions such as low back pain and knee pain. Up to now, the thinking has been that it was all that pressure on the joints—from gaining weight—that caused the pain.

But that's only part of the story.

While losing weight—and getting exercise—remain key anti-pain tactics, a recent study suggests that you may also be able to reduce your pain simply by changing what you eat even if you don't eat less or lose weight.

***Background:*** Over the years, a number of studies have established a connection between obesity and chronic pain, yet what's behind that connection wasn't fully understood. It was thought that the increased load on joints was the only factor to blame—a mechanical thing. But what you eat affects much more than just your weight—so could there be other factors at work?

***Study:*** Researchers at The Ohio State University evaluated 98 men and women who were already participating in a larger study of the effect of the home environment and eating patterns on health and weight. The participants ranged from normal weight to overweight to obese. Each completed a pain survey and was interviewed by a trained assessor to evaluate the healthfulness of his or her diet.

***Findings:*** Obesity was related to joint pain—no surprise there. But what was also found was that participants who ate anti-inflammatory diets reported less pain—regardless of weight. In other words, the nature of the diet was an independent factor in how much pain these men and women had.

Foods associated with less pain included...

- **Fruit (but not fruit juice)**
- **Whole grains**
- **Seafood**
- **Plant proteins** (such as from nuts, seeds, beans, legumes and soy foods)
- **More polyunsaturated and monounsaturated fats and fewer saturated fats**

Foods associated with more pain included...

- **Refined grains**
- **Excess sodium**

The most powerful anti-pain foods? Seafood and plant proteins.

***Bottom line:*** Eating more seafood, beans and tofu may ease joint pain even if it doesn't lead to weight loss. If your joints are painful, it makes sense to try eating more anti-inflammatory foods such as those found in the Mediterranean diet.

# Does It Seem Like You're Always Chilly?

Michael Aziz, MD, a board-certified internist and attending physician at Lenox Hill Hospital and founder and director of Midtown Integrative Medicine, both in New York City. Dr. Aziz is also author of *The Perfect 10 Diet.*

You find yourself reaching for a sweater when everyone else is comfortable in short sleeves. Your hands and feet often feel like ice. What's going on? Could something be wrong with you?

It could be perfectly normal. Some people are naturally more prone to feeling chilled—especially women. Ironically, it stems from the way women's bodies keep internal organs warm, which protects the uterus and future generations. In women, insulating body fat is concentrated around their core—leaving toes and fingers in the cold. Plus, when women are exposed to cold, their blood vessels contract more dramatically than men's, which sends more blood to protect inner organs—but leaves their hands and feet colder.

***Result:*** While a woman's core body temperature tends to be slightly warmer than a man's (97.8°F versus 97.4°F), her hands register about three degrees colder—87.2°F versus 90°F. But it isn't just being a woman that makes you feel a chill. It might be your health. *Here's why...*

## Medical Conditions That Can Leave You Cold

The following two medical conditions often go undiagnosed. *They can affect both genders, although they're more common in women...*

- **Underactive thyroid.** A telltale symptom of hypothyroidism—when the thyroid gland does not produce sufficient thyroid hormone—is feeling constantly cold. Other symptoms can be weight gain, constipation and fatigue. Your doctor can diagnose a low-thyroid condition with a simple blood test. Once your thyroid levels have been normalized, usually by taking daily thyroid hormone medication, your tolerance to cold should improve.

- **Raynaud's disease.** Cold fingers and toes are also symptoms of Raynaud's disease. It's a usually benign condition in which the small blood vessels in the extremities overreact to cold, as well as stress. This causes fingers and toes to feel cold to the touch and, in many cases, to change color—from white to blue or red and back to normal again.

While Raynaud's has no cure, lifestyle modifications can help—such as keeping hands and feet warm by wearing mittens (they keep fingers warmer than gloves) and socks...or keeping hand and foot warmers in your boots or pockets.

More cold culprits...

***COLD CULPRIT #1:*** **You're too thin.** Muscle generates heat, and fat acts as insulation. But if you're underweight—with a body mass index (BMI) under 18.5—you may lack sufficient body fat or muscle to maintain a normal core body temperature.

***My advice:*** If your low body weight is the result of extreme dieting, a nutritionist can help you adopt healthier dietary strategies. Also, certain medications, including bronchodilators for asthma and the antidepressant *bupropion* (Wellbutrin), can cause weight loss. If you've shed pounds without trying, see your primary care physician to rule out a possible serious medical condition, such as an overactive thyroid, diabetes or cancer.

***COLD CULPRIT #2:* You're on a low-carb diet.** Diets that severely restrict carbohydrates, such as Atkins and Paleo, are popular for their ability to promote quick weight loss. But one of their downsides is that they can make you feel as cold as a caveman. One reason is that carb-restricted diets are very high in protein and fat, which require more energy to be digested, so after a meal your body directs more blood toward your stomach and intestines. Over the long term, a high-protein diet can also inhibit the conversion of thyroid hormone to its active form, which results in feeling cold…or eventually a full-blown underactive thyroid.

***My advice:*** Rather than omit or limit an entire category of food, stick to a balanced 40/40/20 diet—40% of your calories from carbohydrates…40% from (healthy) fats…and 20% from protein. Aim for three meals and one or two snacks per day, depending on your activity level. Your body needs high-quality whole grains, such as brown rice and quinoa, as well as other complex carbohydrates, such as sweet potatoes and squash, for energy and essential vitamins and other nutrients.

A sample day might include a veggie omelet and two slices of rye toast for breakfast…grilled salmon and a mixed greens salad for lunch…chicken with vegetables and brown rice for dinner…and a few chocolate-covered strawberries for dessert.

***Also:*** Don't skip meals. Being hungry causes the body to conserve energy, producing less heat as a result.

***COLD CULPRIT #3:* You don't get enough sleep.** Lack of sleep disturbs the physiological mechanisms of the brain, especially the hypothalamus, which controls body temperature.

***My advice:*** Aim to get seven to eight hours of sleep a night. Don't keep your bedroom too warm—the National Sleep Foundation puts the optimal room temperature for sleep at around 65°F.

If you have trouble falling asleep, give meditation a try. A *JAMA Internal Medicine* study found that meditating five to 20 minutes a day can help you fall asleep more quickly than using basic sleep-hygiene techniques such as establishing a bedtime routine.

***COLD CULPRIT #4:* You're dehydrated.** Your body is 60% water, and if you are dehydrated, it can affect circulation, making you feel colder.

***My advice:*** Be sure to drink plenty of fluids—and drink even more than usual if you are physically active. Water is best, but contrary to common beliefs, tea and coffee can count—your body still holds onto some of these fluids despite their mild diuretic effect.

***Best self-check:*** If your urine is very yellow and concentrated, you are not drinking enough water and other fluids.

***COLD CULPRIT #5:* You're a vegetarian.** Vegetarians are sometimes deficient in iron. Why? Red meat has plenty of iron and it's easily absorbed, while vegetarian sources, such as beans and greens, have less iron and it's in a less available form. Low iron intake can lead to iron-deficiency anemia—and feeling cold is a common symptom. Vegans, who eat only plant-based foods, may also be low in vitamin B-12, found primarily in animal products, including meat, fish, poultry, eggs and dairy. A B-12 deficiency can lead to "pernicious anemia," which can cause you to feel cold as well.

***Note:*** Antacids and proton pump inhibitors, commonly used to treat acid reflux, also can inhibit iron and B-12 absorption. And people who have Crohn's disease and celiac disease are at risk for anemia.

***My advice:*** If you're a vegetarian or vegan, have your doctor run a simple blood test for iron deficiency.

***Warning:*** Only take an iron supplement if it's prescribed, as too much iron can be dangerous.

Vegans also need a supplementary source of B-12, since it's found only in animal foods. But so do many omnivores and lacto-ovo vegetarians.

***Here's why:*** Between 10% and 30% of older adults have gastritis, which interferes with the absorption of B-12 from food—but they can absorb B-12 from supplements and fortified foods. That's why the Institute of Medicine recommends that adults older than age 50 get much of their vitamin B-12 from vitamin supplements or fortified foods.

***Tip:*** If you rely on antacids or proton pump inhibitors, or have a condition such as Crohn's or celiac, get your B-12 levels tested.

## Is a Drink Warming?

Alcohol, in moderation, dilates blood vessels, making you feel warmer quickly. But here's the rub—the effect is fleeting because your body temperature will drop as heat escapes through those dilated blood vessels.

# What Your Skin Says About Your Health

Jeffrey P. Callen, MD, a professor of medicine and chief of the division of dermatology at the University of Louisville School of Medicine in Kentucky. He is the coeditor of *Dermatological Signs of Systemic Disease*, author or coauthor of more than 400 scientific papers and the recipient of the 2017 Master Dermatologist Award from the American Academy of Dermatology.

Did you know that a skin issue—that red rash or dry, flaky skin—isn't always just about your skin? It might be alerting you to an internal problem, such as a thyroid condition, that your doctor needs to know about and treat.

Plus, some skin conditions may mean that you have an increased risk for other health problems (for example, psoriasis has been shown to increase risk for cardiovascular disease...see chapter 1), and you will want to take measures to reduce these risks.

## Signs of Hashimoto's

Thyroid disease (Hashimoto's thyroiditis) is an autoimmune disease that is one of the most common causes of hypothyroidism, a condition in which the thyroid gland doesn't produce enough thyroid hormone. An estimated 14 million Americans may have the disease—and most don't know it. *But your skin may sound the alarm...*

- **Dry skin.** Hypothyroidism can cause a wide range of symptoms, including fatigue, muscle and joint pain, depression, mental sluggishness, low libido, weight gain, constipation, cold hands and feet, dry, coarse hair—and dry skin, one of the most common red flags.
- **Loss of eyebrow hair.** People with hypothyroidism sometimes lose the outer third of their eyebrows.

When standard treatment for hypo-thyroidism (a thyroid replacement hormone) is given, skin problems typically resolve.

## A Risky Skin Condition

Systemic lupus erythematosus (SLE) is an autoimmune disease in which the immune system attacks various tissues and organs, including the skin. Patients with SLE often develop a "butterfly rash"—a red rash that spreads across both cheeks in the shape of a butterfly's wings. Other skin symptoms can include lesions that worsen when exposed to the sun.

People with lupus are at higher risk for many other health problems, including heart disease, stroke, cancer, kidney disease, bone disease and infections.

***What to do:*** If you have lupus, you and your physician need to create a plan to minimize your risks of developing these other diseases. Elements of the plan should include controlling blood pressure and high cholesterol with lifestyle measures (such as regular exercise) and possibly medications...getting regular cancer screenings...and having regular checkups for kidney function and bone density.

## Check Your Neck for Thyroid Abnormalities

Icahn School of Medicine at Mount Sinai, news release.
Womenshealth.gov

Regular self-exams play an important role in early detection of thyroid disease, a specialist says.

Women are more likely than men to have thyroid diseases, especially right after pregnancy and menopause.

"The number of cases of thyroid cancer is rising, and while in most cases the outcomes of treatment are favorable, some patients present with disease that has progressed and may be more difficult to treat," said Ilya Likhterov, MD. He is an ear, nose and throat doctor in New York City.

About 200 million people worldwide have thyroid disease. Of more than 20 million Americans with thyroid disease, only four out of 10 know they have it, according to the American Thyroid Association.

"While in most patients thyroid cancer develops without signs or symptoms, patients who have had significant exposure to radiation or who have first-degree family members with a history of thyroid cancer need to be especially cautious, since they are at a higher risk," Dr. Likhterov added.

All patients must pay attention to sudden voice changes or masses in the neck, said Dr. Likhterov, an assistant professor of otolaryngology at Icahn School of Medicine at Mount Sinai in New York City.

If undetected and untreated, thyroid disease can cause depression, constant exhaustion, joint pain, muscle aches, weight gain and hair loss, according to a Mount Sinai news release.

To perform a thyroid self-exam, use a mirror to view the lower middle area of your neck, above the collarbones, and below the larynx. This is where the thyroid is located.

While focusing on this area, tip your head back, take a drink of water and swallow. As you swallow, watch for any bulges or protrusions, Dr. Likhterov said.

It's important not to confuse the Adam's apple with the thyroid, which is located farther down on your neck, closer to the collarbone.

If you detect any bulges or protrusions in this area, see your physician, Dr. Likhterov said. You may have an enlarged thyroid or a thyroid nodule. A doctor can determine if cancer is present or if you require treatment for thyroid disease.

The U.S. Office on Women's Health has more about thyroid disease at Womens health.gov

## How a Doctor Beat Her Hashimoto's

Susan Blum, MD, assistant clinical professor in the department of preventive medicine at the Icahn School of Medicine at Mount Sinai in New York City, and an integrative medicine specialist in the medicine department at Greenwich Hospital in Connecticut. The founder and director of the Blum Center for Health in Rye Brook, New York, Dr. Blum is also author of *The Immune System Recovery Plan*. Blum CenterForHealth.com

More than a decade ago, I was diagnosed with Hashimoto's thyroiditis (HT), the most common cause of hypothyroidism, a condition in which the thyroid gland doesn't produce enough thyroid hormones.

Hypothyroidism is more widespread than many people realize, affecting about 14 million Americans. And because thyroid hormones regulate metabolism—key functions such as breathing, heart rate, digestion and body temperature—symptoms are wide ranging. They can include daylong fatigue, weight gain, constipation, low libido, weakness, muscle cramps and aches, cold intolerance, dry skin, poor memory and depression.

HT is typically diagnosed with the same blood tests used to diagnose other causes of hypothyroidism (including those that measure thyroid hormone levels and antithyroid antibodies). With HT, however, an imaging test, such as ultrasound, might also be used to identify the characteristic inflammation of the thyroid gland that occurs with this disease.

***My story:*** When I was diagnosed with HT, my primary care physician said, "No big deal. You'll just take thyroid hormone replacement medication and be fine." I disagreed. As a doctor board-certified in preventive medicine, I wanted to discover the causes of HT, an autoimmune disease in which the immune system mistakes the thyroid for a foreign invader, attacking it and destroying thyroid cells.

For years, I've researched HT for myself and for my patients. With the help of an increasing body of scientific evidence, I have identified key factors that often trigger and worsen most cases of HT—and the natural therapies that can help...

## Mercury

When I began to investigate my disease, I discovered that my body had trouble excreting mercury—a toxic metal that can damage tissues and cause autoimmune disease. I've now found that many patients with autoimmune disease have a high mercury level, based on blood and urine tests. One main source of mercury toxicity—eating lots of fish.

***My advice:*** Large fish at the top of the food chain, such as swordfish and tuna, contain the most mercury, but all fish deliver some levels of the toxic metal. That's why I recommend eating fish only twice a week. Opt for varieties that are low in mercury (such as anchovies, sardines, salmon, sole, trout and Arctic char). If you limit your intake of mercury, your body will start to eliminate the excess stored in tissues via urine and stool.

## Missing Nutrients

Two nutrients are key for preventing or healing HT...*

*Check with your doctor before taking these supplements—they can interact with some medications and affect certain medical conditions.

- **Selenium.** This mineral helps create thyroid hormone...helps convert T4 (the less active form of thyroid hormone) to T3 (the active form)...and protects the thyroid gland from oxidative damage. Selenium is so important for thyroid health that several studies suggest that a deficiency of the mineral might trigger HT.

***My advice:*** Each day, take 400 micrograms (mcg) of selenomethionine (the form found in food, which is easier to absorb) for three to six months, then switch to a maintenance dose of 200 mcg.

***Important:*** Selenium is therapeutic when taken in the appropriate dose but toxic in high doses. Never take more than 400 mcg daily. Once selenium levels are restored, you may be able to maintain adequate levels by eating selenium-rich foods (such as Brazil nuts, shrimp and sardines) instead of taking a supplement.

- **Vitamin D.** Researchers have linked low levels of this immune-strengthening nutrient to many autoimmune diseases, including multiple sclerosis, rheumatoid arthritis, lupus, inflammatory bowel disease—and now HT.

***Recent research:*** Greek scientists studied 218 people with HT and found that 85% of them had a vitamin D deficiency.

***My advice:*** Start by getting your vitamin D level checked. If your level is low, take a vitamin D-3 supplement. Most people can safely take up to 4,000 international units (IU) daily, but get your vitamin D level checked every three months. Once you reach an optimal vitamin D level (about 50 ng/mL), cut back to 1,000 IU to 2,000 IU daily.

## Gluten

This protein, found in wheat, barley and rye, can damage the intestinal lining, triggering increased intestinal permeability (also known as leaky gut), in which gluten and other undigested proteins enter the bloodstream.

Once these undigested proteins are in the bloodstream, the immune system attacks them as if they were foreign invaders. People with gluten sensitivity can end up with leaky gut syndrome...diarrhea, bloating and/or fatigue...an immune system in constant overdrive...and an autoimmune disease such as HT.

***Recent research:*** A study published in the journal *Gastroenterology* showed that people who were sensitive to gluten were seven times more likely to develop HT and other types of autoimmune disease compared with people who did not have gluten sensitivity.

***My advice:*** Eliminate gluten for three weeks—and then eat gluten-containing foods for two or three days. Nine out of 10 of my HT patients feel a lot better after the three-week elimination period, with more energy and mental clarity—and their symptoms return after they reintroduce gluten. This is how you will know whether you are gluten sensitive.

Rice, buckwheat, millet and quinoa are gluten free. Gluten-free breads are often in the frozen section because they are not made with the usual chemical preservatives. For more on gluten-free foods, go to MassGeneral.org/digestive/assets/pdf/gluten_free_diet.pdf.

## Fibromyalgia Options

People with fibromyalgia should not pin their hopes on hyperbaric oxygen therapy. A preliminary study found that women who received the high-pressure oxygen treatments five times weekly for two months showed significant reduction in pain.

***But:*** Insurers may not reimburse treatment costs, which can be tens of thousands of dollars...and the effects are temporary.

***Better:*** Exercise...vitamin D supplements ...*pregabalin* (Lyrica), *duloxetine* (Cymbalta) and other medications.

Anne Louise Oaklander, MD, PhD, associate professor of neurology at Harvard Medical School and director of the nerve injury unit at Massachusetts General Hospital, both in Boston.

## Better MS Treatment

Yoga or water exercise can dramatically reduce common multiple sclerosis (MS) symptoms, such as fatigue, depression and paresthesia (pins and needles tingling), a recent study of women with MS found. Those who did these forms of exercise for at least 30 minutes three times a week had a 35-fold lower risk of developing moderate-to-severe depression, as well as less fatigue and paresthesia, than those who did no exercise.

Serge Brand, PhD, professor of affective, stress and sleep disorders, University of Basel, Switzerland.

## When Low Thyroid Symptoms Don't Go Away...Even on Synthroid

Jacqueline Jonklaas, MD, PhD, associate professor of endocrinology and medicine, Georgetown University Medical Center, Washington, DC, and author of a study titled "Risks and safety of combination therapy for hypothyroidism," published in *Expert Review of Clinical Pharmacology*.

Is your doctor giving you Synthroid to treat low thyroid hormone levels (hypothyroidism)—but you still have disturbing symptoms? You're tired...struggling with weight gain...perhaps especially sensitive to cold. Yet your doctor doesn't have a solution.

You're not alone. As many as 15% of patients taking meds to correct hypothyroidism continue to suffer the same symptoms that brought them to their physicians in the first place.

And nearly half of them have normal thyroid hormone levels on blood tests.

What's a suffering patient to do? There is another approach—one your doctor may not tell you about. It's one that combines the storage (or "pro-hormone") form, T4, and the active form of thyroid hormone, T3. To learn more, we spoke with Jacqueline Jonklaas, MD, PhD, associate professor of endocrinology and medicine at Georgetown University Medical Center in Washington, DC, who recently reviewed the scientific literature about this approach.

## When Synthroid Leaves You Cold

As many as 27 million Americans have low thyroid levels. It's more common in women than in men. In many cases, the cause is an autoimmune disease (Hashimoto's), in which the body produces antibodies to the thyroid gland. Medical procedures, including treatment of thyroid cancer, can also bring on a low thyroid condition.

The majority of people with hypothyroid disease are successfully treated with a drug called *levothyroxine* (Synthroid). It's a synthetic form of T4, the pro-hormone that the body converts to T3, the active thyroid hormone the body can use. "The vast majority of patients feel pretty good on levothyroxine, but there is a percentage of patients—between 5% and 15%—who don't," says Dr. Jonklaas.

Why doesn't T4 work for them? One explanation is that some people's bodies are not efficient at converting T4 to T3. Indeed, about 15% of the population, notes Dr. Jonklaas, has a genetic abnormality that, to one degree or another, may interfere with the conversion of T4 to T3.

One obvious solution is to simply give patients T3. There are therapies that contain T3 either on its own or in combination with T4. Medical groups, including the American Thyroid Association, are very wary of these alternatives to levothyroxine because of their potential side effects (which we'll discuss below). Some physicians and patient advocates believe that T3 therapies can be used safely in patients who do not respond well to levothyroxine alone. Mary Shomon, a patient advocate and author of *The Thyroid Diet Revolution: Manage Your Metabolism for Lasting Weight Loss*, has hypothyroid disease herself. "The medical world pushes Synthroid to the exclusion of any other options," she says. "My battle cry is not that any one drug is better than the other, but that patients need to know about all of the options."

## T3 Pros and Cons

One of the concerns with taking T3 is that the available pills are short-acting medications. This results in high levels of T3 right after the drug is taken and low levels when it wears off. High levels of T3 can be harmful—they're associated with insomnia and anxiety and can lead to dangerous rapid heart beat. Prolonged high T3 levels can even harm the heart and the bones. One way to avoid these peaks and troughs in T3 levels is to cut pills into smaller sizes and take these smaller amounts of the medication at more frequent intervals during the day. Another solution is to have a compounding pharmacy make lower-dose capsules—though there is a concern about the potency of such capsules, since these pharmacies are only partly regulated by the Food and Drug Administration along with a patchwork of state regulations, some more stringent and some less so.

In the past, most patients did in fact take a drug that was a combination of T4 and T3 hormones. The drug, Armour Thyroid, is a dried form of pig thyroid. But pig thyroid has a high proportion of T3 to T4 and was found to increase risks for heart and bone disease. Although doctors almost universally now prescribe synthetic T4 (Synthroid) instead, Armour Thyroid is still available and some "nonresponders" to T4 swear by it.

Although recent studies have not shown that a T3/T4 combination is more effective than T4 alone, Dr. Jonklaas says that many of those studies had shortcomings. For instance, in some of the studies, T3 was given only once a day, and most of the studies were short-term and so unable to assess long-term effects—good or bad. "We don't really know whether taking T3 for five years will hurt bone density or increase the risk of having cardiac problems," she says. "We do have anecdotal and common experience of patients about how they feel better."

## What to Do Now

Until more research is conducted, Dr. Jonklaas advises trying to tweak T4 therapy as much as possible before trying combination T3/T4 therapy. If you do try combination therapy, your doctor will need to closely monitor your TSH (thyroid-stimulating hormone, a measure of your pituitary assessment of your thyroid status), thyroid hormones, heart rate, bone density—and any other side effects (such as rapid heart beat, insomnia or anxiety) you might experience.

***Bottom line:*** If you don't feel well even with Synthroid and your endocrinologist is not willing to consider other options, it may be time to find a new physician—someone who is less focused on lab results, more focused on symptom resolution...and open to discussing alternative treatments.

# Headaches Linked to Hypothyroidism

In hypothyroidism, the body does not produce enough thyroid hormone. This can lead to mood swings, weight gain, fatigue and other symptoms.

***Recent finding:*** People with a history of headache had 21% greater risk for hypothyroidism than people without a headache history...and people with migraines had 41% greater risk.

***If you have headaches:*** Talk to your doctor about being screened for hypothyroidism.

Vincent Martin, MD, professor of medicine and codirector of the Headache and Facial Pain Center, Gardner Neuroscience Institute, University of Cincinnati, and coauthor of a study of 8,400 people, published in *Headache: The Journal of Head and Face Pain.*

# When Exercise Harms Your Thyroid

Brooke Kalanick, ND, a naturopathic doctor in private practice in New York City. She is coauthor of *Ultimate You: A 4-Phase Total Body Makeover for Women Who Want Maximum Results.* BetterByDrBrooke.com

There are a few things to think about with autoimmune diseases and exercise, especially with Hashimoto's. You might have a hard time recovering from strenuous workouts and you are more prone to injury.

But strength training is important. What you want is lean metabolic mass. Many women are just not strength training—and I don't mean with two-pound weights. Woman should have a whole workout plan that includes squats, serious weights and deadlifts. Of course, you have to work at your fitness level and, hopefully, with some personal coaching. Bigger movements with heavier weights is not a thing most women gravitate toward.

## Trade Some Cardio for Weights...But Take Care

The goal is getting more lean mass with larger muscle groups involved through full body exercise. A good template is doing that three times a week. But moving toward a point where you're using heavier weights is very important for your metabolism. Leave the lighter stuff and leave the excessive cardio behind and trade that for some weights if you want to get a jump on the fat loss.

Now, that said, if someone is strength training with Hashimoto's or another thyroid condition and she's doing a lot of repetitions—let's say her trainer or her workout routine has got her doing 20 of something with a light weight—there's a good chance she'll have a really hard time recovering. Her metabolism just does not respond as well as someone without this condition. And sometimes those constant repetitions cause serious tendonitis. You'll see almost everyone with Hashimoto's has a shoulder problem or Achilles tendonitis. The high repetition, high volume strength training can really exacerbate certain conditions.

The other thing is overtraining. When you've got someone with Hashimoto's, you've got a lot of inflammation and they have a really difficult time recovering from anything. I've got patients who can't walk more than 20 minutes or they spend two days in bed after overexerting themselves. Then someone else might be training for a power lifting competition. These are very unique situations, but they show the care that you have to take if you have a thyroid condition. You have to be extra careful to build yourself up slowly.

If you're someone with Hashimoto's trying to get more exercise and you're falling apart, dial it back. Rather than dialing back the frequency—let's say you're committed to going three times a week—just dial back the time or the intensity a little bit, and get yourself to a place where you can recover from those workouts before you start adding more on.

Obviously if you're really struggling, you want to stay away from the higher reps and go toward heavier weights. But again, you've got to work yourself into that. So just gauge yourself, and if your particular regimen is that you work out five days a week and you're falling apart after two days, you know you have to take down the volume or the intensity. Just listen to your body.

## What Recovery Means

Some soreness is normal from strength training and exercising. What I'm talking about when I say recovery is when you feel wiped out. You may have gone for a 30-minute strength-training session or may have just gone for a 40-minute walk, and the next day you can barely get out of bed or really dreading just the thought of working out again. That's how you know that you're overtraining and you're not achieving adequate recovery.

So pay attention to how fatigued you are—how achy, how swollen, how difficult it is to get up and get going the next day. And take note how much effort it takes to get to your next workout session.

# Chapter 11

# EMOTIONAL RESCUE

## The 10 Very Best Foods to Prevent Depression (and Build a Healthier Brain)

Here's a startling statistic—studies show that people who consume a healthy diet are 40% to 50% less likely to develop depression.

What are the absolutely best nutrients—and most nutrient-packed foods—to protect your brain from depression and other ailments?

What protects mood also protects against dementia and other brain-related conditions. The brain is the biggest asset we have, so we should be selecting foods that specifically nourish the brain.

Here's how to build the healthiest brain possible—starting in your kitchen.

### Nutrients Brains Need Most

These key nutrients are the most important...

- **Long-chain omega-3 fatty acids.** There are two major ones. Docosahexaenoic acid (DHA) creates hormones called "neuroprotectins and resolvins" that combat brain inflammation, which is implicated in the development of depression (as well as dementia). Eicosapentaenoic acid (EPA) protects the cardiovascular system, important for a healthy brain.
- **Zinc.** This mineral plays a major role in the development of new brain cells and can boost the efficacy of antidepressant medications.
- **Folate.** Also known as vitamin B-9, folate is needed for good moods and a healthy brain. It helps produce defensin-1, a molecule that protects the brain and increases the concentration of acetylcholine, a neurotransmitter that's crucial to memory and cognition.
- **Iron.** This essential element is a crucial cofactor in the synthesis of mood-regulating neurotransmitters including dopamine and serotonin.
- **Magnesium.** This mineral is required to keep myelin—the insulation of brain cells—healthy. It also increases brain-derived neurotrophic factor (BDNF), which promotes the growth of new neurons and healthy connections among brain cells. A deficiency in

Drew Ramsey, MD, psychiatrist, Columbia University Medical Center, and assistant professor, Columbia University College of Physicians and Surgeons, both in New York City. His latest book is *Eat Complete*. DrewRamseyMD.com magnesium can lead to depression, anxiety, symptoms of ADHD, insomnia and fatigue.

• **Vitamin B-12.** This vitamin, which often is deficient as we age, helps makes neurotransmitters that are key to mood and memory.

• **Vitamin E.** This potent antioxidant vitamin protects polyunsaturated fatty acids in the brain—including DHA. Vitamin E–rich foods, but not supplements, are linked to the prevention of clinical depression as well as slower progression of Alzheimer's disease. One reason may be that most supplements contain only alpha-tocopherol, while other vitamin E compounds, particularly tocotrienols, play important roles in brain function.

• **Dietary fiber.** A high-fiber diet supports healthy gut bacteria (the gut "microbiome"), which growing evidence suggests is key for mental health.

## Boosting Your Mood at the Supermarket

The best brain foods are mostly plant-based, but seafood, wild game and even some organ meats make the top of the list, too...

• **Leafy greens** such as kale, mustard greens and collard greens

• **Bell peppers** such as red, green and orange

• **Cruciferous vegetables** such as cauliflower, broccoli and cabbage

• **Berries** such as strawberries, raspberries and blueberries

• **Nuts** such as pecans, walnuts, almonds and cashews

• **Bivalves** such as oysters, clams and mussels

• **Crustaceans** such as crab, lobster and shrimp

• **Fish** such as sardines, salmon and fish roe

• **Organ meats** such as liver, poultry giblets and heart

• **Game and wild meat** such as bison, elk and duck

Eating these nutrient-dense foods is likely to help prevent and treat mental illness. When someone with depression is treated, the real goal is to prevent that person from ever getting depressed again.

## Everyday Brain Foods

Not into eating beef heart? Having a little trouble stocking up on elk? When it comes to meat, wild game may not be widely available, but grass-fed beef, which is higher in omega-3 fatty acids than conventionally raised beef, is stocked in most supermarkets—and may be independently associated with protection from depression.

Other foods that didn't make it to the top of the Brain Food Scale but that still are very good for the brain include eggs (iron, zinc), beans (fiber, magnesium, iron) and fruits and vegetables of all colors (fiber, antioxidants). Plus, small quantities of dark chocolate, which gives you a little dopamine rush. Dopamine, he explains, is a neurotransmitter that provides a feeling of reward.

# Do This to Beat the Blues

Christopher Martell, PhD, clinic director of the Psychological Services Center at the University of Massachusetts, Amherst, author of two textbooks on behavioral activation (BA) for therapists and coauthor (with Michael Addis, PhD) of the client workbook on BA, *Overcoming Depression One Step at a Time: The New Behavioral Activation Approach to Getting Your Life Back.*

If you think of therapy for depression as all talk and no action, here's a pleasant surprise—a simple, short-term and inexpensive new form of therapy helps people with depression feel better and improve their states of mind by "doing." Doing what? *You'll see...*

## Treating Depression from the Outside In

Behavioral activation (BA), as the approach is called, helps people reengage with others and with activities that they enjoy—or used to enjoy—rather than focusing on their inner thoughts and feelings.

When people are depressed, they naturally withdraw socially and from activities they used to enjoy—and get pulled in by their negative moods. This sets up a bad cycle.

That's where BA comes in—breaking this negative cycle. It targets inertia, encouraging people to treat their depression through their behavior.

Let's say you enjoy, or used to enjoy, quilting. (In fact, it could be any activity you like, either alone or with others—cooking with friends, hiking, playing piano, being in a book club, drawing, etc.) With BA therapy, you would be encouraged to pursue that pastime in a small, incremental way—perhaps, say, by searching online for local quilting clubs to join. The next step might involve choosing a particular club and making inquiries about when it meets and whether it's open to new members. When internal barriers arise—if you can't mobilize your efforts because you feel so down and tired, for example—you and the therapist would try to identify what's really standing in your way and what you can do to get around those obstacles.

## How Well Does BA Work?

BA therapy has developed in its current form only within the past 20 years, so it is not as thoroughly researched as other forms of therapy. *But there's a growing body of supportive evidence...*

- **It works as well as cognitive behavioral therapy (CBT),** according to a recent study published in *The Lancet.* When 440 adults who met a primary diagnosis of depression but who were not yet getting any treatment received at least eight weekly sessions of CBT—a well-established approach that focuses on changing thought patterns and behaviors—or BA, the therapies were found to be equally effective.

- **It works in older people.** A recent study from the Weill Cornell Institute of Geriatric Psychiatry in White Plains, New York, published in *The American Journal of Geriatric Psychiatry*, looked at 48 adults over age 60 with mild-to-moderate depression. After the patients were treated with nine weekly sessions of BA, they were engaged, participating in many more personally rewarding activities—and they experienced a sharp decline in their depressive symptoms.

## The Exercise Connection

There's another potential benefit offered by BA. If this therapy could help people with depression become more physically active, the effects could be profound.

***Here's why:*** According to a recent study published in *Psychosomatic Medicine*, 30 minutes of brisk exercise three times a week is not only as effective in treating depression as major antidepressants but also much more effective in preventing the return of depression. Six months after treatment ended, only 8% in the exercise-only group had their depression return, compared with 38% in the drug-only group.

## Should You Try It?

Even though BA isn't successful for everyone, when it works, it can work very quickly. The exact mechanism of action isn't clear, but reengaging in activity can increase positive feelings—and the negative thinking that's associated with depression can change as you change your behavior.

While each patient and each therapist is individual, a typical course of BA consists of weekly 50-minute sessions for up to 24 weeks. It is a nondrug approach but can also work for individuals who are being treated with psychiatric medications, such as antidepressants.

To find a BA therapist, the best place to start is with a therapist trained in CBT (most therapists trained in CBT can do BA). To find a CBT therapist, click on "Find Help," then on "Find a CBT Therapist" at ABCT.org, the site of the Association for Behavioral and Cognitive Therapies. Like other psychotherapies, BA is generally covered by insurance.

And the good news is that the key to this therapy is doing what you enjoy!

---

# The Menopause Depression Trap

Study titled "Independent Contributions of Nocturnal Hot Flashes and Sleep Disturbance to Depression in Estrogen-Deprived Women," by researchers at Brigham and Women's Hospital and Harvard Medical School in Boston, Massachusetts, published in *Journal of Clinical Endocrinology and Metabolism.*

JoAnn E. Manson, MD, MPH, DrPH, chief, division of preventive medicine, interim executive director, Connors Center for Women's Health and Gender Biology, Brigham and Women's Hospital and professor of medicine and Michael and Lee Bell Professor of Women's Health, Harvard Medical School, Boston. She is author of *Hot Flashes, Hormones & Your Health.*

---

If you're a woman, there's a 25% chance that you'll experience depression some time in your life. One vulnerable time is adolescence. Another is menopause.

In fact, a clear risk is emerging. A particular combination of menopausal symptoms may increase your chances of falling into a depressed state, according to recent research.

Most women sail through perimenopause and into postmenopause without a hint of depressive symptoms. But if you personally have any particular reason to be wary of depression—or even if you just want to be extra careful—you should know which menopausal symptoms put you at greatest risk.

***Hint:*** It happens at night.

## Depression Risk and Menopause

What triggers a slide from menopausal moodiness to spirit-sapping depressive symptoms or depression—but only in some women? Certainly a history of depression increases your risk. But some women who've never been depressed experience it for the first time during perimenopause or in the first few postmenopausal years. Hormones are part of the story. It's not just the sometimes wildly fluctuating hormones of early perimenopause that are the culprit. Depression often strikes toward the end of perimenopause and in the first years of postmenopause when estrogen levels are low but stable.

To tease out how hormones, symptoms and moods interact, researchers at Harvard Medical School actually studied 29 young, premenopausal women (average age 27). Why? That way, they could temporarily induce menopause and readily study the "before" and the "after" in the absence of other changes of "aging." Each woman got a single dose of a medication that suppresses estrogen production for four weeks.

Beforehand, the women underwent sleep studies and psychiatric testing to make sure that none had sleep disturbances or depression. Each woman then kept a record of how many hot flashes she got during the day and how many at night (when they're often called night sweats). After four weeks, the women repeated the psychiatric testing and sleep study—this time with a test that objectively gauged hot flashes by measuring skin temperature.

## Depressing Duo: Night Sweats and Disturbed Sleep

Nearly 70% of the women experienced hot flashes—about the same percentage as with women who go through natural menopause. Some had most of their flashes during the day, others, at night. Mild depressive symptoms emerged for about 60% of the women, although only one showed signs of full-blown clinical depression.

Did daytime hot flashes give the women the blues? Not at all! While undoubtedly bothersome—especially if you're 27!—daytime hot flashes had nothing to do with an increase in depressive symptoms for these women.

Nor did night sweats—unless they messed up sleep.

In women whose night sweats woke them up, depressive symptoms reliably went up. That was especially true for women who woke up and couldn't get back to sleep for a while—in some cases, the women were unhappily awake for more than two hours a night. Not being able to fall into that deep, restorative phase of sleep called REM also upped the chance of feeling depressed.

## Getting the Sleep You Need to Feel Good

Getting a good night's sleep, undisturbed by night sweats, is very important if you want to safeguard your emotional health throughout the menopausal transition. JoAnn E. Manson, MD, DrPH, a professor of women's health at Harvard Medical School in Boston and a member of the panel of experts for Bottom Line's Menopause Center, has this advice…

• **Don't ignore bothersome hot flashes,** especially if they happen at night and disturb your sleep.

• **Don't let your health-care provider ignore them, either.** Bring them up so that, together, you can find ways to manage them that work for you.

• **Avoid triggers.** Although hot flashes seem to come out of nowhere, many women notice that they seem tied to a particular activity or situation. Common night sweat triggers include a warm room (see below), feeling stressed, eating spicy food and drinking alcohol. The best way to find your triggers? Keep a hot flash diary (see page 287).

• **Sleeping in a warm room or under blankets is a particular trigger for night sweats.** Make your room cooler, and consider sleeping with a fan or, in the summer, with the air conditioner running. (The ideal sleeping temperature is between 60F and 67F, according to the National Sleep Foundation.)

• **Get educated about your treatment options.** Download the MenoPro app (available on both iTunes/IOS and Android/Google Play) created by The North American Menopause Society. It's free and not supported by industry, so you won't see any drug advertisements.

• **Consider mind-body approaches.** There is evidence from randomized controlled trials that both cognitive behavioral therapy and hypnosis help reduce hot flashes/night sweats.

• **Consider medication options.** Hormone therapy is effective in reducing hot flashes and night sweats, as are SSRIs and other antidepressants. Women in early menopause without elevated breast cancer or cardiovascular risk are usually good candidates for hormone therapy.

***Bottom line:*** If night sweats are keeping you up at night, it's a serious health threat. Get help. It's an investment in your emotional well-being.

---

# More Older Women Hitting the Bottle Hard

Rosalind Breslow, PhD, MPH, epidemiologist, U.S. National Institute on Alcohol Abuse and Alcoholism.

J.C. Garbutt, MD, professor, psychiatry, and medical director, Alcohol and Substance Abuse Program, University of North Carolina, Chapel Hill.

*Alcoholism: Clinical and Experimental Research.*

---

More older American women than ever are drinking—and drinking hard, a recent study shows.

Most troubling was the finding that the prevalence of binge drinking among older women is increasing dramatically, far faster than it is among older men, the researchers noted.

***The difference was striking:*** Among men, the average prevalence of binge drinking remained stable from 1997 to 2014, while it increased an average of nearly 4% per year among women, the researchers found.

## Alcohol's Effects on Women

Increased drinking and binge drinking can be a serious health problem for women, said study author Rosalind Breslow, PhD, MPH, an epidemiologist at the U.S. National Institute on Alcohol Abuse and Alcoholism.

Women don't tolerate alcohol as well as men, and they start to have alcohol-related problems at lower drinking levels than men, Dr. Breslow explained.

She pointed out that on average, women weigh less than men, and have less water in their bodies than men do. (Alcohol dissolves in water.)

"So, after a man and woman of the same weight drink the same amount of alcohol, the woman's blood alcohol concentration will tend to be higher, putting her at greater risk for harm," Dr. Breslow said.

## The Study

For the study, Dr. Breslow and her colleagues collected data on more than 65,000 men and women aged 60 and older who were current drinkers. Among these, more than 6,500 men and 1,700 women were binge drinkers.

Older adults, in general, are at greater risk of the effects of alcohol than younger adults, Dr. Breslow noted. "They're more sensitive to the effects of alcohol, which can contribute to falls and other injuries, a major problem in older people," she said.

As the US population ages, the number of men and women 60 and older who drink will likely increase further, bringing with it more alcohol-related problems.

In the study, said Dr. Breslow, "we found that between 1997 and 2014, the proportion of older male drinkers in the US population increased about 1% per year, and female drinkers increased nearly 2% per year."

The report was published in the journal *Alcoholism: Clinical and Experimental Research*.

A study published last year also found the gap in drinking between men and women is closing.

Women across the globe are now nearly as likely as men to drink and to engage in excessive drinking, according to researchers with the National Drug and Alcohol Research Center at the University of New South Wales in Australia.

## Implications

It's not clear why this is happening, Dr. Breslow added.

"There is a great deal of speculation that baby boomers drank more when they were young and continue to drink more as a group. There is some limited evidence to support this speculation," she said.

"We did find that more younger boomers, ages 60 to 64, both men and women, were drinking than people of the same age in past generations," Dr. Breslow added.

Whether drinking is increasing among certain racial or ethnic groups isn't something the researchers analyzed, she said.

But alcohol can have devastating consequences, particularly for older adults, Dr. Breslow said.

"Too much drinking increases your chances of being injured or even killed. Alcohol is a factor, for example, in about 60% of fatal burn injuries, drownings and homicides; 50% of severe trauma injuries and sexual assaults; and 40% of fatal motor vehicle crashes, suicides and fatal falls," she said.

In addition, heavy drinkers have a greater risk of liver disease, heart disease, sleep disorders, depression, stroke, bleeding from the stomach, sexually transmitted infections from unsafe sex, and several types of cancer, Dr. Breslow said. They may also have problems managing diabetes, high blood pressure and other chronic conditions.

## Expert Reaction

Another alcohol abuse expert also felt that the rise in binge drinking among older women was the most concerning finding in the study.

"We know that, overall, women are more sensitive to the negative health consequences of alcohol than men," said J.C. Garbutt, MD, medical director of the University of North Carolina Alcohol and Substance Abuse Program, in Chapel Hill.

"These consequences include liver disease, high blood pressure, stroke, heart disease and cognitive impairment—serious problems—and addiction to alcohol is possible as well," he said.

Dr. Garbutt said he couldn't explain the increase in binge drinking among older women.

"One would have to think there are major cultural factors at work, including the greater acceptability for women to drink, family structural changes, and perhaps greater access. But we really don't know so it would be premature to speculate," he said.

### Advice

"Regardless, this speaks to the need to continue to educate the public about the harms of alcohol, including the increased risk to women and older individuals," Dr. Garbutt said.

"Think before you drink," Dr. Breslow said. Adults over age 65 who are healthy and do not take medications should not have more than three drinks a day or seven drinks in a week, she said.

"Based on your health and how alcohol affects you, you may need to drink less or not at all," she added.

For more on women and drinking, visit the U.S. National Institute on Alcohol Abuse and Alcoholism, Niaaa.nih.gov. Search "women and drinking."

## Are You Addicted to Your Cell Phone?

Peter J. Papadakos, MD, director of critical care medicine at the University of Rochester Medical Center and professor of anesthesiology, neurology, surgery and neurosurgery at the University of Rochester, both in Rochester, New York. Dr. Papadakos was one of the first experts to identify the potential for distraction from smartphones and to popularize the term "distracted doctoring."

Researchers at the University of Rochester modified the widely used CAGE survey for alcoholism by replacing the term "drink" with "personal electronic device" to help identify addiction to a smartphone or other devices.

**1. Have you ever felt you needed to cut down on your personal electronic device use?**

**2. Have people annoyed you by criticizing your use of your personal electronic device?**

**3. Have you felt guilty about your overuse of your personal electronic device?**

**4. Do you reach for your personal electronic device first thing in the morning?**

Two or more "yes" answers suggest an addiction. Recognizing that you have a problem is the first step to cutting down on excessive use of technology.

## How to Stop Your Worst Memories from Tormenting You

Ronald A. Ruden, MD, PhD, an internist on the clinical staff at NYU Langone Medical Center and Lenox Hill Hospital. He sees patients at his private practice in New York City. He created Havening Techniques to eliminate the consequences that arise from stressful or traumatic events. He is author of *Havening Techniques: A Primer* and *When the Past Is Always Present: Emotional Traumatization, Causes and Cures*. Havening.org

What can you do if you suffer from phobias, panic attacks, traumatic memories or other emotional disturbances? Like millions of Americans, you might choose to see a psychiatrist or other therapist. You could engage in some form of talk therapy to gain a fuller understanding of your emotions. You might take an antidepressant or other medication. Both talk therapy and medication (often used together) are helpful, but they may not eliminate the root causes of your distress.

***New approach:*** Havening. It's a technique ("havening" means to put into a safe place) that uses touch to change how electrical signals are transmitted in the brain. After a successful havening session, the traumatic memory is viewed as distant and detached from the emotions, such as fear and anger, that are generated during the event—that is, it no longer causes distress. The havening technique still is considered experimental and is not scientifically proven, but it is inexpensive, safe, rapid and gentle, and there is growing anecdotal experience suggesting that it works.

## Emotions Linger

To understand the theory behind the havening technique, it helps to understand what happens when we experience a traumatic event. Let's say, for example, that you get mugged in an alley—if you're lucky, you'll put it behind you over time. But for some people, the event may be encoded in the brain as a trauma. When you perceive a threat, your brain activates neurons in the amygdala, the region of the brain associated with threat detection and other emotions. If certain criteria are met, cell receptors in the amygdala are potentiated. In other words, they increase in number and remain permanently primed for activation by related stimuli.

Because the encoded receptors are always present, the emotions associated with traumatic memories can be reactivated over and over again. Individuals might experience nightmares, worry every time they walk past an alley or even stop leaving the house altogether. This leads to a worsening of emotional distress.

Experts used to think that traumatic events caused lifelong distress because the memories—and associated emotions—could never be erased. But the brain is essentially an electrochemical system. The theory behind havening is that if you change the brain's circuitry, you can eliminate the response to signals that have been causing emotional pain—even if the memory originally associated with that pain is not gone.

## Havening Touch

The goal of havening therapy is to delink the emotions from the encoded traumatic event. The therapy is designed to generate brain waves that remove the potentiated receptors so that the individual won't experience again those fears or other emotional disturbances associated with the event.

During a typical havening session, a patient is asked to recall the painful memory. This activates the potentiated receptors. He/she then is exposed to "havening touch"—gentle, soothing stroking of the arms, face and hands. At the same time, the patient distracts himself from the memory by counting or singing a song.

***How it works:*** Touching triggers the production of low-frequency delta waves in the brain. Delta waves open calcium channels in the amygdala. The influx of calcium sets off an enzymatic reaction that causes "trauma" receptors to disappear. A patient might still remember the details of the traumatic event, but he will no longer feel disturbed by the memories.

## Does Science Support It?

Only one peer-reviewed, published scientific study has examined the effects of havening. Two others are completed and awaiting publication. The published study, which appeared in *Health Science Journal*, looked at workers in the UK who self-reported that they suffered occupational impairments because of depression and/or anxiety due to a traumatic event. After a havening session, participants showed improvements in tests that measured depression, anxiety and work and social adjustment.

***Important caveats:*** The study was small (27 participants) and didn't include a control group...and the participants weren't randomly selected. In addition, the workers were all health-care professionals, so they might have been more open to—and affected by—psychotherapy than other adults.

## What to Do

In the US, there are only about 40 havening practitioners who have participated in courses and trainer events and have been certified by a Havening Techniques trainer. These practitioners are mainly in New York City and on Long Island and in Chicago and Los Angeles…and there's one in the Louisville, Kentucky, area. Worldwide there are about 140 certified practitioners. The average cost for a havening session is about $200 to $400. But because there are only a small number of havening professionals, some people choose to practice the therapy on their own. In our experience, self-havening often is as effective as practitioner-guided sessions.

What happens in a session…

• **Activate the emotion.** You'll be asked (or you'll ask yourself) to recall the distressing event and all of the details. It might be a street crime…a memory of childhood abuse…even a cruel thing you yourself once did…or another memory that causes you repeated distress. You'll rate the distress that the memory causes on a scale of 0 to 10.

• **Apply havening touch.** The practitioner (or you or a loved one) will offer comforting touch that involves stroking the arms from shoulder to elbow, stroking the forehead and rubbing palms.

• **Distraction.** Simultaneously, with your eyes closed, you will distract yourself by imagining that you're climbing a staircase with 20 steps. Count the steps aloud. With each step, you'll imagine that your distress is diminishing.

After the twentieth step, with eyes still closed, you'll hum two rounds of "Row, Row, Row Your Boat" or another neutral song. You'll open your eyes, look to the right and left, and inhale and exhale deeply. If your distress level is still high, you should repeat the touch/distraction components (using different visualizations and tunes) until the level of distress is zero or remains fixed after two rounds.

The distraction is important because your mind can't process two thoughts at the same time. The idea is that distracting yourself from the memory displaces the recalled event and prevents it from continually activating the amygdala. At the same time, the touch part of the therapy produces the brain waves that de-link the memory from your emotions.

A single session can last for minutes to hours, but a typical session lasts 60 minutes. In my experience, many people will notice permanent improvement after a single session.

# New Moms Need Me Time

New mothers who take time just for themselves are 40% less likely to have signs of major depression six months after a baby's birth than mothers who get no time off. The effect was seen regardless of how much support the first-time mothers received from spouses and partners. In all, 9.1% of new mothers reported symptoms of major depression—but only 5.8% of those who had time off at least once a week reported symptoms, compared with 15.2% who never had time off.

Study of 1,392 women by researchers at Murdoch Childrens Research Institute, Melbourne, Victoria, Australia, reported in *The Wall Street Journal.*

# Antidepressant Helper

Some psychiatrists are beginning to use natural medicines to help prescription antidepressants work better. Deplin is a prescription form of a natural B vitamin called L-methylfolate. Studies of patients who did not respond well to antidepressants found that those who took 15 mg of Deplin daily responded much better to antidepressant medication.

It appears that folate, which is found in foods like leafy green vegetables, helps to balance levels of the neurotransmitters that regulate mood. Low folate levels can result from poor eating habits, aging, certain drugs, such as antiepileptic medication, and excessive alcohol intake.

Peter Bongiorno, ND, LAc, naturopathic doctor in New York City and author of *How Come They're Happy and I'm Not?*

## Laughing Gas for Depression?

Adults with hard-to-treat depression who inhaled nitrous oxide showed improvement within hours. Some had complete relief from depressive symptoms with this experimental treatment.

*Biological Psychiatry.*

## High-Status Job Is Hard on Depression

Treatment for depression is less effective for people with high-status jobs than for people in lower-status positions, reports Siegfried Kasper, MD.

***Recent finding:*** 55.9% of people with the highest-level jobs did not respond to the standard treatment of medication plus psychotherapy...compared with 40.2% of midlevel workers and 44.3% of low-level employees.

***Possible reason:*** People with high-level jobs—and the resulting stress and responsibilities—may find it more difficult to accept or cope with illness.

Siegfried Kasper, MD, professor and chair of the department of psychiatry and psychotherapy at Medical University of Vienna, Austria.

## Empathy: Do You Need a Little More?

Nancy Eisenberg, PhD, Regents' Professor in the department of psychology at Arizona State University in Tempe. Her research interests include empathy and altruism. She is a former editor of the journal *Psychological Bulletin* and editor of several books, including *The Caring Child.*

When it comes to personality traits, empathy—the ability to feel another person's experiences and emotions—is one of the least understood.

We think of empathy as an admirable trait that gives us the ability to "walk in another's shoes." But some people are better at expressing empathy than others.

***Why it matters:*** With so much tragedy around us—whether it's mass shootings, floods, wildfires...or even a serious health threat in a loved one—how do we strike the right balance when it comes to being empathetic?

To learn more, we spoke with Nancy Eisenberg, PhD, a leading psychologist who has written extensively about empathy and similar traits.

*How is empathy different from sympathy?*

Empathy is more than just listening and relating to someone's concerns. You experience empathy when you understand (or intuit) someone's feelings so completely that their feelings become your own. If you feel sad when watching a sad child, for example, that's empathy.

A person who feels empathy may also feel sympathy. In that case, you may feel sorry for a sad child but also want to help—"I'm so sorry you feel sad. What can I do to help?"

*Does being empathetic and/or sympathetic give a person more personal happiness?*

Individuals who are inclined to be helpful tend to be better adjusted overall and get along better with others than those who are less helpful. In general, people who participate in "prosocial" activities—such as volunteering and community service—will be happier and experience more empathy/sympathy than those who aren't socially engaged.

When empathetic/sympathetic individuals want to help, they are generally motivated by their concern for others, with little regard for concrete or social rewards.

Consider a child who stands up for a bullied classmate. The defender faces physical or social risk but does so out of concern for the other child. Research has shown that this type of "defending behavior" is associated with high levels of sympathy, which often stems from empathy.

*Are empathetic people born that way—or is it something that we learn?*

A bit of both. Studies involving twins suggest that genetics, as well as environment, play a large role in empathy, altruism and similar traits.

Neurochemistry also comes into play. Oxytocin, for example, is widely known as the "love" hormone, but it is also called a "bonding" hormone because it's released when people get close emotionally. When test subjects are given oxytocin, they exhibit more generosity, cooperation and empathy. In one study, women who watched emotional film clips showed an increase both in oxytocin and empathy.

Parental influences are critical, too. Children who grow up with warm, empathetic parents are more likely to develop the same traits than children who come from households where there is less empathy. Children can also learn not to be empathetic. Adolescents who have experienced difficult childhoods, for example, and feel less secure with parents and friends tend to be less empathetic than those with closer relationships.

*So some people have a distinct lack of empathy?*

Yes. They're called psychopaths. Those with antisocial personality disorders don't respond to the distress of others, and they have little empathy or remorse.

Without empathy, as well as sympathy, people are more likely to behave violently... have poor relationships...and show little or no regard for other people. Some of the most notorious criminals (including serial killers) fall into this category.

*Is it possible to become more empathetic?*

Perhaps, but empathy is largely developed in childhood. Children as young as age two to three become aware of other people's feelings (and realize that the feelings might be different from their own). Empathy begins even earlier than that. Infants will look more uncomfortable when their mothers show sadness—and express more joy when their mothers are happy.

*What specific steps can a person take to become more empathetic?*

It's largely a matter of heightening your own awareness. When you read or hear about a news event, think about the emotions that are likely affecting those who are involved instead of seeing it simply as a news report. It's easy to imagine that a person who has just lost his/her home in a flood, for example, would be experiencing sadness, anger and any number of other strong emotions.

This is good training for situations that may come up in your own life. Let's say that a spouse is upset after learning that a good friend has betrayed him/her. The first step is to really listen to and acknowledge your spouse's hurt feelings...accept those feelings without judging them...and resist the temptation to try to talk your spouse out of having those feelings. All these steps will go a long way toward strengthening the relationship via empathy.

*In general, do women have more empathy than men?*

People tend to think so. Women themselves often believe it. But it's not clearly supported by the research.

A recent study in the journal *Psychoneuroendocrinology* found that women given high doses of testosterone had reduced activity in the brain regions involved in empathy and processing emotional cues, but the correlation to empathy isn't conclusive. Does the finding mean that girls/women are more empathetic than boys/men? Not necessarily. The differences could have more to do with presentation than biology. An empathetic man might simply be less likely to express it.

What's more, the capacity for empathy is not all-or-nothing...everyone is a mix. You might be highly empathetic one day and less so the next. It depends on how you're feeling, what you're going through, etc. No one's empathetic all the time.

# Hours of Power...Use the Science of Chronobiology to Harness Your Peak Times

Michael Breus, PhD, board-certified sleep specialist, Manhattan Beach, California, and author of *The Power of When: Discover Your Chronotype—and the Best Time to Eat Lunch, Ask for a Raise, Have Sex, Write a Novel, Take Your Meds, and More.* TheSleepDoctor.com

Imagine what your day would be like if you did everything at the best time—when your body clock is naturally most in tune with what each kind of activity requires and rewards. The reality is, the way you feel and function changes throughout the day, hour by hour, based on your body's daily (circadian) rhythms. These physiologic ups and downs are orchestrated by 24-hour fluctuations in hormones (such as serotonin, cortisol, dopamine and melatonin), blood pressure and body temperature.

The trick is to match each activity to your appropriate biological peak. Then you'll find the best time to eat, think, exercise, daydream, talk to friends—even see your dentist—for you. "There's a never-ending set of peaks, depending on what you want to accomplish. It's all about riding the wave and jumping from one peak to another.

## Dolphins, Lions, Bears and Wolves

The "power of when" works whether you're an early-morning lark or a night owl—it's just that your peaks will come at a different times of the day for you. Most of us are one of four "chronotypes.

The following "best time to" routine is based on the chronotype called "Bears." It's the most common one, describing about 50% of the population. Bears tend to wake up in a daze after hitting the snooze button once or twice, start to feel tired by mid-to-late afternoon and sleep deeply but not as long as they'd like.

To adjust to an earlier schedule or later schedule, just shift the numbers to be closer to your starting wake and sleep times.

## The Best Activity to Plan When the Clock Says...

You won't be able to do each of these activities every day—after all, if you have a job, shopping and napping in the afternoon aren't daily options! Yes, there's no TV time here, either, but then there's no ideal time to watch—although there's an ideal time not to watch (right before bedtime). So don't consider this an actual schedule. *Rather, it's a guide to the best times to do these activities...*

***7:00-8:00 am:*** **Wake up—and have sex.** While many people have sex before bedtime, sexual desire actually peaks in the morning for most people. That's when testosterone, which affects sex drive in both men and women, is at its highest. Plus, having sex in the morning, which can put you in a good mood and flood your brain with feel-good hormones such as oxytocin (the "love hormone"), is a great way to start your day.

***8:00-9:00 am:*** **If you need to schedule something that's uncomfortable, do it now.** On most days, you'd eat a hearty breakfast about now, but if you need to have a tooth drilled or get a mammogram, now's the best time. Pain tolerance peaks in the early morning—no one knows exactly why, but it may be related to the lingering analgesic effects of cortisol, which tends to rise just after you wake up. So if you have any kind of physically uncomfortable or potentially painful event to schedule, get it over with early in the day.

***9:00-9:30 am:*** **Organize your day.** Alertness and attention build slowly after you wake up and tend to be at a high level by mid-morning—which makes this the perfect time to map out what you plan to accomplish for the rest of the day. Instead of just jumping into the routine task that you didn't finish yesterday—something you may be able to do when you're less primed for alertness—step back and think strategically. It's a great time to make lists.

***9:30-11:30 am:*** **Tackle your hardest work problems now.** During this window of opportunity, your intellectual capabilities are the highest they'll be all day. This is an ideal time to learn new information or work through a complicated project.

***11:30 am-1:00 pm:*** **Get aerobic exercise such as a walk or do yoga—and then have lunch.** If you exercise first before you eat, you'll speed up your metabolism—and decrease your appetite at the same time. Plus, it's a great way to stave off that afternoon lull. Your core body temperature dips between 1:00 and 3:00 pm—that may make you feel a little sleepy, but getting a little exercise beforehand can rejuvenate you.

***1:00-3:00 pm:*** **Do chores—especially shopping.** You're less susceptible to overspending now. Why? Chances are you're not hungry and your energy is slightly low. Shopping in this state can help you avoid impulse purchases—which are more common when adrenalin levels are up.

***2:30 pm:*** **Take a (short) power nap.** A 20-minute nap can restore your energy and alertness. Set an alarm so you don't sleep longer than that—or else you could wake up with a case of sleep inertia (aka, brain fog).

***3:00-5:00 pm:*** **Make important decisions.** Your alertness picks up again in the later afternoon. Now you'll be better able to make logical, less risky decisions rather than being emotionally reactive when faced with choices. If you're a little hungry, have a light snack—no more than 250 calories—with some protein, since eating too much can dampen your alertness.

***Examples:*** An apple with a tablespoon of almond butter...or a handful of whole-grain crackers with an ounce of cheese.

***5:00-7:00 pm:*** **Didn't exercise at lunch? Go now!** Consider a run, a bike ride, lifting weights—or playing a team sport. Why? Your body temperature is higher in the early evening, which means your strength, hand-eye coordination and aerobic capacity are at their peak. This is a great time to get physical.

***7:00-8 pm:*** **Eat dinner.** Make it the smallest meal of your day—a vegetable-rich stew and a salad, for example—so your body isn't overwhelmed with digestion when you need to start winding down. You'll want to finish eating at least three hours before your bedtime.

***8:00-9:00 pm:*** **Call a friend or brainstorm.** Your alertness and concentration now start to wane, but that means creativity starts to peak. Now is also a good time to play games. So now's your best time to come up with innovative ideas or have fun conversations with friends and family.

***9:00-10:00 pm:*** **Power down.** Create a "digital sunset"—power off all screens—at least one hour before bed to help you get in the mood to snooze. This way, the blue light from your screens won't interfere with the release of melatonin, which helps you fall asleep.

***9:00-11:00 pm:*** **Read for pleasure, not purpose.** As you power down, reading an engrossing or comforting book lowers your cortisol level—reducing stress—and your heart rate, which helps relax your body and mind. Your mind will wander a bit and bring the imagery of a book to life. That'll put you in a great state for drifting off to sleep.

***10:00-11:00 pm:*** **Go to bed.** Your pillow unlocks your potential. If you know when the right time to sleep is, everything else falls into place. Try to keep your bedtime and wake-up time fairly consistent to anchor your body's rhythms and help you enjoy these hours of power, day after day.

## Can't Sleep?

Get up! In a recent study of more than 400 adults, researchers found that those who try to make up for lost sleep by napping and/or staying in bed longer in the morning reinforce poor sleeping patterns, which can lead to chronic insomnia.

***Better:*** If you intend to wake up at 7:30 am, for example, but find yourself wide awake at 5 am and unable to fall back to sleep, get up and start the day.

Michael Perlis, PhD, director, University of Pennsylvania Behavioral Sleep Medicine Program.

## This Blanket May Help You Sleep

Study titled "Positive Effects of a Weighted Blanket on Insomnia" by researchers at University of Gothenburg, Sweden, published in *Journal of Sleep Medicine & Disorders.*

Michael J. Breus, PhD, a sleep specialist in Manhattan Beach, California. His latest book is *The Power of When.* TheSleepDoctor.com

Brett Scotch, DO, an osteopathic physician specializing in sleep medicine and otolaryngology and director of Scotch Institute, Wesley Chapel, Florida.

Karen Moore, OTR, an occupational therapist and founder of The Sensory Connection Program in Franconia, New Hampshire.

Move over sleep meds—there's a new solution in town. Weighted blankets. The comforting heavy covers, filled with small plastic balls that are sewn into compartments for even distribution, have been used for years to treat children with anxiety, ADHD, autism spectrum disorders and other disorders. Parents swear by them, especially to help kids sleep.

Now they're catching on as a simple DIY solution for healthy adults with sleep problems. The theory is that they provide "deep pressure" that helps you feel calmer and more relaxed, making it easier to fall asleep and stay asleep. Think of it as a kind of swaddling for grown-ups.

### Lessons from Insomniac Swedes

A recent study from the University of Gothenburg in Sweden looked at the effect of weighted blankets in 33 normal healthy adult men and women with chronic insomnia. Participants wore "actigraph" watches, which recorded the pattern of their movements when they went to bed, and they also kept sleep diaries. In the first week, they slept their usual way. Then for two weeks, they slept under weighted blankets of their choice, which ranged in weight from 13 pounds to 22 pounds—at least 12% of their body weight. During the fourth week, they went back to their normal sleeping conditions.

***Results:*** When they used the weighted blankets, the sleepers spent more time in each phase of sleep, including truly restful deep sleep, and they moved around less during the night. According to their diaries, they found it easier to settle down to sleep, had better quality sleep and felt more refreshed in the morning.

While the Swedish study didn't take anxiety into account, the blankets have a documented calming effect, which may help explain how they enhance sleep, according to sleep expert Michael Breus, PhD. "Most people who have insomnia have some level of anxiety," he said. The sympathetic nervous system, which regulates the "fight or flight" reflex, is often easily aroused in people who have trouble sleeping, he explained. "A weighted blanket puts pressure on the mechanoreceptors—nerve endings under the skin—which sense pressure and signal muscles to relax. That makes us feel safe and supported."

### Snuggling Tips

Who's a good candidate to try a weighted blanket? Anyone who is in good health but has trouble falling asleep or staying asleep, according to Dr. Breus.

***Who isn't:*** Anyone with a respiratory disorder (such as severe asthma) or a circulatory disorder, according to Brett Scotch, DO, an osteopathic physician specializing in sleep medicine and otolaryngology in Wesley Chapel, Florida. "The weight on your chest may impede your ability to breathe or decrease circulation to your extremities," he warned. (If you have any serious health condition, consult your doctor before sleeping with a weighted blanket.)

If you do decide to try getting under heavy covers, look for a blanket that weighs about 10% of your body weight or more, has a material that feels good to you and distributes the weight evenly to provide firm, constant tactile stimulation across your body. The blankets are widely available online, from companies such as Sommerfly (Sommerfly.com) and Mosaic Weighted Blankets (MosaicWeighted Blankets.com), and cost around $140. "If you're claustrophobic, you may want to start with a lighter one and give it a chance," said Karen Moore, OTR, an occupational therapist.

Will it work for you? The Swedish study is relatively small and short-term, so this is not the definitive solution to insomnia. Ultimately, the only way to find out if a weighted blanket will help you get better shut-eye is to try it.

***The good news:*** It's safe and free of side effects. And unlike with prescription sleep medications, there's no "rebound" problem—except, perhaps, to your wallet—if you decide it's not for you.

---

## It's 3 am and You're Awake...Again!

Michael Breus, PhD, a sleep specialist with a private practice in Los Angeles. Dr. Breus is also author of *The Power of When: Discover Your Chronotype—and the Best Time to Eat Lunch, Ask for a Raise, Have Sex, Write a Novel, Take Your Meds, and More.* TheSleepDoctor.com

In the world of sleep disorders, having difficulty staying asleep is just as troubling as having difficulty falling asleep.

Both sleep problems rob us of the consistent, high-quality rest that helps protect against high blood pressure, obesity, diabetes, stroke and depression.

Plenty of people who have nighttime awakenings turn to a prescription sleep aid, such as *zolpidem* (Ambien). But these pills are only a temporary fix and can cause prolonged drowsiness the next day or, in rare cases, sleepwalking or sleep-eating within hours of taking them.

***A better option:*** Cognitive behavioral therapy for insomnia, known as CBT-I, is now recommended as a first-line treatment for chronic sleep problems.* With CBT-I, you work with a specially trained therapist (typically for six to eight sessions) to identify, challenge and change the patterns of thinking that keep you awake at night. A 2015 study found CBT-I, which is typically covered by health insurance, to be more helpful than *diazepam* (Valium), commonly used as a sleep aid, in treating insomnia.

But if you are not quite ready to commit to a course of CBT-I—or even if you do try it—there are some simple but effective strategies you can use at home to help you stay asleep and get the deep rest you need.

Best approaches to avoid nighttime awakenings...

- **Get more omega-3 fatty acids.** While the research is still preliminary, a recent study published in *Sleep Medicine* found that the more omega-3–rich fatty fish adults ate, the better their sleep quality.

***My advice:*** Eat fatty fish...and to ensure adequate levels of omega-3s, consider taking a fish oil supplement (one to two 1,000-mg capsules daily).**

- **Avoid "blue light" at night.** Exposure to blue light—the kind emitted by smartphones, computers, tablets and LED TVs—disrupts sleep patterns by blocking the release of the sleep hormone melatonin. Even if you do fall asleep fairly easily, blue light exposure may

*To find a CBT-I therapist, consult the Society of Behavioral Sleep Medicine, BehavioralSleep.org. You can also try the free CBT-i Coach app, available at iTunes or Google Play.

**Consult your doctor if you take medication.

come back to haunt you in the form of a middle-of-the-night wake-up.

If you can't force yourself to power down your electronics within two hours of bedtime, try positioning handheld devices farther away from your eyes than usual.

In addition, consider various apps that filter blue light on your smartphone or tablet. Some operating systems are automatically programmed with this feature—Apple's iOS 9.3 offers Night Shift, for example. Using your device's geolocation and clock, the colors of your display are automatically shifted to the warmer end of the spectrum (which is less disruptive to sleep) around sundown. Free apps for Android devices include Night Shift: Blue Light Filter and Twilight.

• **Use special lightbulbs.** If you wake up in the middle of the night and make a trip to the bathroom, the glare of the bathroom light tells your brain "It's morning!"

***What helps:*** Use low-blue lightbulbs in your bathroom and bedroom that don't block the release of melatonin. A variety are available from Lighting Science (LSGC.com). Or look online for night-lights designed to emit low levels of blue light.

## If You Do Wake Up

Even if you follow the steps described above, you may still have occasional nighttime awakenings with trouble falling back asleep (meaning you are awake for at least 25 minutes).

Experiment with the following strategies to see what works best for you…

• **Resist the urge to check e-mail or do anything else on your phone.** Even short exposures to blue light are enough to suppress melatonin. Mentally stimulating activities, such as loud TV, are also best avoided. (However, a TV at low volume with the setting adjusted to dim the screen can be a great distractor for an active mind at night.)

***My advice:*** Choose a relaxing activity like reading, listening to soothing music or knitting. If you read, use a book light or a bedside-table lamp that has one of the special bulbs mentioned earlier.

• **Don't look at the clock.** If you do, you'll start doing the mental math of how many hours you have left until you need to wake up. This will cause anxiety that will spike your levels of cortisol and adrenaline, sleep-disrupting hormones that make you feel wide awake!

***My advice:*** Turn your clock around, and try counting backward from 300 by threes to distract yourself and promote drowsiness.

***Also helpful:*** Try the "4-7-8 method"—inhale for four seconds…hold your breath for seven…and exhale slowly for eight. Breathe in this manner for up to 15 to 20 minutes or until you fall asleep. Inhaling and holding in air increases oxygen in the body, which means your body doesn't have to expend as much energy. The slow exhale helps you unwind and mimics the slow breathing that takes place during sleep, which will help you fall asleep.

• **Turn on some pink noise.** The well-known "white noise"—used to mask conversations and potentially startling sounds—is comprised of all frequencies detectable by the human ear. Pink noise, on the other hand, has a lower, softer frequency. Pink noise is generally considered more relaxing and has a steady sound like gentle rain.

Sleep experts believe that our brains respond better to the lower spectrum of pink noise than to the fuller spectrum of white noise. The result is a more peaceful and sleep-conducive feeling.

***My advice:*** Search for a free app that contains pink noise, and listen to it with earphones on your smartphone, laptop or tablet if you wake up in the middle of the night. Just be sure to glance only briefly at the screen when turning on the device, and turn off the screen light while listening. You can set the pink noise to play for a set amount of time, such as 30 minutes. As an alternative, you can purchase a pink-noise generator online.

## Online Therapy Can Relieve Insomnia

After one year, 57% of people using the focused online behavioral-modification program SHUTi were sleeping normally, versus 27% who had received only advice and education. Online programs are based on cognitive behavioral therapy and have proved effective among adults ages 18 to 65. Online programs include SHUTi, $135 for 16 weeks of access, and Sleepio, $300 for one year of access.

Lee M. Ritterband, PhD, director of Center for Behavioral Health and Technology, University of Virginia School of Medicine, Charlottesville.

## Don't Stay Online Too Long

People who spent significant time online, especially those who stream video, use instant messaging or frequent social networking sites, had higher rates of depression, anxiety, impulsiveness and inattention, and difficulty with planning and time management. Internet use may not cause these problems—more study is needed—but it could be a red flag for mental health issues.

***Takeaway:*** Spend no more than an hour or two a day using the Internet for reasons other than work or school.

Michael Van Ameringen, MD, professor of psychiatry and behavioral neurosciences, McMaster University, Hamilton, Ontario, Canada.

## Do You Have a Short Fuse?

Bernard Golden, PhD, a psychologist and founder of Anger Management Education, a clinical practice in Chicago. He is author of *Overcoming Destructive Anger*. Anger ManagementEducation.com

Here are a few questions worth asking yourself...Do you often snap at people and later regret it...or continue to stew after a disagreement has passed? Do friends or loved ones ever call you a hothead? Does the intensity of your anger sometimes escalate from 0 to 10 in a matter of seconds?

If any of these situations ring true, then you may be experiencing destructive anger.

And it's hurting you!

### Healthy or Harmful?

Like all emotions, anger can express itself in good or bad ways. Healthy anger motivates us to make important changes in our lives...challenges us to overcome unfairness and social injustices...and is a signal to look inward to identify our core desires, needs and values.

Destructive anger is another story. Whether you quietly simmer with rage or erupt at even slight provocations, destructive anger has been shown to increase one's risk for health problems such as high blood pressure, heart attack, stroke, digestive ailments and depression.

***The unfortunate truth:*** Far too many people assume that they can simply turn off their anger like a spigot. But it doesn't work that way.

### The Tool That Works

If you want to reduce your anger, the first step is to realize that out-of-proportion or out-of-control anger stems from a chain of internal experiences and is almost always not just a reaction to whatever has set you off.

For example, you might experience intense anger when someone cuts in front of you in the checkout line, but this triggering event may evoke past anger as well.

To better understand your anger, it helps to complete an anger log, identifying the interplay of your thoughts, feelings and body sensations that occurred before and during your episodes of anger. By doing this, you'll start to see patterns and can interrupt the cycle.

Ideally, you will complete a log entry every time you get angry—but you should wait at least an hour or two so you're calm enough to recognize all of the important elements.

Key aspects to write down...

• **Motivating forces.** People experience anger when they're feeling threatened or when a need—for safety, for respect or to feel important, for example—isn't being met.

Let's say that you shouted an obscenity while arguing with your spouse. Maybe he/she had scolded you for something you did—but did it really warrant that level of verbal retaliation? You might realize that the motivation behind the anger was your (unmet) need for love and connection and respect.

• **Expectations.** We get angry when things run counter to our expectations. In the example above, one expectation might be, "We're a couple, so we should care about each other's feelings." But your conflict is putting that basic expectation into doubt.

• **Triggering event.** Sometimes it's obvious what makes you angry—the car that cuts in front of you...a negative job review...or a curt reply from a store clerk. But sometimes it's less clear—for example, the triggering event could be something that you anticipate will happen. You might, for example, become angry because you anticipate not getting a job for which you interviewed.

• **Body reactions.** Anger evolves in the body. Identifying a pounding heart, sweating palms and other such reactions will help you become more alert to anger in its initial stage.

## Give It Time

You may be surprised by the range of feelings that accompany a "simple" episode of anger.

***Example:*** A client sought my help because of conflicts with her teenage daughter. When she first completed her anger log, she wrote that the motivating factor was "to be respected." Her main expectation was that "she should listen to me."

But the more my client thought about it, the more she realized that the real motivating factor was her desire for closeness and a meaningful relationship with her daughter. She also had the expectation that "our closeness will never change."

Emotional discoveries don't happen all at once. Keeping a log will help you understand the trajectory of your anger—and become much more skillful at altering its course. You'll know you're making progress when there's a decrease in the intensity, duration and/or frequency of anger episodes.

***For additional help:*** Consult The National Anger Management Association, NAMASS.org, for a referral to a therapist.

# How Marital Fights Hurt Your Health... and What You Can Do

Claudia Haase, PhD, assistant professor of human development and social policy at Northwestern University, Evanston, Illinois. She is one of the authors of the *Emotion* study featured in this article.

It's no secret that arguing with your husband can cause stress. Nor will it come as a shock that that stress can be bad for your health, particularly if the marital discord is chronic. But a recent study published in *Emotion* introduced an interesting new twist to this story—it turns out that how you argue with your spouse could determine what sort of health problems you are likely to endure.

Researchers at Northwestern University tracked 156 married couples for more than 20 years and found compelling evidence that spouses who fly off the handle during arguments are prone to cardiovascular problems such as high blood pressure and chest pain... while spouses who shut down and bottle up their feelings tend to develop muscular problems such as back or neck pain.

That makes some intuitive sense. Yelling and screaming makes one's heart rate accelerate, which can do damage to the heart muscle when it occurs frequently. Holding in emotions makes the body tense, which over time can lead to muscle and joint issues.

The good news is that it might be possible to reduce the odds of these future health problems by modifying your arguing style. Hotheads could go for a walk when they feel their temperature rising, for example, and return to resume the difficult discussion only when they've cooled down. If they continue to get excessively worked up during marital disagreements, they could seek anger-management counseling.

Stonewallers must come to terms with the fact that in the long term, not voicing their feelings is not good for their relationships or their health. If you tend to withdraw during a conflict, you can benefit from learning to resist the impulse to bottle up your emotions. The Gottman Institute, which features a research-based approach to strengthening relationships, has an excellent blog post about stonewalling at Gottman.com/blog/the-four-horsemen-stonewalling/.

To have healthier spats, though, it takes more than working on your own emotional reactions. It takes two. Discover measured, constructive ways to argue with your spouse. It might be worth going for individual or couple's therapy.

Change is hard, especially in long-term relationships. But learning new ways to resolve the inevitable conflicts of even the strongest marriage may benefit not just your marriage but also your health.

---

# Write Your Way to Better Health

James W. Pennebaker, PhD, the Regents Centennial Professor in the department of psychology at The University of Texas at Austin. He is author of numerous books, including *Expressive Writing* and his most recent, *Opening Up by Writing It Down*.

When it comes to staying healthy (or getting healthy), most people are willing to do whatever it takes—whether it's changing their diet, getting more exercise, using supplements and/or taking medication. But there's another way to improve your health that doesn't get nearly the attention it deserves.

Writing down your feelings not only helps you feel better mentally but also results in beneficial physiological changes, including reduced blood pressure and strengthened immune function. Now researchers are uncovering the best ways to get the greatest health benefits from therapeutic writing.

This may all sound great if you're a would-be novelist or poet. But what if writing has never been your thing...or the rules of grammar leave your head spinning? Don't worry. You can still realize the health benefits of this powerful technique.

## How Secrets Harm Us

Therapeutic writing got started when my colleagues and I became intrigued by a landmark study that found that people who suffered a trauma (such as the death of a loved one, a breakup of an important relationship or a sexual or physical assault)—and kept it a secret—were at higher risk for illness (ranging from colds and flu to ulcers and elevated blood pressure) compared with those who talked about their traumatic experiences.

***This finding led us to wonder:*** If not talking about traumatic events harms health, would asking people to talk—or write—about emotional upsets improve health?

To test this hypothesis, we asked college students to write for 15 minutes a day for four consecutive days on a nonemotional topic or to write about their deepest thoughts and feelings related to a traumatic experience—or a current major conflict or stressor—in their lives. (The latter approach is known as "expressive writing.")

***Result:*** By the last day, most of those who did expressive writing said that the experience was important to them...and four months later, those students had made 43% fewer (onetime) visits to the doctor for sickness than those who wrote about superficial topics.

Since our first study, a growing body of research has revealed specific physiological changes that occur after writing expressively.

The benefits include faster healing following surgery...lower blood pressure...strengthened immune function...reduced physical symptoms as well as better sleep and daytime functioning in cancer patients...and less fatigue in rheumatoid arthritis patients.

## Getting Started

To harness the health benefits of expressive writing, plan to write for a minimum of 15 minutes a day for four consecutive days.

***Day one:*** Write your deepest thoughts and feelings about a past trauma or a current emotional upheaval that may be influencing your life now. This could include major life experiences or traumas, such as divorce, a death or a long-lasting conflict in your life.

Simply write about the event itself—how you felt when it was happening and how you feel about it now. Do not worry about grammar, sentence structure or spelling.

***Days two, three and four:*** For the next three days, continue to write about the same trauma, upheaval or major life conflict, digging even deeper into your feelings and thoughts. Write about how this trauma affects all aspects of your life, including your relationships. *Other considerations...*

- **Type or write longhand?** Studies have not found a significant difference in effectiveness. Do whichever you find more comfortable.
- **Plan to throw away your writing.** What you write is for your eyes only. Feel free to destroy or hide it each day when you are done.
- **Don't worry if you initially feel sad.** Give yourself some time after your writing session to reflect on what you've written and to relax. Any sadness usually lifts after an hour or so as you move on to other activities. This exercise helps you to get some emotional distance from the trauma. If the sadness doesn't lift, you may want to consider seeing a therapist.

***Also:*** Feel free to experiment. The four-day method, as used in our study, works for many people, but you may prefer writing about your feelings for two days...or six days. You may find it easier to talk into a tape recorder about your deepest emotions rather than writing about them. See what works for you!

# Take a Deep Breath to Cure What Ails You

Jane Pernotto Ehrman, MEd, lead behavioral health therapist at the Cleveland Clinic Center for Lifestyle Medicine. Ehrman is also the owner of Images of Wellness, LLC, which teaches stress management to individuals and corporate groups. A variety of her guided meditations can be found on iTunes.

What do stubbing your toe, getting cut off in traffic and worrying about an ill friend have in common?

All these experiences cause us to hold or restrict our breath. When this happens, you are likely not even aware of it, but your breathing becomes shallow...and too little oxygen flows to the body and the brain. You may suffer from poor concentration, memory problems and low energy—or even a panic attack, as shallow breathing triggers the body's fight-or-flight response.

On the other hand, deep, purposeful breathing can have an incredibly positive impact on your well-being. It stimulates the parasympathetic part of your involuntary nervous system, slowing a rapid heartbeat and lowering blood pressure. And now, there's even more proof to back up its benefits.

***Recent scientific evidence:*** Deep breathing, as practiced in meditation, has been linked to a lengthening of people's telomeres (the protective caps on chromosomes that impact aging and longevity), according to research conducted at the University of California, San Francisco.

The benefits don't stop there. *Deep breathing has also been shown to help with the following...**

• **Pain.** When we hurt, our muscles often tighten up and we breathe shallowly. In addition to depriving the brain and body of oxygen, this increases inflammation, slowing the healing process and triggering pain-promoting anxiety.

***What helps:*** Combining deep breathing with positive imagery can relax muscles in the affected area, which also decreases inflammation and pain.

***What to do:*** Find a quiet spot, and sit or lie in a comfortable position. Picture a place where you feel calm. Close your eyes and begin breathing using a "1:2 inhale-to-exhale ratio." For example, on the inhale, you can count to four and breathe in a feeling of calm, cooling energy...on the exhale, you can count to eight and imagine the painful area getting smaller and smaller and leaving your body.

• **Sleep.** The use of deep breathing with "body scans" (an exercise designed to create awareness of the body) has been shown to improve sleep in older adults—half of whom report sleep troubles.

***What to do:*** While lying comfortably in bed, begin the same 1:2 inhale-to-exhale ratio described above—long, slow exhalations stimulate the brain's vagus nerve, which tells the body: "It's time to relax."

To begin the body scan, concentrate on your feet—wiggle and scrunch your toes, then relax them and notice how comfortable your feet feel simply resting on the bed. Move on to your ankles, perhaps rolling them in circles... then your calves...knees...thighs, etc.

***Remember:*** Keep breathing deeply, and focus on how relaxed and heavy each body part feels, allowing it to become soft and limp like a cooked noodle. You should be asleep before you reach your head! If you're feeling particularly tense, you can tighten each body part before relaxing it.

*Unless noted otherwise, start with five minutes and work up to 15 to 20 minutes daily.

• **High blood pressure.** For many people, stress can cause the amygdala, the region of the brain that processes danger signals, to activate the release of stress hormones that raise blood pressure.

***What to do:*** Sit tall, with your head held straight, looking forward. Close your eyes or gaze at a single point straight ahead. Breathe in naturally...then exhale more slowly while silently repeating, "I let it go." When your mind wanders, simply refocus on your breath and mantra. By practicing mindful breathing, you will learn to become less reactive to daily stressors.

***Extra move:*** Gratitude breath. As you breathe, focus on a person, place or thing for which you are thankful. Research has linked the positive energy and uplifting mood that results from gratitude with a healthier heart rate.

• **Depression.** This breathing technique activates the parasympathetic nervous system while rewiring the brain for positivity. Consistent practice will heighten your awareness of negative thinking so it will be easier to shift your focus away from sadness and pull yourself out of a downward spiral.

***What to do:*** Breathe in for a count of four...breathe out slowly, counting to eight. Add a mantra that you say silently to yourself. *Possibilities...*

*Inhale:* In this moment.
*Exhale:* I am OK.

*Inhale:* Peace.
*Exhale:* Calm.

***My advice:*** Whenever you can, do this exercise in a peaceful outdoor setting—nature has a calming, antidepressant effect.

---

## Best Way to Make Up

***Best way to make up after an argument:*** Address the underlying issue instead of apologizing quickly and trying to move on.

## It Gets Better

Happiness increases with age. Even though aging is tied to declines in physical health and cognition, older people report more satisfaction, happiness and well-being than younger ones, on average...and less anxiety, stress and depression.

Study of 1,546 people ages 21 to 99 led by researchers at University of California, San Diego, published in *The Journal of Clinical Psychiatry.*

***Reason:*** If you both don't come to a resolution about what started the argument, you will end up getting upset over the same thing later.

Hal Shorey, PhD, associate professor of clinical psychology, Widener University, Chester, Pennsylvania, quoted in *The Wall Street Journal.*

## Fun Way to Stop Cravings

Playing Tetris may reduce cravings for food, cigarettes, alcohol, coffee, sleep and sex by up to 21%.

***Reason:*** Playing Tetris affects the parts of the brain involved with visual imagery, keeping the imagination on a single track and distracting it from cravings.

Study of 31 people by researchers at Plymouth University, Devon, UK, and Queensland University of Technology, Brisbane, Australia, published in *Addictive Behaviors.*

## Happy Husband

A happy spouse is good for your health. People with unhappy partners have more physical problems, engage in less exercise and rate their health worse than people with happy partners.

***Possible reason:*** Happy spouses are more likely to offer social support and to encourage exercise and eating right.

Study of 1,981 heterosexual couples led by researchers at Michigan State University, East Lansing, published in *Health Psychology.*

## Stop the Twitch

Twitching eyelids usually are caused by stress or fatigue. Getting rest should stop the twitch. Sometimes twitching results from eyestrain after spending a long time looking at a computer or smartphone screen, so look away at least every 20 minutes.

***And:*** A warm compress can help soothe the area.

Shilpi Agarwal, MD, family physician, Washington, DC, quoted in *Better Homes and Gardens.*

## Happiness Is a Snap

Regularly snapping selfies of yourself smiling and sharing the photos with friends can help make you a happier person, according to a recent study.

Study conducted at University of California, Irvine, published in *Psychology of Well-Being.*

## Grief Hurts Your Heart

Grief may cause irregular heartbeat. Atrial fibrillation (AF), which can lead to stroke or other cardiovascular problems, was 41% more common among people mourning the death of a partner than among other people. The effect was even stronger in people younger than age 60—they were more than twice as likely to have AF after a partner's death. The risk was greatest eight to 14 days after a death and then gradually subsided.

Study by Danish researchers of 88,612 people newly diagnosed with AF between 1995 and 2014... and 886,120 people without the diagnosis, published in *Open Heart*.

## Depression in the ICU

One-third of intensive care patients become depressed. That is three to four times the prevalence of depression in the general population. Patients with pre-ICU psychological symptoms and ones who had psychological distress while in the ICU are at greatest risk. Families and caregivers should be alert if patients talk about the ICU being stressful, have flashbacks or delusional memories, act angry or nervous, or exhibit emotional detachment.

Dale M. Needham, MD, PhD, professor of medicine at Johns Hopkins University School of Medicine, Baltimore.

## Shocking Treatment to Eliminate Bad Habits

The wristband Pavlok (Pavlok.com, $199) encourages you to break bad habits by delivering a noticeable, but safe, electric shock of varying intensity, loud beeps, vibrations and other means. The device pairs with your phone. You can have the device give you a jolt if you oversleep, or tap the screen to shock yourself if you eat a donut. Online user feedback for Pavlok has been enthusiastic, although there is no scientific evidence supporting the long-term success of this device.

*The New York Times.*

## Tanning's Allure Tied to Other Addictions

Brenda Cartmel, PhD, senior research scientist, Yale School of Public Health, New Haven, Connecticut.

Bryon Adinoff, MD, professor of psychiatry, University of Texas Southwestern Medical Center, and director of mental health research, Dallas VA Medical Center.

*Journal of the European Academy of Dermatology and Venereology*, online.

People who seem to have a deep tan year-round—whether from the sun or indoor tanning—may be "addicted" to tanning. And recent research suggests there's also a link between such tanning and other addictions.

"People who were tanning-dependent were six times as likely to have a history of alcohol dependence, and were almost three times as likely to have seasonal affective disorder (SAD)," said study leader Brenda Cartmel, PhD. She is a senior research scientist at the Yale School of Public Health.

SAD is a type of depression related to the shorter, darker days of winter.

Dr. Cartmel said previous smaller studies have also suggested these associations.

### The Study

Dr. Cartmel's team surveyed nearly 500 people who had previously sunbathed or used an indoor tanning bed. All of the participants had also been part of a study on early onset skin cancer among those under age 40 in Connecticut.

Just about one-quarter of the group surveyed was categorized as tanning-dependent based on their answers to two questionnaires.

Dr. Cartmel pointed out that, unlike alcohol dependence, tanning dependence isn't an official psychiatric diagnosis.

People were classified as tanning-dependent if they answered "yes" to five or more questions out of 13 on the two different questionnaires.

***The survey included questions such as:*** Do you feel guilty about tanning? Are you annoyed when people say you tan too much? Do you feel guilty about continuing to tan despite knowing that tanning can increase the risk of skin cancer?

Other questions evaluated SAD, depression, nicotine dependence, alcohol dependence and exercise "addiction."

Those addicted to tanning were mostly women. Being female was linked to a nearly seven times higher risk of tanning-dependency, the study found.

Tanning-dependency was also tied to a higher risk of SAD or alcohol dependence, as well as exercise addiction.

However, the study only found an association between tanning dependency and the other behaviors; it did not prove cause and effect.

The study was published in the *Journal of the European Academy of Dermatology and Venereology.*

## Explanation

Dr. Cartmel cited other research that said exposure to ultraviolet light triggers production of endorphins, a "feel good" hormone.

"The reward of endorphins might play a role," she suggested.

Bryon Adinoff, MD, a professor of psychiatry at the University of Texas Southwestern Medical Center, has studied brain changes associated with tanning.

"We have found that UV light activates areas of the brain and chemicals in the brain that are known to be involved in other rewards and other addictions," said Dr. Adinoff, who is also director of mental health research at Dallas VA Medical Center.

Those with tanning dependence and other addictions may have an environmental or genetic predisposition to those behaviors. This study adds new information about the crossover between tanning and other addictions, said Dr. Adinoff, who was not involved with the recent research.

The pull of tanning seems quite strong for some. Past research has found that even those who survive the deadly skin cancer melanoma often continue to tan.

Dr. Cartmel and Dr. Adinoff both said they don't know of any treatment to reduce tanning dependence.

To learn more about tanning addiction, visit the Skin Cancer Foundation at SkinCancer.org. Search "tanning addiction."

# APPENDICES

## APPENDIX I: DIET, NUTRITION AND FITNESS

### What's the Perfect Diet? That Depends on You

Paleo. Mediterranean. Vegetarian. High-protein. Low-carb. Gluten-free. Low-glycemic. Intermittent fasting. Organic. Probiotic. DASH. MIND. Detox.

Help!

If you want to eat in a healthier way to prevent or cure health problems, you have a dizzying number of choices. Unfortunately, those choices are confusing—and conflicting.

The truth is, no one diet is perfect for everyone. Some people have specific food sensitivities and respond well when they eliminate their "trigger" foods, while others do fine on a wide variety of healthy foods. Some thrive on moderate portions of high-carb whole foods, while others really need a low-carb approach. And so on.

What we really need are core principles for a healthy diet—and then ways to tailor them to our personal health needs. That is exactly what the Institute for Functional Medicine (IFM)—an organization that trains health professionals to treat the underlying causes of diseases—has developed. In a heroic attempt to bring clarity to the dietary "Tower of Babel," the IFM interviewed nutrition-oriented physicians, health-care practitioners and nutrition researchers and crossed-referenced the results with the scientific literature.

***The good news:*** The IFM's Core Food Plan fits just about any healthy person's needs and is very customizable—in fact, it's designed to be customized. Read on to get the details of a healthy eating pattern that's good for nearly everyone—and ways you can work with a health professional to get it tailored for you.

#### An Evidence-Based Approach to a Healthy Diet

Why do we need a new way to eat? It's because in our society today, to a large extent, we don't eat real food. It's that simple. Add in our sedentary lifestyles, polluted environment and lack of sufficient sleep, and it's no wonder so many of us have high blood pressure, heart disease, diabetes, headaches and other chronic pain, chronic infections and too much body fat.

To break this cycle, the IFM's Core Food Plan can be a good place to start. IFM's director of medical education, Kristi Hughes, ND, emphasizes that it's not necessarily better than other well-established evidence-based

Kristi Hughes, ND, naturopathic physician, director of medical education, Institute for Functional Medicine, Federal Way, Washington.

Margaret Mills, MS, functional nutrition clinical coordinator, Institute for Functional Medicine, Federal Way, Washington.

Mary Willis, RD, LD, CDE, nutrition services director, College Park Family Care Center, Overland Park, Kansas.

dietary plans such as the Mediterranean Diet. Indeed, it derives some of its principles from that approach (as well as from Paleo). But the beauty of the Core Food Plan is that it provides dietary guidance that can be easily tailored to individual needs. And it does go a step beyond the official US dietary guidelines. For example, research suggests that consumption of high-glycemic grains and low-fat dairy, which are promoted by the US dietary guidelines, are not consistent with overall health. In contrast to those guidelines and most conventional nutrition advice, the IFM Core Food Plan emphasizes fresh whole foods with high phytonutrient diversity.

Nutritionist Mary Willis, RD, CDE, who helped develop the Core Food Plan, says the challenge was to create a healthy eating plan that would help transition people away from the standard American diet (or what nutritionists fittingly call "SAD"). One key problem with SAD is the preponderance of highly-refined carbs with little or no nutritional value. Many people transitioning from SAD are consuming more than 50% of their calories from carbs, Willis says, and most of those carbs are refined carbs from sugar and grains, not from vegetable or fruit sources.

The Core Food Plan, in contrast, is a balanced "plant-dominant" approach. It does include meat (if you want it to). But you can still think of Core as everything SAD isn't—high in vegetables (and fruits) from across the rainbow spectrum...low or moderately low in grain-based carbohydrates...low in sugar...and devoid of processed foods.

## The Core Food Plan: What to Eat Every Day

The Core Food Plan is not a deprivation diet—in fact, it's actually pretty balanced when it comes to protein (25% of calories), fat (30%) and carbohydrates (45%). That all comes from nine distinct food groups (listed in next column). The appropriate servings are based on calorie needs and therapeutic considerations. To get an idea of what's included, consider the recommendations for the 1,800-to-2,200 calorie range, which is appropriate for an average man or a woman who is physically active. ***Here's what you would eat each day...***

- **Proteins.** Seven or eight small "portions." This category, which includes animal and plant protein, is measured in "portions" rather than "servings." Each portion is small—just one ounce of meat, fish or poultry, one egg or one-half ounce of hard cheese, for example—but you can mix-and-match sources and have multiple portions at a meal. (A four-ounce filet mignon, for example, would be four portions.) The plan stresses "clean" sources of animal protein—lean, free-range, grass-fed, wild-caught. It can also be tailored to vegetarians—and vegans—with portions such as one ounce of tempeh or two ounces of firm tofu. According to Willis, when you eat your protein is an important factor. In her 30 years of clinical experience, she has found that Americans do not eat enough high-quality protein at breakfast and/or lunch—and then overeat protein at dinner.

- **Legumes.** Two or three servings. One-half cup of cooked beans or lentils is one serving, so the total is one to one-and-a-half cups a day. Vegetarians and vegans, however, may want to increase their daily servings of legumes as a substitute for animal protein.

- **Dairy and dairy alternatives.** Three servings. Fermented dairy foods such as yogurt and kefir are emphasized over, say, milk, as they feed the "good" bacteria in the gut, which in turn help turn down inflammation, explains Dr. Hughes. Nondairy alternatives such as almond and soy milk are also encouraged. One serving is eight ounces of milk or six ounces of Greek yogurt. In the Core Food Plan, "dairy" doesn't include cheese, which is in the protein category.

- **Nuts and seeds.** Three to five snack-sized servings.

***Examples:*** 10 peanuts, six almonds, one tablespoon of sunflower seeds or one-half tablespoon of nut butter would each be considered one serving.

- **Fats and oils.** Four to five small servings.

***Examples:*** One teaspoon of butter or olive oil or two tablespoons of an oily food, such as avocado (one-eighth whole fruit). If you eat butter—which is considered a fat rather than a dairy food—choose butter made from the milk of grass-fed cows, which has a healthier balance of fats.

• **Nonstarchy vegetables.** 10 servings.

***Example:*** One-half cup of cooked broccoli or spinach or one cup of salad greens. This is a big increase in veggies for many people. "Most Americans get only two to four servings a day—and most are fried," says Dr. Hughes.

• **Starchy vegetables.** One or two servings.

***Examples:*** One cup of cooked squash or one-half a medium potato.

• **Fruit.** Two or three servings.

***Examples:*** One small apple, three-quarter cup of blueberries, one cup of melon. Including fruit in your diet provides antioxidants, fiber and key vitamins. The fiber blunts the body's response to sugar, so whole fruit, compared with foods with added sugars, is a lower-glycemic source of natural sweetness.

• **Grains.** Two servings.

***Examples:*** One-third cup of cooked rice, one slice of bread. "Grains are de-emphasized in the IFM food plans," says Willis. Why? "To make room for a robust amount of colorful plant foods from other food categories that are overlooked in the grain-dominant standard American diet. Americans put a bun or wrap or breading on everything!" For people who need to avoid gluten, the IFM plan also includes many gluten-free grain picks including oats, quinoa, rice and millet.

The core plan emphasizes organic foods to reduce exposure to pesticides. It can be tailored to accommodate people who are avoiding gluten, dairy or animal foods. It can be customized for athletes, who may, for example, need extra protein. It can also be tailored for people who want to experiment with "intermittent fasting," which calls for certain very low-calorie days followed by normal eating days as a way to improve body composition, enhance metabolism and control weight.

Some people lose weight on the IFM Core Food Plan, but that's not the primary goal—or even the best measure of success. Rather, the emphasis is on improving health and maintaining a healthy way of eating for life. A person who transitions from SAD to Core can expect to have more energy, which in turn may motivate him or her to get more physically active. Those lifestyle changes could then lead to improvements in metabolic fitness and a reduced risk for chronic disease. Clinically, adds Dr. Hughes, patients who switch to this eating style often report more focus and concentration, enhanced sleep, greater daily stamina and an improved sense of well-being.

## If You Want to Try One of the IFM's Customized Food Plans...

While adopting the Core Food Plan itself would bring a world of improvement for many people, the IFM also has developed other plans to allow health professionals—including MDs, osteopaths, naturopaths, nutritionists, nurse practitioners and others—to help patients with specific, identified needs.

Some IFM plans are "first step" diets, while others are more advanced interventions for people with certain medical conditions. Some are designed to be short-term. As the IFM practitioner's guide states, "Nutritional and dietary needs may change or evolve as a patient moves through a layered healing process."

The first step interventions are...

***Cardiometabolic Food Plan:*** This is for people with cardiovascular and blood sugar–related issues such as insulin resistance and the problems that often go with them, including unhealthy cholesterol ratios, excess abdominal fat and high levels of inflammation. It emphasizes low-glycemic foods (which help keep blood sugar stable), increased fiber, meal timing and ideal serving sizes. Compared with the Core Food Plan, the macronutrient balance is slightly lower in carbohydrates and higher in protein—30% protein...30% fat...40% carbs.

***Elimination Diet:*** Pinpointing the foods causing food allergies, intolerances or sensitivities and eliminating them (and eventually reintroducing some) is the goal. According to the practitioner's guide, "Often, symptoms that have failed to respond to conventional medical therapy will resolve by following an elimination diet. After the initial period of eliminating foods, many chronic symptoms should improve or disappear."

One example of an advanced intervention is the Detox Food Plan, which builds on the Elimination Diet by eliminating certain trigger foods but then goes a step further by emphasizing avoidance of environmental toxins (in plastics for example), consumption of organic foods and consumption of specific therapeutic foods that support the gut, liver and kidneys. These emphasize cruciferous vegetables such as broccoli and cauliflower, dark leafy greens and bitter greens, for example.

There are also customizable "GI specific dietary interventions" for people with gastrointestinal complaints who have followed the elimination diet but are still experiencing symptoms. They include an antifungal (anti-Candida) diet, a low-FODMAP diet and others. The Mito Food Plan ("Mito" is short for mitochondria, the "energy factories" inside each cell) is designed to nutritionally support people with pain and fatigue syndromes as well as those who are at risk for autoimmune conditions or those experiencing neurological concerns. It is a strict anti-inflammatory, low-glycemic, gluten-free, low-grain, high-quality-fats approach to eating. There's also a ReNew Food Plan, which can be used as a modified elimination diet and is designed to be "a whole systems reboot and system detox." It's geared toward people with autoimmune, gastrointestinal, neurological and other chronic health conditions. It eliminates sugar, dairy, grains (including gluten-free), alcohol, caffeine, artificial sweeteners, processed foods that contain heavy metals and foods high in pro-inflammatory saturated animal fats.

Do these customized versions really work? To be clear, they have not been studied in clinical trials but rather are based on clinical practice in functional medicine and related nutrition research. Various research projects are in the works—the Cleveland Clinic, for example, collaborated in the creation of the ReNew plan and is using it with some of its patients. The Cleveland Clinic is also using the Mito plan for certain patients of the clinic's Center for Functional Medicine.

While the Core Food Plan is fine for anyone who's generally healthy, the more personalized and specific versions are really designed to be undertaken with the supervision of a medical professional, nutrition professional or functional medicine health coach trained to customize the food plan to the individual. To find a health-care professional who is trained in the IFM approach, go to FunctionalMedicine.org and choose "find a practitioner." Additionally, the Functional Medicine Coaching Academy trains health coaches in collaboration with the IFM, and you may be able to find a nutrition coach through it.

# 11 Surprising Ways to Shed Pounds

Brian Wansink, PhD, director of the Food and Brand Lab at Cornell University, Ithaca, New York. In 2007, the White House named him the US Department of Agriculture executive director in charge of Dietary Guidelines for 2010. He is author of *Slim By Design: Mindless Eating Solutions for Everyday Life.* SlimByDesign.org

If you store boxes of breakfast cereal in the wrong spot in your kitchen, you could end up 20 pounds heavier. If you set serving dishes in the wrong spot at mealtimes, you could consume 20% more calories than you otherwise would have. If you get seated at the wrong table in a restaurant, the odds that you will order a dessert could leap by 73%.

People tend to think that avoiding overeating is mainly a matter of willpower. But willpower alone is never enough. Almost all of us have moments when willpower wavers... and moments when we eat irresponsibly because we are not paying enough attention to eat properly.

The good news is that there are clever, surprising things you can do to avoid overeating without relying on superhuman willpower and vigilance...

## Food Storage Tricks

• **Segregate snack food.** Each time you open a cupboard that contains empty-calorie snack food, there's a reasonable chance that you will indulge—even if you originally opened the cupboard to retrieve something else.

To avoid this, it's best to just not buy unhealthy snack food. But if that's not in the cards, store all unhealthy snacks, such as potato chips and cookies, in a single cupboard rather than spread them throughout the kitchen as is common. (The typical US kitchen has five cupboards—and snack food is stored in the majority of them.) Do not store anything but snacks in your snack cupboard so that you never accidentally stumble upon temptation.

Healthy snacks such as fruit or wholegrain rice cakes can remain elsewhere in the kitchen—there's nothing wrong with stumbling upon these.

***Next step:*** To reduce snacking even further, store unhealthy snacks in a cupboard located in a room that you enter less often than your kitchen, such as the basement or the laundry room.

• **Store snacks in single-serving portions.** When snack foods leave the kitchen, they rarely come back. Carry a family-size bag of chips to the living room, for example, and if you're like most people, there's a good chance that you will eat the entire thing...and even if you don't, you likely will eat more than you meant to.

One solution is to buy snacks pre-packaged in single-serving portions—but these tend to cost much more per ounce than larger sizes. Instead, buy economy-size bags, but immediately repackage these snacks into single-serving-size plastic bags or other small containers as soon as the snacks enter the house.

• **In the refrigerator, store healthy snacks in clear containers...unhealthy ones in opaque ones.** Remove fruit from the crisper drawer, and store it in clear plastic bags or storage containers at eye level in your fridge. Meanwhile, wrap unhealthy snacks in tin foil or put them in opaque food containers. The snacks that people are most likely to eat are not the ones they think taste best...they are the ones that they happen to see first.

• **Store cereal boxes out of view.** It probably comes as no surprise that people are especially likely to eat foods that are "on display" on countertops or exposed shelves in their homes. But what is surprising is that this seems to matter most not with candy but with breakfast cereal.

People who keep candy on display in their homes are, on average, three pounds heavier than people who do not...people who have cookies or crackers on display are about eight pounds heavier...while people who have cereal boxes out where they can be seen are in excess of 20 pounds heavier.

The most likely explanation is that people realize that snacking on candy and cookies is bad for them, so they often manage to stop themselves from grabbing these sugary treats...but breakfast cereal has the aura of healthfulness—even though it usually is quite sugary and fattening—so people who have it out on display are less likely to stop themselves from indulging.

## Meals

• **Leave serving dishes and pots on the kitchen counter or stove while you eat.** People who fill their plates at least six feet from the table tend to eat around 20% fewer calories at mealtime than people who bring serving dishes or pots to the table. The reason—having additional food within easy reach greatly increases the odds that people will help themselves to seconds or thirds.

Men are particularly likely to do this. They tend to eat faster than their wives and children, so they finish meals first—then take extra helpings even when they are not very hungry because they get bored sitting around doing nothing.

• **Eat off slightly undersized plates, and use undersized serving spoons.** You might have heard that people eat less when they eat off small plates—small plates make modest amounts of food look more substantial. It turns out that this can be taken too far. If you try to eat dinner off a very small plate, it only increases the odds that you will go back for more. The ideal dinner plate size is around nine inches in diameter—smaller than the typical 10-to-12-inch dinner plate but not so small as to encourage the taking of seconds.

***Also:*** Using serving spoons of modest size reduces consumption, too...as does replacing serving tongs with serving spoons. (Do use tongs to serve salad. Taking large servings of salad makes people less likely to fill up on more fattening foods.) An undersized ice-cream scoop is an especially worthwhile investment—people tend to pay attention to the number of scoops of ice cream they take, not the total amount of ice cream they eat.

But do not try to eat with undersized utensils. It turns out that doesn't make people eat less—it just annoys them.

• **Put on slow music, and turn down the lights.** These things tend to calm people down—and people who feel calm at mealtimes tend to eat more slowly and eat less.

## Dining Out Tricks

It's easy to overindulge when you eat out. *These strategies will help...*

• **Ask to be seated at a well-lit table...by a window...at a table that is higher-than-normal table height...or in a bustling part of the dining room.** When people feel on display in restaurants, they tend to order healthier meals, such as fish or salad. When they are seated in booths or dark, private corners, they are more likely to order fattening things such as ribs and desserts.

***Example:*** People seated at the table farthest from a restaurant's front door are 73% more likely to order a dessert than people seated near the entrance.

• **Ask to be seated at least three tables away from the bar.** When people eat dinner at a restaurant's bar—or within two tables of its bar—they order three-and-a-half more alcoholic drinks per party of four. This applies only at dinner, however—people do not drink significantly more when they eat lunch near a restaurant's bar.

• **Adopt trim people's habits at buffets.** Trim people and heavy people tend to exhibit significantly divergent behavior when they dine at buffets—generally without even realizing they are doing so. Thin buffet diners choose tables far from the food (when given a choice of table)...they choose seats that face away from the food...they use smaller plates if multiple plate sizes are available...they use chopsticks (if this is an option)...and they scout out the entire buffet before taking any food. Heavy people tend to do exactly the opposite of each of these things. Act trim, and it will help you be trim!

• **Be aware of your waiter's weight.** If your waiter is overweight, you're more likely to overindulge. In a study of 497 people at 60 full-service restaurants, diners ordered more food—especially dessert—and more alcohol when the waiter had weight to lose than when the waiter was thin. This was true regardless of how much the diners themselves weighed. It's likely that the presence of a heavy person made the diners feel as if they had "permission" to indulge.

You can't control who your waiter is, but just recognizing the effect that a heavy waiter could have on your ordering can help you resist temptation. It's also helpful when eating out to have a "predetermination strategy," such as deciding in advance what you'll order (you usually can view menus online). Or you can have "rules" in place such as only one glass of wine with dinner.

## Diet Soda–Weight Gain Link

Diet soda is linked to weight gain. People who drank one or more cans of diet soda every day for nine years added 3.2 inches to their waistlines versus only 0.8 inches for people who did not drink diet soda. People who drank diet soda only occasionally expanded their waists by 1.8 inches.

Study of 749 people over age 65 by researchers at University of Texas Health Science Center at San Antonio, published in *Journal of the American Geriatrics Society.*

## Stress Can Wreck Your Healthy Diet

Stress may undo benefits of a healthful diet.

***New research:*** Women who ate a healthful unsaturated-fat meal and had a highly stressful day had identical levels of inflammatory markers as women who ate a saturated-fat meal of biscuits and gravy but reported no stress.

***Self-defense:*** Take steps to manage stress—for example, do yoga or meditation, exercise regularly and get enough sleep.

Janice Kiecolt-Glaser, PhD, director, Institute for Behavioral Medicine Research, The Ohio State University, Columbus.

## Danger of the Paleo Diet

Joseph Feuerstein, MD, assistant professor of clinical medicine at Columbia University, New York City, and director of integrative medicine at Stamford Hospital, Connecticut. He is author of *Dr. Joe's Man Diet: Lose 15-20 Pounds, Drop Bad Cholesterol 20% and Watch Your Blood Sugar Free-Fall in 12 Weeks.* DrFeuerstein.com

Recent research has cast doubt on the trendy Paleo diet, an eating plan that encourages consumption of meat and discourages consumption of grains and other processed foods.

The Paleo diet has become popular in part because it makes some intuitive sense. Humans were hunter-gatherers long before the advent of farming, so it is not unreasonable to speculate that our bodies might be well-suited to subsist on the meats, vegetables and nuts that our Paleolithic hunter-gatherer ancestors ate for all of those millennia.

Proponents of the Paleo diet argue that modern humans are prone to packing on excess pounds in part because we now eat processed foods and farm products such as grains that our early ancestors did not eat.

But while the Paleo diet is a compelling theory, there has never been much research to back it up. And now a study has cast doubt on whether the Paleo diet even was healthy for people who lived during Paleolithic times. When researchers at St. Luke's Mid America Heart Institute in Kansas City conducted CT scans on 137 ancient mummies from four different parts of the globe, they discovered that more than one-third of them showed signs of heart disease (though it is worth noting that Paleolithic people probably smoked most or all of their meat over fires, a preparation technique that likely exacerbates heart disease dangers).

Meanwhile, a long-term study conducted in China by researchers from Cornell, Oxford and the Chinese Academy of Preventive Medicine found a strong correlation between the consumption of meat (as well as dairy products) and coronary heart disease, casting further doubt on the healthfulness of meat-heavy diets.

***Advice:*** Exercise caution in trying the Paleo diet (or any other meat-heavy diet) if you have a history of heart disease and/or if heart problems run in your family. But this diet might be a reasonable option if your doctor confirms that your heart is in good shape and if you choose grains high in soluble fiber, such as oats or flax, which have been shown to help lower blood pressure and stroke risk.

# Avoid This Food/Sleep Trap!

Study titled, "Fiber and Saturated Fat Are Associated with Sleep Arousals and Slow Wave Sleep" by Marie-Pierre St-Onge, PhD, FAHA, research associate, New York Obesity Research Center, College of Physicians and Surgeons, Columbia University, New York, and colleagues, published in *Journal of Clinical Sleep Medicine.*

You know that when you sleep poorly, it's easy to overindulge in junky snacks the next day. It's one of the reasons why problems sleeping are associated with an increased risk for obesity.

But the opposite is true too—eating poorly can interfere with the quality of your sleep.

Researchers have long suspected this, but now they have shown that it happens—and what nutrients are the worst culprits.

Researchers at Columbia University College of Physicians and Surgeons studied 26 normal-weight men and women in their 30s and 40s. None had insomnia or other sleep problems. For one part of the study, participants ate a balanced, healthy diet provided by the researchers. For the next part, they were given an allowance to buy their own food, which the researchers then weighed before and after consumption so that they knew what and how much the participants ate.

***Results:*** Diet didn't affect how long participants slept—the average was about seven-and-a-half hours—but it had a big effect on how well they slept. Those who ate the most fiber-rich foods (think fruits and vegetables) fell asleep more quickly and spent more time in the truly refreshing deepest stage of sleep. Conversely, those who ate the most high-sugar, high-saturated-fat foods (think cookies and ice cream) spent less time in that oh-so-healthy deep sleep. Refined carbs, such as white bread and white rice, also were linked with poorer sleep.

Sounds like a vicious cycle? Right you are! Sleep poorly because you ate poorly…then eat poorly because you slept poorly…then sleep poorly again…and so on. This may describe you or someone you know right now.

The solution to this vicious cycle, according to study author Marie-Pierre St-Onge, PhD, is to start by practicing the best sleep habits you can at night and then use the benefits of a good night's sleep to eat better the next day. You probably already know what to do—a really dark room, a comfortably cool room temperature and no electronics use right before bedtime.

The better the quality of your sleep—what sleep researchers call the architecture of sleep—the easier it should be to make smart, healthy food choices the next day.

If you do eat right, the result should be better sleep quality that next night.

Which then makes it easier to eat right the next day.

# The Real Benefits of Mindful Eating

Study titled "Effects of a Mindfulness-Based Weight Loss Intervention in Adults with Obesity: A Randomized Clinical Trial" by researchers at University of California, San Francisco, et al. published in *Obesity.*

Does "mindful eating" help you lose weight? That's what researchers at the University of California set out to find out. It is common knowledge that stress can lead to overeating, especially mindless eating when you're not even hungry. Stress is linked to weight gain, especially belly fat, plus increases in blood sugar and blood fats.

And it is also common knowledge that learning mindfulness helps people regulate their emotions, including eating habits, especially when they're stressed.

But whether mindfulness training actually helps people lose more weight than regular dieting hasn't been rigorously studied in a double-blind randomized controlled trial.

Until now. And there are indeed benefits to dieters—just not the ones that were expected.

## Protein Helps Sleep

In a recent small study, researchers found that middle-aged adults slept better after four months when consuming 750 fewer calories daily on a high-protein diet. Up to 30% of their calorie intake was from protein sources, including beef, pork, soy, legumes and/or milk.

***Theory:*** Protein boosts neurotransmitters needed for sleep.

***Important:*** If you have kidney disease or another chronic condition, consult your doctor before increasing your protein intake.

Jing Zhou, PhD, nutrition researcher, Purdue University, West Lafayette, Indiana.

## Breathe Deeply, Feel Your Hunger

The California researchers studied about 200 obese men and women with an average age of 48. Participants didn't have diabetes, nor were they taking any medications that affected weight. About half of them entered into a standard weight-loss program for 16 weeks—healthy food choices leading to cutting calories by about 500 calories a day plus daily exercise such as walking and strength training. Once they completed the program, they were followed up over the next 14 months.

The second group went through the same diet/exercise program but also worked with a trainer on mindfulness-based eating awareness, including meditation, with specific emphasis on becoming aware of the feelings of hunger, taste, cravings, emotions and other eating triggers.

Results...

- **The mindful dieters did lose a little more weight than the regular dieters**—more than one year after the study ended, they weighed about nine pounds less than at the beginning, compared with about five pounds less for the regular dieters. However, it wasn't statistically significant, which means it may have been due to chance.
- **Much more statistically significant were differences in cardio-metabolic health.** Fasting blood sugar for the regular dieters crept up about 4 mg/dl, but it dropped about 4 mg/dl for the mindful group.
- **Triglycerides**—blood fats associated with diabetes risk—went down for only the mindfulness group, too.
- **The triglyceride/HDL ratio,** an indicator of metabolic syndrome, which raises the risk for both heart disease and diabetes, improved only for the mindfulness group.

There was also a hint in the data that those who meditated the most lost the most weight and had the best improvements in health measurements. Interestingly, those who liked their mindfulness trainer—did better than those who didn't feel good about the trainer.

Bottom line? Mindfulness-based eating might help you lose a little extra weight. But even if it doesn't, there's a good chance that it'll make you significantly healthier.

# Beware the New Normal for Average Weight

Donald Cutlip, MD, Harvard Medical School, with Rebecca Shannonhouse, editor, *Bottom Line Health.*

Most Americans have obviously gotten heavier over the years. What's shocking is how much heavier. A few decades ago, the typical man weighed 181 pounds...now he's 196, according to a recent report from the CDC. For women, the average weight has gone from about 153 to 166.

The dangers of this alarming trend are not new—we all know that being overweight or obese is a risk factor for diabetes, heart disease, stroke and other serious conditions.

So why are so many people still tipping the scales? Part of the problem is how we see ourselves. Now that more than two-thirds of American adults are overweight or obese, "big" has become the new normal. We've simply stopped noticing.

To make matters worse, the main tool for assessing obesity—a weight-to-height ratio known as the body mass index (BMI)—doesn't distinguish patterns of obesity. For example, visceral (abdominal) obesity—often evident from the size of one's belly—is the pattern that's linked to the greatest health risks.

For that reason, a waist-to-hip measurement can also be useful for people who suspect that they may be gaining too much weight, says Donald Cutlip, MD, of Harvard Medical School. All you need is a tape measure.

***What to do:*** Measure your hips...measure your waist just above your belly button...and divide the waist number by the hip number. For women, a good reading is 0.8 or below... men should be 0.9 or under.

***Important:*** Being underweight—a BMI below 18.5—or suffering unexplained weight loss can be harmful, too.

# Help for Holiday Weight Gain

Weight gained from Thanksgiving until around New Year's takes five months to lose.

***During the holiday season:*** Except for salad and vegetables, keep all other serving dishes off the table when eating. Place them on a counter. That way you have to leave the table to get seconds—and so are less likely to do so.

***To limit the temptation of leftovers:*** Keep them out of sight by freezing them or wrapping them in aluminum foil.

Brian Wansink, PhD, director of Cornell Food and Brand Lab, Ithaca, New York, and author of *Slim by Design* and coauthor of a study of holiday weight gain, published in *The New England Journal of Medicine.*

# Eating in Moderation? It's a Weight Trap

Michelle vanDellen, PhD, associate professor, behavioral and brain sciences, The University of Georgia, Athens, lead author of study titled "How Do People Define Moderation?" published in *Appetite.*

Susan McQuillan, MS, RDN, registered dietitian based in New York City and author of *Low-Calorie Dieting for Dummies.*

"Eat in moderation." It's the new clarion call for healthy eating, even touted as the new way to lose weight—especially now that there's a big trend in the US away from restrictive weight-loss diets.

***The idea:*** Depriving yourself of foods that you love is old-fashioned advice. It's better to eat what you like, including your favorite high-calorie foods—but not too much.

***Here's a tip:*** It's a trap. And it may be making you fat.

So finds a recent paper entitled "How do people define moderation?" published in the respected peer-reviewed journal *Appetite.*

## Let's Feel Good About Eating Too Much

On the fast-food chain Chick-fil-A's bags for takeout food, according to the paper, there's this statement...

***"Moderation Is Key:*** All foods can fit within a healthy diet if consumed in moderation. With appropriate portion sizes and physical activity, you can enjoy treats like our Frosted Lemonade."

Moderation is one of many myths that Big Food uses to rationalize their calorie, fat and sugar bombs. (That Frosted Lemonade from Chick-fil-A contains 63 grams of sugar, the equivalent of 16 teaspoons.) But according to this recent research, food companies cynically proselytizing moderation is not the core of the problem with that seemingly healthy concept.

The real problem is you. Chances are that you have no idea what moderation in eating really means—and that you might find it easy to twist the idea unconsciously to help feel good about yourself while you overeat. To learn more, we spoke with the lead study author, psychologist Michelle vanDellen, PhD, an associate professor in the behavioral and brain sciences program at The University of Georgia, and to registered dietitian Susan McQuillan, MS, RDN, author of *Low-Calorie Dieting for Dummies.*

## What Moderation Means in Real Life

In a series of studies, Dr. vanDellen and colleagues examined how people think about moderation, especially when it comes to foods that they know they should limit such as cookies, fruit-shaped gummy snacks, soda, pizza and fast food. *Her findings held true for both men and women...and normal-weight and overweight people...*

- **Most people define "eating moderately" as eating a bigger amount than they think they should eat.** For example, in one study, subjects were presented with a big plate with 24 cookies and asked how many a person should eat—and how many would constitute eating in moderation. On average, they said a person "should" eat about two cookies, but that "moderation" was a little more than three cookies.

- **The more you like a food, the bigger a "moderate" portion will be for you.** In another study, subjects were shown a picture of gummy snacks and asked to specify "should eat" and "moderation" portions. Once again, "moderate" portions were the larger portions. But the more a person liked gummy snacks, the researchers found, the bigger the "moderate" portion tended to be.

- **The more often you eat a particular kind of food, the more frequent you'll consider eating it in moderation to be.** Eating in moderation isn't just what you eat at any given meal—it's also how often you eat it in a day, a week or a month. After all, eating ice cream daily is less "moderate" than eating it weekly or a few times a month. But here, too, perception was malleable—and (literally) self-serving. In a third study, the researchers asked subjects how often over two weeks they ate 12 different high-calorie foods, including pizza, soda, fast food and ice cream. No matter how often people ate a particular food, they consistently defined "moderate" frequency as more frequent than what they themselves did! Thus, if you eat ice cream once a week, you might define moderate as twice a week. But if you eat ice cream three times a week, you might define moderate as four times a week—so you're still off the hook!

Dr. vanDellen believes that these malleable definitions are contributing to the obesity epidemic—by encouraging overeating. One way it happens occurs at the exact moment when you've eaten a portion of a food that you know isn't really good to eat a lot of. That's when you have a decision to make about whether eating more would be going overboard. To gain control over overeating, explains Dr. vanDellen, you need to recognize that you have a conflict at that moment—for example, that you'd really like to eat another piece of pie but you know you shouldn't. Only then can you muster the motivation to override your immediate desire—for example, you know that you'll feel good about yourself if you stick to your eating plan. But if you delude yourself that you're eating "moderately," you'll never feel that conflict—and you'll just keep eating.

## How to Really Eat in Moderation

The solution? Pay attention to good old-fashioned serving sizes—and calories. While there are many contributors to our obesity epidemic, including sugar and other low-fiber refined carbs, there is strong evidence that the increasing size of portions is a major culprit.

That's not to say you should radically cut down on how much you eat, a dieting mentality that almost always backfires. "Severe food restriction is both physically and psychologically unhealthy," says McQuillan. "But knowing your calorie limits and recognizing the calorie count of the various foods you eat is still important when you try to lose weight or maintain it."

Ironically, paying attention to the actual amounts of foods that you eat may be the best way to actually eat in moderation. To illustrate this, let's go back to that 16-ounce Chick fil-A Frosted Lemonade. It's a 16-ounce, 330-calorie cup of lemonade blended with ice cream. It's 63 grams of sugar is more than the 50 grams from added sugar maximum that the US Dietary Guidelines recommends for average Americans for the entire day.

But if you think of it as ice cream, and know your serving sizes, you'd realize that a serving size for ice cream is one-half cup—four ounces. For juice, a serving size is six ounces. So instead of drinking that entire thing, let's say you enjoy six ounces—three quarters of a cup. You'll get about 125 calories and 24 grams of sugar. That's about half the added sugar daily maximum for an average American. So it's a still a high-sugar treat, but a more manageable one...perhaps even "moderate."

# To Lose Weight, Cut Carbs...Just Twice a Week

Louis Aronne, MD, professor of medicine, Weill Cornell Medical College, director, Comprehensive Weight Control Center at Weill Cornell Medicine and New York-Presbyterian, both in New York City.

There are many popular ways to lose weight. Lots of people try cutting calories across the board, but then they are hungry a lot of the time. Others dramatically cut carbs, which often helps with hunger, but that is hard to stick with if you love "carb-y" foods. Some people practice intermittent fasting, eating only 500 or 600 calories on certain days, but you might find that overly restrictive, too.

Fortunately, there is another, little-known approach that's just as effective as any of the above—and a whole lot easier for many people to stick with. Like intermittent fasting, it involves restrictive days, and like low-carb dieting, it involves drastically cutting carbohydrates.

***But here's the big difference:*** All you do is go low-carb twice a week, without counting calories at all. The rest of the week you eat as much of a normal healthy diet as you want. It may work by "resetting" the brain so that you're not as hungry—not just on low-carb days but even when you go back to your "normal" way of eating the rest of the week.

Here's how to make it work for you.

## The Two-Day Low-Carb Diet

At the Comprehensive Weight Control Center at Weill Cornell Medical College, we became interested in this new approach when we reviewed a four-month British study of 115 overweight women. *The women were divided into three groups...*

- **Daily dieters cut their calories by 25% to an average of 1,500 a day on a balanced healthy Mediterranean-style diet.**
- **A second group did intermittent fasting on two consecutive days.** It was pretty intense—low-carb and no more than 600 calories a day...and then repeat the next day. The rest of the week, they ate as much as they wanted from a balanced diet.
- **The third group of women also went on an intermittent low-carb diet for two consecutive days, but they didn't have to restrict calories.** It was a big carb reduction—to just 40 grams, slightly less than the amount in one cup of rice. On those days, they were allowed unrestricted protein and healthy fats. The rest of the week they ate as they wanted from a balanced diet.

***Results:*** The two-day-a-week low-carb dieters lost just as much weight as the intermittent fasters...and lost more weight than the everyday dieters. And besides losing more weight (11 versus eight pounds), the two-day-a-weekers also lost more body fat, becoming lighter and leaner.

What was even more intriguing was that just cutting carbs on those two days—and not counting overall calories—was as effective as intermittent fasting. In fact, neither group tended to overeat on days when they weren't, respectively, cutting carbs or fasting.

Could it really be that easy to lose weight—just cut carbs two days a week? Yes, it could—because carbs do some very particular things to the brain.

## The Carb-Brain-Appetite Connection

When you eat a lot of carbohydrates, especially simple starches and sugars, it can literally damage neurons in the hypothalamus, a part of the brain that helps regulate appetite. The nerve cells in the hypothalamus become surrounded by inflammatory cells, and then they don't function as well as they should.

Quality of fat matters, too. In animal studies, for example, high-saturated-fat diets—the kind of fats that are very prevalent in a typical Western diet—have also been shown to disrupt the appetite-signaling pathways. So the emphasis on healthy, mostly unsaturated fats in the diet may contribute to its effectiveness.

In effect, the brain becomes resistant to input from hormones, including leptin and ghrelin, which play key roles in regulating appetite. The hypothalamus mistakenly sends out signals to eat more. You feel hungrier, you eat more, and you create more damage—and so on.

The secret of the two-day-a-week carb-cutting diet is that the hunger-signaling pathway can be "reset" by giving the damaged neurons a break by cutting carbs, which also tends to cut calories, and by your eating healthy polyunsaturated and monounsaturated fats. When the oxidative load that's hitting those nerves decreases, the whole system can work much better.

That explains why people on this diet don't go crazy with overeating on their "off diet" days. Even after just one day of going very low carbohydrate, the signaling system between the appetite hormones and the hypothalamus works much more efficiently. That effect can last for a few days.

### Better Lunch Choices

Cutting calories? Order lunch (or make it) at least one hour before eating.

***Recent findings:*** People who ordered lunch (including a beverage) in advance made more healthful choices and ate about 10% fewer calories than those who ordered just before eating.

***Why:*** When you're not hungry, it's easier to make wise choices—the same reason that experts suggest not grocery shopping on an empty stomach.

Eric VanEpps, PhD, postdoctoral research fellow, Center for Health Incentives and Behavioral Economics at the Leonard Davis Institute, University of Pennsylvania, Philadelphia.

Steven P. Cohen, MD, professor of anesthesiology, The Johns Hopkins University School of Medicine, Baltimore.

## Ready to Try the Intermittent Low-Carb Diet?

In our clinical experience, we have found that there is no need to avoid carbohydrates two days in a row. We tell dieters that they are free to restrict their carbohydrates on any two days of the week.

For a lot of people, just eliminating bread, pasta and sweets (sugars are carbs) gets most of the job done. *But for a little more detail, here's a sample one-day low-carb menu...*

- **Breakfast:** Two or three eggs with spinach and mozzarella cheese, made with one teaspoon of oil.
- **Lunch:** A large vegetable salad with one-third of an avocado, five or more ounces of chicken or grilled shrimp or cheese, and one or two tablespoons of Italian dressing.
- **Snack:** Six to eight ounces of Greek yogurt (0% to 2% fat) with eight walnut halves.
- **Dinner:** Five or more ounces of grilled poultry, fish or red meat, roasted vegetables

(such as cauliflower, Brussels sprouts or broccoli) with one or two tablespoons of olive oil, a tossed salad with one tablespoon of oil-and-vinegar and one cup of berries.

True, there's no linguine with clam sauce... no bread-and-jam. But it's only for a few days a week—and on the other five days, you may find that you're not craving carbs as much as you do now. You're almost sure to lose weight.

# Diet-Free Weight Loss

Reduce clutter to make weight loss easier. People who live with extreme clutter are 76% more likely to struggle with weight issues than those who keep their homes orderly. Clutter causes stress that can lead to overeating and makes it harder to make healthy food choices.

***Self-defense:*** Clear kitchen counters and tables regularly, and throw out anything that makes you feel stressed or guilty, such as expired, never-used spices.

Peter Walsh, professional organizer, Los Angeles, and author of *Lose the Clutter, Lose the Weight*, quoted in RedbookMag.com.

# When Weight Loss Is Worrisome

Robert Wergin, MD, the immediate past board chair of the American Academy of Family Physicians and a volunteer faculty member in the department of family medicine at the University of Nebraska Medical Center in Omaha.

If you start losing weight without even trying, it may at first seem like a dream come true. But if the number keeps on dipping, your excitement should turn to worry.

Unintentional weight loss is when you lose weight (5% or more of your normal weight within six to 12 months) without dieting or increasing physical activity. It may occur following a loss of appetite or when you're consuming the same number of calories as usual. In either case, it is often a warning signal that something serious is going on with your health. While older adults are at greater risk for unexplained weight loss—it occurs in 15% to 20% of adults age 65 and older—people who are in their 50s or even younger can also be affected.

A thorough checkup is critical to determine the cause of unintentional weight loss. I recommend starting with your primary care physician or family doctor, who will take a detailed history and order blood work and urine tests based on other symptoms. Armed with the results, he/she can direct you to an appropriate specialist if necessary.

Many people know that cancer can cause unintentional weight loss (more on this below), but there are other underlying causes as well...

## GI Disorders

If you have diarrhea, abdominal pain, bloating and/or gas in addition to unintentional weight loss, you could have a gastrointestinal (GI) disorder, such as celiac disease or inflammatory bowel disease (IBD). *The facts you need...*

- **Celiac disease is a genetic autoimmune disorder affecting one in 100 people.** When an affected individual consumes gluten (a protein found in wheat, rye and barley), the immune system launches a response that attacks the lining of the small intestine.

This can trigger a number of unpleasant GI symptoms, such as pain, bloating and diarrhea, all of which can lead to weight loss. Repeated exposures to gluten eventually damage the intestine enough to compromise nutrient absorption, further contributing to weight loss.

A simple blood test done by a primary care physician can screen for celiac disease, but the diagnosis is confirmed by a small bowel biopsy done by a gastroenterologist. There's no cure, but adhering to a strict gluten-free diet should bring relief and halt excessive weight loss.

***Caution:*** There are many foods you would be surprised to learn contain gluten—these can include soups, potato chips, granola bars, rice mixes and salad dressings. Gluten can also be found in some supplements, medications and personal-care products like lip balm. Be sure to check food, drug and product labels.

***Best:*** Opt for naturally gluten-free whole foods such as produce, fish, chicken, nuts, beans, dairy and certified gluten-free whole grains such as brown rice, buckwheat and quinoa. For more on gluten-free foods, consult the Celiac Disease Foundation, Celiac.org.

• **Inflammatory bowel disease (IBD) includes Crohn's disease,** which affects the entire GI tract… and ulcerative colitis, which is limited to the colon. Symptoms can include abdominal pain, diarrhea (which may have blood in it), fatigue, low-grade fever and weight loss. If you have any of these symptoms, it's useful to keep a detailed diet journal (record food/drinks you consume and the symptoms you experience), which will help with diagnosis and symptom relief.

The cause of IBD is not known, but there seems to be a genetic, dietary and stress component. It is diagnosed definitively by a colonoscopy, usually done by a gastroenterologist. Treatment for IBD includes various medications to reduce inflammation and suppress the immune system…stress management…avoiding certain medications, such as nonsteroidal anti-inflammatory drugs, which can irritate the bowel, and antibiotics, which can alter bacteria in the colon…and forgoing foods that you have linked to flare-ups while keeping a journal.

## Hyperthyroidism

If unintentional weight loss is accompanied by nervousness, irritability, sleep problems, racing heart, increased perspiration and/or frequent bowel movements (but not diarrhea), hyperthyroidism (overactive thyroid) could be the cause.

Thyroid hormones regulate your metabolism—too little can result in weight gain…too much in weight loss. The more severe the hyperthyroidism, the more extreme the weight loss. A primary care physician can diagnose hyperthyroidism by checking for an enlarged thyroid gland, a rapid pulse and trembling hands. Lab tests to measure the amount of thyroid hormones in your blood will help confirm a diagnosis—a combination of high T3 and T4 thyroid hormones plus low thyroid stimulating hormone (TSH) is common in hyperthyroidism.

An endocrinologist will map out a treatment plan, which may include medication, surgery and/or radioactive iodine to damage or destroy thyroid hormone–producing cells. In most cases, any weight that was shed will be regained once thyroid levels normalize.

## Cancer

Unexplained weight loss might be the first sign of cancer, particularly cancers of the pancreas, stomach, esophagus or lung. The reasons for weight loss due to cancer include changes in metabolism, depression (see below) and reduced appetite.

Treatment works best when cancer is found early, so don't hesitate to make an appointment with your doctor to discuss concerns, especially if you're also experiencing nausea or loss of appetite (frequent symptoms of lung, stomach or ovarian cancer)…shortness of breath or coughing up blood (lung cancer)…fatigue (leukemia)…pain (bone or testicular cancer)…or night sweats (lymphoma). Your doctor will most likely order blood tests and conduct appropriate cancer screening, then refer you to an oncologist if needed.

## Depression

Nearly one in 10 Americans is battling depression at any given time. Symptoms of depression can include feeling sad, worthless or guilty…loss of interest in activities you usually enjoy…difficulty concentrating…sleep disturbances…and, yes, unexplained weight loss.

***Why:*** The loss of energy and interest in life commonly associated with depression can severely weaken one's appetite (however, some people overeat when depressed) and also cause someone to lose enjoyment in cooking or exercising.

A primary care physician can screen for depression and develop a treatment plan, which may include medication and/or a referral to a mental health professional for therapy. People with depression-related weight loss also can improve mood and appetite with regular exercise and better eating and sleep habits.

## Other Causes

Widows sometimes find themselves suddenly responsible for single meals after decades of cooking for their spouses. As a result, they skip meals or don't take in enough calories. In this case, a nutritionist can help by offering advice on meal choices and preparation. Widowed individuals can also be depressed and lose weight as a result (see above).

A loss of smell (due to nasal polyps, Alzheimer's disease, advanced age or certain medications, such as many blood pressure and thyroid drugs) can cause appetite loss and unintentional weight loss, too. An otolaryngologist can identify and treat a smell disorder by changing a drug, lowering a dosage or removing nasal polyps, for example.

# Cooking Tricks for Much Healthier Foods

Lisa R. Young, PhD, RD, a nutritionist in private practice and an adjunct professor in the department of nutrition and food studies at New York University in New York City. She is author of *The Portion Teller Plan: The No-Diet Reality Guide to Eating, Cheating, and Losing Weight Permanently.*

Loading up your grocery cart with fruits and vegetables is a great start to a healthful diet. But even if you hit the produce section on a regular basis, chances are you're not getting the same level of nutrients in your fruits and vegetables that earlier generations did.

Modern agricultural methods have stripped soil of important nutrients, so produce that is eaten today may be less healthful than it used to be.*

***Troubling findings:*** A study published in the *Journal of the American College of Nutrition* found "reliable declines" in the amount of key vitamins and minerals in 43 fruits and vegetables compared with nutrient levels of those foods in 1950.

Other research has found that the levels of calcium in 12 fresh veggies dropped, on average, by 27%...iron by 37%...and vitamin C by 30% over a 22-year period. Such changes in nutrient values can have a hidden danger by contributing to nutrition deficiencies, which are more common than one might imagine finding in the US.

For these reasons, it's crucial for you to do everything you can to squeeze all of the available nutrition from your foods. Besides stocking up on fruits and veggies, studies have shown that how you store, prepare and cook foods—and even how you combine them—can make a difference. *Six tricks that will help you get the greatest nutrition from your foods...*

• **Make steaming your first choice.** Vegetables are good for you no matter how they're prepared. But to get the most nutrients, steaming is the best choice.

***Scientific evidence:*** Steamed broccoli retained virtually all the tested antioxidants in a study published in the *Journal of the Science of Food and Agriculture*, while microwaved broccoli lost 74% to 97% of these disease-fighting nutrients—possibly because microwaves can generate higher temperatures than other cooking methods.

Boiling is also problematic. The liquid—combined with the high heat and lengthy cooking time—strips out significant levels of important nutrients.

***Example:*** Broccoli that's been boiled loses large amounts of glucosinolate, a

*Organic fruits and vegetables may have more nutrients than those that are conventionally grown.

compound that's been linked to cancer prevention.

***Helpful:*** The liquid does retain nutrients, so consider using it in a soup.

***A caveat:*** If you simply don't have time to steam your veggies and, as a result, risk not eating them, microwaving can be an acceptable option—if you add only a teaspoon or so of water and cook for the shortest time possible to retain nutrients.

Even though microwaving has been found to remove certain nutrients, it can be one of the best ways to preserve vitamin C and other water-soluble nutrients because the cooking times tend to be shorter. Other methods, such as sautéing and roasting, retain nutrients if you don't cook vegetables at high temperatures or for too long.

• **Cooked beats fresh.** Fresh, minimally processed foods should usually be your first choice—but not with tomatoes. Cooked tomatoes or canned tomato sauce or paste (best in a BPA-free can or glass jar) provides more lycopene than fresh tomatoes. Lycopene is a well-studied antioxidant that's been linked to reduced risk for prostate and other cancers, along with reduced risk for stroke.

***Scientific evidence:*** A study in *The American Journal of Clinical Nutrition* found that the lycopene in tomato paste has 2.5 times the bioavailability of the lycopene in fresh tomatoes.

***Why:*** The heat used during processing breaks down cell walls and releases more of the compound. Also, the oils that are added to processed tomatoes make it easier for the body to absorb lycopene.

• **Cook first, chop later.** Many people chop their veggies first, then add them to dishes before they go on the stove or into the oven.

***Smart idea:*** Chop most veggies after you've done the cooking.

***Here's why:*** Vitamin C and other nutrients oxidize when they're exposed to air for an extended period of time. An oxidized vitamin loses some of its bioactivity. In addition, chopped or diced vegetables have a greater surface area than whole ones, which allows more nutrients to leach into cooking liquids.

***Exception:*** Onions and garlic should be chopped first (see below.)

***Scientific evidence:*** A recent study found that carrots, chopped before cooking, had 25% less falcarinol, a natural anticancer compound, than cooked whole carrots.

• **Try lemon (or lime) to boost iron levels.** Iron deficiency is among the most common nutrition deficiencies in the US, particularly among women of childbearing age. Meats are high in iron, but women with heavy periods might need more.

Low iron can also be a problem for vegetarians/vegans. That's because the non-heme iron in plant foods isn't as readily absorbed as the heme iron in meats.

***Helpful:*** Add a little vitamin C–rich lemon or lime juice to recipes. Research shows that vitamin C can boost the absorption of nonheme iron by fourfold.

• **Add a spoonful of fat.** A garden-fresh salad or a plate of steamed broccoli is undoubtedly healthy. But for an even greater nutrient boost, add a teaspoon of olive oil.

You need fat to absorb vitamin E, beta-carotene, vitamin A and other fat-soluble nutrients/antioxidants. The average meal contains more than enough fat to get the job done, but simpler, fat-free meals won't provide that extra boost.

***My advice:*** Add a little bit of olive oil to dishes...or dress up fat-free dishes with ingredients that contain healthy fats, such as nuts, olives, feta cheese or a hard-boiled egg.

• **Chop garlic, and let it sit.** Many people love the robust flavor of whole garlic cloves that are roasted to buttery smoothness. But you'll get more health benefits from garlic that's been chopped.

Garlic (as well as onions) contains alliin and other sulfur-containing compounds that are locked within cell walls. The cells rupture when these foods are minced or chopped (or well-chewed), which releases enzymes that transform alliin into allicin, a compound with cardiovascular and anticancer benefits.

***Good rule of thumb:*** Chopping and letting garlic or onions sit for about 10 minutes will allow the enzyme to make the healthful conversion. Heating garlic or onions before the completion of the enzymatic reaction will reduce the health benefits.

## Get Some Cauliflower Power!

Janet Bond Brill, PhD, RDN, FAND, a registered dietitian nutritionist, a fellow of the Academy of Nutrition and Dietetics and a nationally recognized nutrition, health and fitness expert who specializes in cardiovascular disease prevention. Based in Allentown, Pennsylvania, Dr. Brill is author of *Blood Pressure DOWN, Cholesterol DOWN* and *Prevent a Second Heart Attack*. DrJanet.com

Cauliflower is one of my all-time favorite vegetables. Once revered by the French king Louis XIV, this royal vegetable should be a frequent addition to everyone's plate for better health and weight control.

***Here's why:*** Cauliflower is loaded with nutrition and is a powerful cancer-fighting vegetable that tastes great and is ridiculously low in calories. Botanically speaking, cauliflower is a cruciferous vegetable from the Brassicaceae family. It is a rich source of certain "anticancer" phytochemicals, especially a sulfur compound called *isothiocyanate*. Cauliflower is also an excellent source of vitamin K, as well as B vitamins including folate, *pantothenic acid* (vitamin B-5) and *pyridoxine* (vitamin B-6). A single cup will provide you with a healthy dose of fiber, potassium and more than half of your daily quota of vitamin C—and all for just 27 calories!

Cauliflower is available year-round but is best when harvested in winter months. There is also no need to buy organic—cauliflower is one of the few vegetables that has a low pesticide residue due to its thick outer covering. I recommend choosing fresh heads with compact florets that are not bruised. Cauliflower can be stored in the refrigerator for about a week. When you're ready to eat it, remove the tough stem and outer leaves and wash the head well, upside down, rinsing numerous times in a bowl of cold water.

The versatility of recipes in which cauliflower can be used is remarkable. Pizza crust and other baked goodies, soup, fritters, tabouli, mac and cheese, veggie burgers, barbecued cauliflower steaks—the list is an endless universe of deliciousness. *Simple ways to enjoy this nutritional powerhouse...*

- **Pizza crust.** Cooked and mashed cauliflower works well as a pizza crust, but just make sure to cook the cauliflower until it's really soft and tender and then squeeze every last drop of water out so that the mash is completely dry. (Use a stainless steel bowl that fits snugly inside a sieve, and press down on the mash to squeeze out every last drop!) To finish your crust, simply combine with mozzarella cheese, Parmesan, dried oregano, basil, garlic powder, onion powder, salt, pepper and eggs (two per head of cauliflower). Then transfer to a baking sheet, form into a flat circle and bake for 20 minutes at 400°F. After baking the crust, add desired toppings and rebake for 10 minutes.

- **Purée.** Chop the florets and steam the cauliflower. Then place in a blender to form a smooth cauliflower purée. You can use the purée instead of starches to thicken chowders and potato-based soups—a great way to add nutrition and cut the calorie count.

- **Seasoned cauliflower.** One of the simplest ways to cook cauliflower is to just roast it in a hot oven. Preheat the oven to 425°F, toss cauliflower florets with chopped onion and garlic, drizzle with extra-virgin olive oil and season with fresh thyme, salt, pepper and Parmesan cheese. Roast, tossing occasionally, until tender and golden brown—usually 25 to 30 minutes.

***Buffalo-style cauliflower "wings":*** Looking for a light and delicious alternative to greasy, calorie-laden buffalo-style wings? Try buffalo cauliflower "wings"!

***What to do:*** Preheat the oven to 450°F, and line a baking sheet with parchment paper. Coat cauliflower florets with batter (a mixture of flour, seasonings and water or soy milk for moisture). Then roast the florets for 30 minutes (flipping halfway). Dip cooked florets in your favorite buffalo hot sauce, and bake for an additional 20 minutes until the pieces are crispy. Remove from the oven, and serve with a side of light blue-cheese dressing for dipping.

## The Extra-Virgin Olive Oil Hoax

Larry Olmsted, author of *Real Food, Fake Food: Why You Don't Know What You're Eating & What You Can Do About It.* Based in Hartland, Vermont, he also writes the "Great American Bites" column for *USA Today.* RealFoodFakeFood.com

The "extra-virgin olive oil" in your kitchen is probably not extra-virgin at all. To qualify as extra-virgin, olive oil is supposed to be subjected to minimal processing and be made exclusively from fresh, high-quality olives. But a highly publicized research report from the Olive Center at University of California, Davis, found that 69% of the olive oil sold as "extra-virgin" in the US does not meet those standards. The flavor of these fakes typically falls well short of the real thing. Also, a diluted or heavily processed olive oil might not provide the same cancer- and heart disease–fighting benefits of a true extra-virgin olive oil.

Producers get away with selling fake extra-virgin olive oil because the US government does little to enforce olive oil standards...and because most Americans have never tasted a true high-quality, extra-virgin olive oil, which makes it difficult to spot fakes.

***What to do:*** Buy from trustworthy brands, such as California Olive Ranch (from $12.59 for a 500-ml bottle, CaliforniaOliveRanch.com)...Cobram Estate (from $12.99 for a 375-ml bottle, CobramEstate.com)...Whole Foods' 365 Everyday Value brand (from $6.99 for a 500-ml bottle)...and Oro Bailén (often $20 or more for a 500-ml bottle, OroBailen.com).

Or buy from an importer or a distributor of high-quality olive oils, such as Oliviers & Co. (OliviersAndCo.com) and Zingerman's (Zingermans.com). Alternately, you could join the Fresh-Pressed Olive Oil Club and receive three bottles of stellar olive oil four times a year ($99 per quarter for three 250-ml bottles, FreshPressedOliveOil.com).

Other good bets include any US-produced olive oil that has the "COOC" seal of the California Olive Oil Council on its label...or any Italian olive oil that says "100% Qualità Italiana." Extra-virgin olive oil produced in Australia is a reasonable choice, too—Australia enforces the world's strictest extra-virgin olive oil standards.

***Note:*** To read research results from the University of California, Davis, go to OliveCenter.UCDavis.edu and click on "Research" and then "Reports."

## Small Fish—Big Benefits!

Janet Bond Brill, PhD, RDN, FAND, a registered dietitian nutritionist and health and fitness expert who specializes in cardiovascular disease prevention. Dr. Brill is author of *Blood Pressure DOWN, Cholesterol DOWN* and *Prevent a Second Heart Attack.* DrJanet.com

When it comes to fish that people either love or hate, sardines are among the top contenders. Iridescent and tiny, these oily fish within the herring family are oh so flavorful when being enjoyed by their fans! But what if you can't imagine savoring sardines? Well, don't be so quick to swear off this miniature but mighty nutritional powerhouse. Keep reading, and you may just end up with an entirely new appreciation for this budget-friendly, convenient and superbly heart-healthy food.

Fresh sardines are tough to find and are highly perishable, so canned sardines are the go-to option for most people. Because canned sardines generally include the fishes' organs, skin and bones, they are a concentrated source of vitamins and minerals (especially calcium). You may already know that these petite fish are excellent sources of omega-3 fatty acids...are packed with vitamin D...and are rich in protein. But did you realize that one can (3.75 ounces) contains a whopping 1.4 g of heart-healthy omega-3 fat (that's about the same as a serving of sockeye salmon or tuna!) and 23 g of lean protein? Available just about anywhere (even at some gas stations and convenience stores), a can of sardines will cost you a paltry $3.50 or even less on sale.

***And if that's not enough, consider this:*** Sardines are very low in heavy metal contaminants such as mercury—they feed on plankton, ranking them very low on the aquatic food chain.

The only bad news is that sardines from certain areas have been overfished and, as a result, appear on the "Avoid" list at SeafoodWatch.org, created by the Monterey Bay Aquarium, a nonprofit educational group that makes science-based recommendations for seafood sustainability. Since 2007, the Pacific sardine population has plunged by 90%—a decline that is believed to have contributed to the deaths of sea lions and brown pelicans across the West Coast. As a result, federal fishery managers have banned nearly all sardine fishing off the West Coast (as of early 2017). The good news is that you can still purchase sardines that were canned before the ban—the FDA says sardines from an undamaged, properly stored can are safe to eat for up to five years after packing. You can also find sources of approved sardines from areas not affected by overfishing—they are certified by the Marine Stewardship Council (MSC), MSC.org, an international nonprofit organization established to address the problem of unsustainable fishing and safeguard seafood supplies for the future.

When choosing canned sardines, check the package label. Buy the kind packed in water or extra-virgin olive oil (stay away from those packed in other oils or sugary tomato sauce) and look for the MSC certification. On the convenience scale, sardines rate high because they can be served straight out of the can (or mashed with mustard and onions for a quick and delicious spread on crackers). *You can also try my favorite serving suggestions...*

- **Broiled.** Place your drained can of sardines on a baking tin lined with aluminum foil. Season with a drizzle of extra-virgin olive oil and one-half teaspoon of a fresh herb (such as rosemary), a few capers, a fresh garlic clove (minced) and a spritz of fresh lemon juice. Broil for a few minutes and serve.
- **Sardine-lemon-garlic pasta.** Fry one can of sardines (chopped) with two cloves of fresh garlic, juice from half a lemon and one-half cup of bread crumbs in extra-virgin olive oil. Add your own tomato sauce to the pasta bowl along with the sardine mixture, parsley and fresh Parmesan.

## Powdered Eggs as Nutritious as Fresh

Powdered eggs have almost as much protein as the real thing and the same vitamins and minerals. Made from whole eggs using a process called spray drying, powdered eggs have a long shelf life and can stand in for fresh eggs in cooking and baking, although the result could have a different texture. Powdered eggs are also a good substitute for raw eggs, which can cause food poisoning, in recipes such as hollandaise sauce.

***Egg safety:*** All egg products (including powdered eggs) are pasteurized to destroy salmonella. For extra protection, the USDA recommends that egg products be thoroughly cooked (to an internal temperature of 160°F) when served to young children, pregnant women, older adults or those with cancer, diabetes, kidney disease and/or other conditions that weaken the immune system.

Julie Garden-Robinson, PhD, RD, professor of nutrition and food safety, North Dakota State University, Fargo.

# Get a Bigger Health Boost from Dark Chocolate

Michael F. Roizen, MD, chief wellness officer of the Cleveland Clinic and chief medical consultant to *The Dr. Oz Show.* He is author of *This Is Your Do-Over: The 7 Secrets to Losing Weight, Living Longer, and Getting a Second Chance at the Life You Want.*

As chief wellness officer at the Cleveland Clinic, there are two things I do every day to protect my health—I really get my heart pumping...and I eat three small pieces of 72% cacao dark chocolate!

By now, most of you know that dark chocolate offers many health benefits. Enjoying an ounce a day correlates with less depression, better heart health, fewer strokes and reduced rates of system-wide inflammation.

***Latest research findings:*** Dark chocolate even curbs appetite and improves gut health. But which forms of chocolate and which products are the most healthful?

## Cacao or Cocoa?

Lots of people get tripped up when chocolate products are labeled either cacao or cocoa. *What these terms mean...*

Cacao beans are what's used to make chocolate products. These beans are brimming with polyphenols (including flavanols and resveratrol), which act as antioxidants. Polyphenols enhance the production of artery-relaxing nitric oxide, blunt the effects of free radicals and turn on beneficial genes.

Once cacao beans have been fermented, dried and roasted, they're chopped up into cacao nibs (which are like chocolate chips minus the added sugar and fat). Cacao in this form is fairly bitter due to its high concentration of polyphenols, so manufacturers sometimes decrease the polyphenol content. The nibs are then mixed with sugar, milk and other ingredients—milk chocolate has more of these ingredients...dark chocolate has less.

Cacao nibs can also be ground into raw cacao powder, a fiber- and nutrient-rich superfood. Cacao powder often undergoes additional processing to give it a smoother taste, but this processing strips it of much of its nutrients and fiber (this is known as Dutch-processed cocoa).

***Bottom line:*** The higher percentage of cacao beans in a chocolate product and the less processing involved, the higher the polyphenol content. To maximize the health benefits from chocolate, the key is to choose chocolate (nibs, powder or bars) with 70% or more cacao and little or no added sugar.

## Get the Most from Your Daily Chocolate

Simple ways to maximize the health benefits of chocolate...

• **Get a boost by adding apples, walnuts and more.** Like dark chocolate, fruit is also high in polyphenols, so eating the two together is extra-healthful...plus, fruit helps to balance out the bitterness of dark chocolate, so less sugar is needed. I particularly like my chocolate with berries, orange slices or apples.

***Recent finding:*** When paired, apples and dark chocolate are uniquely powerful, having been shown to lower blood pressure and inflammation. Be sure to eat organic apples (to avoid pesticides) and consume the peel of the apple, which contains the most beneficial nutrients.

***Also:*** I often eat a small handful of walnuts with my chocolate to add a dose of heart-healthy omega-3s and protein. In fact, some chocolates come fortified with healthful ingredients such as probiotics, fruit and nuts.

***Worth trying:*** Fantasy Candies Sweet Truth 72% Dark Chocolate Roasted Almond Bark with Probiotics ($7.50 for a four-ounce box). The company also makes cinnamon/chia and cranberry/chia dark chocolate bark.

• **Fun ways to incorporate cacao powder into your diet.** I like adding unsweetened dark cacao powder to spicy tomato sauce and to black beans seasoned with cinnamon and hot sauce.

***Also:*** To make a heart-healthy chocolate mousse, I purée six dates, one-half avocado, four tablespoons of high-quality cacao powder and one to two teaspoons of water. It makes two delicious servings. The dates are a rich source of potassium and other minerals, and the avocado provides omega-3 fatty acids.

***Good Cacao powder products:*** CocoaVia Unsweetened Dark Chocolate Powder, which can be mixed into skim milk, coffee or smoothies or used in the recipes above ($44.99 for 30 packs, each pack contains 375 mg of flavanols)...or Navitas Naturals Cacao Powder ($9.99 for eight ounces).

- **For snacking.** My favorite chocolate for eating by itself is Featherss Dark Chocolate. Each disk is 72% dark chocolate and just 22 calories ($18 for a 52-piece box).

***More great chocolate choices:*** Theo 85% Dark Chocolate Black Rice Quinoa Crunch Bar ($4 for a three-ounce bar)...or Lindt 85% Cocoa Extra Dark Excellence Bar ($3.99 for a 3.5-ounce bar).

# The Truth About Yogurt

Leslie Bonci, RD, CSSD, MPH, owner of the Pittsburgh-based nutrition consulting company Active Eating Advice by Leslie. The former director of sports nutrition for the University of Pittsburgh Medical Center, Bonci is author of numerous books, including *The Active Calorie Diet* and the *American Dietetic Association Guide to Better Digestion*.

Yogurt has long been a favorite of Europeans, but this creamy treat is now a staple in more American households than ever before.

***Trap to watch out for:*** With yogurt's increasing popularity in the US, consumers must now be alert for trumped-up claims about the food's healthfulness.

It's true that researchers are uncovering more and more reasons to consume yogurt. For example, a study recently presented at a meeting of the American Heart Association found that women who consumed five or more servings of yogurt weekly lowered their risk of developing high blood pressure by 20% compared with those who ate one serving of yogurt per month.

But anyone who has shopped for yogurt recently knows that the dairy aisle is chock-full of options ranging from Greek yogurt and "yogurt-style" drinks like kefir to coconut and soy yogurts—and even "desserty" yogurts with candy toppings. So how do you know what to believe about all these products? *Beware of these misconceptions...*

***MISCONCEPTION #1:* Greek yogurt is always healthier than regular yogurt.** Yogurt is produced by the bacterial fermentation of milk (usually cow's milk). Greek yogurt takes it a step further by straining out whey (the watery part of milk) and lactose (milk sugar) so that the result is a thick, creamy texture not unlike sour cream.

For the same amount of calories, most Greek yogurt has about twice the protein of regular yogurt...and less carbohydrates, sugar and sodium. Greek yogurt, however, has more saturated fat than regular yogurt. (For more on saturated fat, see the next page.) With regular yogurt, you also get more bone-strengthening calcium, which is partially lost from Greek yogurt when the whey is strained out.

***Important:*** Even though Greek yogurt's processing leaves it with less sugar to start with, some products still add in generous amounts of sugary flavoring. For example, plain, unsweetened Greek yogurt typically contains about 6 g of sugar per eight-ounce serving—thanks to the remaining naturally occurring lactose sugar. When you see a Greek yogurt with 20 g or 25 g of sugar per serving, that means extra sugar has been added, typically in the form of honey or fruit purée.

***Best bet:*** Buy plain yogurt (Greek or regular), and mix in fresh fruit—you'll get an extra serving of produce without all the sugar of a purée. If you like crunch, sprinkle in some seeds (sunflower and pumpkin work well) or nuts (like pistachios). Check labels for sneaky sugar aliases like "evaporated cane juice," date or coconut sugar and high-fructose corn syrup (HFCS).

***MISCONCEPTION #2:*** **Low-fat yogurt is a better choice than full fat.** A 2015 *American Journal of Clinical Nutrition* study made headlines when researchers found that people who ate the most high-fat dairy products had lower rates of type 2 diabetes.

As it turns out, it's not the amount of fat we consume but the type that's important. Full-fat yogurt is high not only in saturated fat but also in conjugated linoleic acid, which may have a protective effect against type 2 diabetes. Also, the full-fat yogurt's rich, thick mouthfeel sends a message to the brain that says, "I'm satisfied. I don't need to keep eating." Once in the stomach, the fat takes time to digest and, as a result, you feel full longer.

So feel free to include a daily serving of full-fat yogurt, but balance it by cutting back on other forms of saturated fat, such as fried foods, meat, eggs and/or butter.

***MISCONCEPTION #3:*** **Yogurt has the most probiotics of all dairy.** Probiotics are "friendly" bacteria that can enhance digestion, relieve constipation and bloating and even improve immune functioning.

While yogurt usually contains a few strains of probiotics, kefir, which is similar to yogurt but drinkable and more tart, offers far more. In fact, some kefir products contain 10 to 12 strains of probiotics! Don't ditch your yogurt entirely, but go ahead and switch things up with some kefir. Try it in a smoothie, swirled in oatmeal or in hummus recipes.

***MISCONCEPTION #4:*** **People with lactose intolerance should avoid yogurt.** The good bacteria in both Greek and traditional yogurt actually predigest some of the lactose in dairy products, lessening the odds of troubling symptoms such as gas, bloating and diarrhea. (Greek yogurt is especially low in lactose due to the straining process.)

In fact, research suggests that these bacteria are so potent that the enhanced lactose digestion may last for weeks following regular consumption. However, the bacteria must be alive for this to happen, so be sure to select products with the words "live and active cultures" on the label.

***Helpful:*** Start out eating only a couple of tablespoons and watch for gastrointestinal symptoms. If there are none, slowly increase your intake over a period of days.

If you still cannot tolerate dairy, there are non-milk-based yogurts, such as soy and coconut. But be aware that they don't have nearly as much protein as Greek yogurt and can be high in sugar (natural and/or added).

Coconut yogurt, with about 4 g of saturated fat per one-half cup, contains fats called medium-chain triglycerides—research suggests that the body may prefer to use these fats for energy versus storing them as fat.

***MISCONCEPTION #5:*** **Yogurt is just a breakfast food.** With the right mix-ins, yogurt (Greek or regular) is a delicious treat any time of day.

***To use plain yogurt:*** Make a higher-protein version of Brie or Rondelé cheese by emptying a large container of unflavored Greek yogurt into a strainer lined with a coffee filter and set over a bowl. Let it drain, refrigerate overnight, mix peppercorns and chives into the resulting yogurt "cheese" and use it as a spread with whole-grain crackers and crudités...or as a higher-protein cream cheese substitute.

Plain (regular) yogurt has a runnier consistency—use it to lighten up mac and cheese, mashed potatoes or your favorite stroganoff recipe (just cut back a bit on the milk, butter and cream, respectively).

For an indulgent-feeling, lower-calorie dessert, top one-half cup of full-fat vanilla Greek yogurt with one-quarter cup of chopped strawberries and a drizzle of chocolate balsamic vinegar. At just 130 calories and 11 g of sugar, this is a refreshing treat with an intense, not-too-sweet flavor.

---

## Sweet Potato—A Real Superfood

Janet Bond Brill, PhD, RDN, FAND, a registered dietitian nutritionist and health and fitness expert who specializes in cardiovascular disease prevention. Dr. Brill is author of *Blood Pressure DOWN, Cholesterol DOWN* and *Prevent a Second Heart Attack.* DrJanet.com

"Don't judge a book by its cover." This well-worn aphorism certainly applies to veggies...especially the sweet potato. This starchy root vegetable is, to be honest, not the most attractive food—with its odd shape, imperfect skin and dusting of dirt. But don't let the appearance stop you from incorporating it into your meals. Chock-full of vital nutrients, including vitamin A, vitamin C, beta-carotene, potassium, folate, fiber, B vitamins and manganese, the sweet potato is one of the healthiest complex carbs around.

Sweet potato or yam? Before we get too far along, let's clear up this confusion about sweet potatoes versus yams.

***Here's the truth:*** Even though they're both tuberous root veggies, a yam is not even botanically related to a sweet potato! Real yams are typically imported from the Caribbean and generally sold only in international food markets in the US. A true yam, which has white interior flesh, is starchier and drier and not nearly as tasty as a sweet potato. It's worth noting, though, that the veggies that are often mislabeled as yams are actually soft sweet potatoes. With their copper-colored skin and orangey flesh, this variety becomes fluffy and moist when cooked. So opt for this one if you want to bake it—and especially if you're looking for that classic roasted sweet potato with the crispy skin and sweet, orange flesh.

Sweet potatoes come in purple, too. Did you know that there's a variety of purple potato that is actually a sweet potato, too? Available commercially in the US for about 10 years now, it is packed with even more antioxidants than its orange cousin. The purple hue is a giveaway that this variety is filled with anthocyanins—the same phytochemicals found in blueberries—which are powerful antioxidant and anti-inflammatory compounds that fight such diseases as heart disease and diabetes. For this reason, it's a good idea to splurge on purple potatoes (they usually cost about twice as much as regular sweet potatoes) whenever possible in lieu of the less nutritious white-fleshed varieties. No matter what type of sweet potato you choose, it's fun to add them to your diet in new ways.

***My favorite spud ideas:*** Cube potatoes, roast them and add to salads or even mac and cheese...bake, scoop out the insides and add to baked goods such muffins or pancake mix. *Or try my sweet potato hummus recipe...*

### Sweet Potato Hummus

Change up your basic hummus by making it sweet...or spicy, depending on your taste preference. *Ingredients...*

1 medium sweet potato, washed

1 15-ounce can of garbanzo beans, rinsed, drained

2 Tablespoons of extra-virgin olive oil

1 Tablespoon of tahini (optional)

*Sweet spices:* 1 teaspoon of cinnamon and 1 teaspoon of pumpkin spice

*Spicy spices:* ½ teaspoon of cayenne pepper, ½ teaspoon of paprika and 1 teaspoon of cumin

***Instructions:*** Preheat oven to 400°F. With a fork, poke holes in the sweet potato all over (both sides). Place the sweet potato on a baking sheet and bake for 45 to 60 minutes (until you can squeeze it). Once cooked, remove the skin and chop the potato into pieces. Add the chopped sweet potato and the other hummus ingredients into a blender, and mix until it makes a smooth consistency with no visible pieces of sweet potato. Add either sweet or spicy spices. Taste and add more spices, if needed.

### Just a Few Nuts a Day...

Just a few nuts a day may lower disease risk. In a review of studies, people who ate nuts had a 29% lower risk for coronary heart disease...21% reduced risk for cardiovascular disease...and 15% lower risk for cancer. Nut eaters also had a 52% lower risk for respiratory disease...39% lower risk for diabetes... and 75% reduced risk for infectious disease. Most risk reduction for all diseases occurred in people who ate just one ounce of nuts per day—about two dozen almonds or 15 pecan halves.

Review of data from 20 prospective studies led by researchers at Imperial College London, UK, and Harvard T.H. Chan School of Public Health, Boston, published in *BMC Medicine*.

## Seeds: The Forgotten Superfood

Janet Bond Brill, PhD, RDN, FAND, a registered dietitian nutritionist and health and fitness expert who specializes in cardiovascular disease prevention. Dr. Brill is author of *Blood Pressure DOWN, Cholesterol DOWN* and *Prevent a Second Heart Attack*. DrJanet.com

When we think of those ultra-healthy foods known as "superfoods," seeds are one of the least talked about. That's a shame because they are among the most nutrient-rich foods you can consume. But with literally dozens of health-promoting seeds to choose from, does it really matter which ones you add to your diet?

Well, yes. When it comes to research supporting health benefits, two of the heaviest hitters are chia seeds and flaxseeds. Both are spectacularly heart-healthy. But in terms of convenience, chia seeds win hands down. These seeds are more stable than flaxseeds, so you don't have to worry about them going rancid. Chia seeds can also be eaten whole or ground, and you'll still get all the health benefits. Flaxseeds, on the other hand, must be ground before the nutrients are released. Chia seeds also win points because they don't need refrigeration, while flaxseeds must be stored in a preferably dark, airtight container in the fridge or freezer so the nutrients aren't destroyed.

Now, for the nitty-gritty nutritional comparison. Here's what you'll get from a serving (one ounce) of chia seeds versus one ounce of ground flaxseeds (the calorie count is roughly the same—138 in chia seeds...and 148 in flaxseeds)...

- **Alpha-linolenic acid (ALA).** Chia seeds and flaxseeds are virtual storehouses of the super-heart-healthy anti-inflammatory omega-3 fat known as ALA. Chia seeds contain 5 g and flaxseeds have 6 g.
- **Fiber.** There's lots of fiber—insoluble and soluble—packed in both of these tiny seeds. Chia seeds edge out flaxseeds—10 g versus 8 g.
- **Protein.** Both seeds contain a respectable amount of vegetable protein (4 g in chia seeds...5 g in flaxseeds). But chia seeds are a "complete" protein because they have all nine of the essential amino acids while flaxseeds do not.
- **Vitamins and minerals.** Both seeds are bursting with vitamins and minerals such as iron, manganese, copper, zinc and niacin, to name just a few. Flaxseeds are higher in folate, magnesium and potassium. But chia seeds, unlike flaxseeds, are a potent source of calcium.
- **Lignans.** When it comes to lignans, a disease-fighting phytochemical, flaxseeds are a much richer source than chia seeds. Lignans may protect against cardiovascular disease and breast and prostate cancers.

Since the nutritional benefits of these two seeds do differ somewhat, how do you choose? To get the best of both worlds nutritionally, I suggest adding both types of seeds to your diet, perhaps alternating days. Both chia seeds and flaxseeds can be sprinkled on yogurt, cereal, oatmeal or salads. Either seed can also be sprinkled on top of one of my favorite snacks—a slice of whole-grain toast topped with peanut butter and banana slices. If you like to bake, replace one-half cup of flour with one-half cup of ground chia seeds or flaxseed meal in muffins, pancake mix or breads. *And for a delicious treat...*

• **Raspberry chia seed pudding.** This festive-looking dessert is perfect for the holidays.

***Ingredients for a single serving:*** One cup of light vanilla soy milk...one-half cup of fresh (or frozen and defrosted) raspberries...one-quarter cup of chia seeds...and mint leaves.

***What to do:*** Mix the raspberries with milk in a blender until smooth. Pour into a mason jar, add chia seeds, cover tightly, give it a good shake and refrigerate overnight. The chia seeds will "gel" to create a pudding-like consistency. (You can add a sweetener of your choice, if desired.) Garnish with mint leaves and enjoy!

## Avocado Pits Are Edible

The pits are packed with antioxidants, monounsaturated fats, vitamin E and plant sterols. Grind the pit in a powerful blender, then add two to three teaspoons of the powder to oatmeal or smoothies.

Ali Miller, registered dietician, quoted in *Prevention.* Prevention.com

## An Insider's Look at the New Food Label

Lisa R. Young, PhD, RD, a nutritionist in private practice and an adjunct professor of nutrition in the department of nutrition, food studies and public health at New York University in New York City. She is author of *The Portion Teller Plan: The No-Diet Reality Guide to Eating, Cheating and Losing Weight Permanently.*

It's hard to believe, but the Nutrition Facts Label—that government-mandated nutritional information box on all food products—only recently got its first overhaul in more than 20 years.

***My take:*** While most of the changes to the Nutrition Facts Label are positive, there are still a few traps that can trip up unsuspecting consumers. *The five most important changes—and what each means for you...**

***CHANGE #1:* More realistic portion sizes.** The updated label will help consumers better understand how many calories they are actually getting in their favorite meals, snacks and beverages.

For example, the current (soon-to-be-outdated) label on a typical 20-ounce bottle of soda might list the calories as 100, but this is misleading because that number represents "calories per serving." Most people consume the full bottle in one sitting, which would technically be 2.5 servings. With the new label, a 20-ounce soda will be listed as a single serving with 250 calories.

***What's good:*** Consumers who mistakenly believed that they were getting fewer calories than what were actually in the food or beverage will now have a much easier time keeping track of their daily calorie intake. This can help with weight control—a crucial factor in minimizing risk for diabetes, heart disease, certain cancers and other chronic illnesses.

***What's still lacking:*** While serving sizes will now more accurately reflect what people are consuming, these amounts are not necessarily what we should be eating. Many people consume supersized portions that are two to five times larger than what they should be, contributing to obesity. I would have loved to have seen a footnote on the new labels clarifying that "the serving size is based upon the amount typically consumed but is not a recommended portion size."

***CHANGE #2:* A new listing for added sugars.** Food labels have traditionally lumped all sugar together. For example, when you buy vanilla yogurt, you may see "Sugars: 22 g" on the label, but you have no way of knowing how many of those grams are from naturally occurring sugar (such as those found in the milk) and how many were added for flavor. For the first time ever, food manufactur-

*The previous deadline for companies to incorporate these changes into their Nutrition Facts Labels was July 26, 2018. At press, the FDA has granted more time with no final date.

ers will be required to disclose *added* sugars on the Nutrition Facts Label. This includes sugars from syrups and honey, as well as white sugar. It does not include 100% fruit or vegetable juice concentrate or some sugars found in jams, jellies, preserves and other fruit spreads.

***What's good:*** On average, Americans get about 13% of their total calories from added sugars—think sugary beverages such as soft drinks and juice...and processed cookies and candy. These sugars provide nothing but "empty" calories with no nutritional benefit.

However, naturally occurring sugars in, say, fruit and milk aren't empty because they are found in foods and beverages that also boast beneficial nutrients such as fiber, calcium, vitamins and minerals.

For optimal health, the FDA advises keeping added sugar to no more than 10% of your total daily calories (50 g of added sugar, based on a 2,000-calorie intake, or less).

***What's still lacking:*** I would have liked to have seen the FDA switch from grams to teaspoons. The latter is a more consumer-friendly measurement (most Americans are unfamiliar with the metric system)...plus, teaspoons are easier to visualize. So if you're advised to limit your added sugar intake to 12 teaspoons (which equals 50 g), that seems much more concrete.

*CHANGE #3:* **New listings for vitamins.** Labels will no longer be required to include amounts of vitamins A and C. They must, however, begin displaying amounts of vitamin D and potassium.

***What's good:*** This change was enacted in response to the growing percentage of Americans who are deficient in vitamin D and potassium. About 40% are deficient in vitamin D, and hardly anyone consumes enough potassium-rich foods. People who don't get enough vitamin D have been shown to be at increased risk for osteoporosis, while those who aren't consuming enough potassium are more likely to develop high blood pressure.

As for vitamins A and C, deficiencies are now rare, but manufacturers can still list these vitamins voluntarily.

***What's still lacking:*** I don't believe that including vitamin D on food labels will prevent deficiencies. Vitamin D deficiency is common, in part, because this vitamin is found in few foods—except for salmon and fortified milk, for example.

The new labeling may also lead to unnecessary fortification as companies race to add the nutrient to foods in an effort to make them appear healthier. As a result, people taking vitamin D supplements may have trouble regulating their actual vitamin D intake, because few of us eat the same packaged foods every day.

*CHANGE #4:* **No more "Calories from Fat."** The scientific community now agrees that the type of fat you consume matters more than the amount. That's why "Calories from Fat" will disappear.

***What's good:*** Fat was vilified for so long that people continue to be frightened off by labels that display higher "Calories from Fat"—even if it appears on such nutritional powerhouses as walnuts and olive oil, which contain mainly the unsaturated, heart-healthy kind of fat.

***Beware:*** Food labels can say a product has "0 g" of trans fats—unhealthy, artificial fats added to processed foods—as long as it contains less than 0.5 g per serving. If you consume more than one serving, you may be getting an appreciable amount of trans fats.

As most people now know, we should try to avoid all trans fats. These fats—commonly found in crackers, various baked foods, fried foods, etc.—increase risk for heart disease and stroke. To determine whether trans fats are included in a product, check the ingredients list for "partially hydrogenated oils," the most common alias for trans fats.

*CHANGE #5:* **A bigger, bolder typeface.** Tired of fumbling with your glasses (or even a magnifying glass) to read the food label? If so, this change should please you.

The calories, serving size and number of servings per container will now be printed in a larger, bolder typeface, so you'll be able to see these crucial items more easily.

## Mediterranean Diet Wins for Breast Health

Women who followed a Mediterranean diet had 68% lower risk for breast cancer than women who did not follow the diet—but whether the diet actually can prevent the disease is not yet clear. The number of people who developed cancer during the study was too small to make definitive comparisons. More research is necessary to clarify any possible link.

***In the meantime:*** Many physicians recommend the Mediterranean diet—which is low in animal fats and rich in fruits, vegetables and olive oil—for its proven heart benefits.

Susan Love, MD, chief visionary officer at Dr. Susan Love Research Foundation, Encino, California, clinical professor of surgery, UCLA's David Geffen School of Medicine, Los Angeles, and author of *Dr. Susan Love's Breast Book*.

## We Do Not Have Healthy Diets

Seventy-five percent of Americans say they eat healthfully—even though they don't. That is the percentage that rated their diets good, very good or excellent.

***But:*** More than 80% of Americans don't eat the recommended amount of fruits and vegetables.

Survey by NPR and Truven Health Analytics of 3,000 US adults, reported at NPR.org.

## How to Get Discount Coupons for Fresh Produce

SavingStar.com/coupons is free to join and gives cash back for items bought at major grocery chains. Earthbound Farm (EBFarm.com) offers recipes and coupons when you sign up for the Organic Bound guide. Fresh Express.com offers coupons if you sign up for the company's newsletter. Target occasionally offers produce coupons, especially through its mobile Cartwheel app, Cartwheel.Target.com (*recent example:* 25% off all produce). Organic Girl (ILoveOrganicGirl.com) offers coupons and promotions when you join its e-mail list.

MoneyTalksNews.com

## Hurrah! High-Fat Cheese Can Be Good for You

High-fat cheese may be as good for you as the low-fat type, when eaten in moderation. In a 12-week study, people who ate three ounces a day of cheese with 25% to 32% fat content had the same blood-chemistry picture—including cholesterol and triglyceride levels—as people who ate three ounces a day of cheese with 13% to 16% fat. And there were no significant differences in body weight change between the groups.

Study of 139 people by researchers at University of Copenhagen, Denmark, published in *The American Journal of Clinical Nutrition*.

## Super-Broth for Super-Health

Sally Fallon Morell, founding president of The Weston A. Price Foundation, which champions nourishing, traditional foods such as bone broths. She is author of the best-selling *Nourishing Traditions* and coauthor of *Eat Fat Lose Fat, The Nourishing Traditions Book of Baby & Child Care* and, most recently, *Nourishing Broth: An Old-Fashioned Remedy for the Modern World*. NourishingTraditions.com

Before the 20th century, almost all soups and stews were made with a stock of bone broth—bones and other animal parts slowly simmered in a cauldron or stockpot, producing a nutrient-rich concoction.

Fast-forward to the 21st century, when food processing has largely replaced home cooking. Today's processed "broth" often is nothing more than a powder or cube dissolved in water and spiked with additives such as MSG that mimic the taste of broth.

The loss of bone broth is a big loss.

***What most people don't realize:*** Traditional bone broth delivers unique, health-giving components that can be hard to find anywhere else in the diet. And a brothless diet may be hurting your health—contributing to arthritis, nagging injuries, indigestion and premature aging.

***Good news:*** Bone broth is simple to make or buy (see next page). The optimal "dose" is one cup daily. If you are trying to heal, increase this to two cups.

## Super-Healthy Ingredients

Bone broth, whether it's made from the bones of a chicken, cow, lamb, pig or the like, is extraordinarily rich in the following...

- **Collagen.** The number-one health-giving component of bone broth is melted collagen, or gelatin. Collagen is the most abundant protein in the body, providing strength and structure to tissue. In fact, microscopic cables of collagen literally hold your body together—in joints, tendons, ligaments, muscles, skin and membranes around internal organs.

Your body makes its own collagen, of course. But it becomes harder for your body to make it as you age, leading to arthritis, wrinkled skin and other degenerative conditions.

- **Glucosamine and chondroitin sulfate.** These two nutrients are well-known for helping to ease arthritis pain—and bone broth supplies ample amounts of both.

Glucosamine is created from glucose (sugar) and glutamine (an amino acid, a building block of protein). It's found in cartilage, the part of the joint that provides cushioning and lubrication between bones.

Chondroitin sulfate is a proteoglycan, a type of molecule that helps hydrate cells. It also supplies sulfur, a mineral that nourishes cartilage and balances blood sugar.

- **Glycine.** This amino acid supports the health of blood cells, generates cellular energy, aids in the digestion of fats, speeds wound healing and helps the body rid itself of toxins, such as mercury, lead, cadmium and pesticides. Glycine also regulates dopamine levels, thereby easing anxiety, depression and irritability and improving sleep and memory.

- **Glutamine.** This amino acid nourishes the lining of the gut, aiding the absorption of nutrients. It boosts the strength of the immune system. It helps the body recover from injuries such as burns, wounds and surgery. It also strengthens the liver, helping the body process and expel toxins. And glutamine boosts metabolism and cuts cravings for sugar and carbohydrates, aiding weight loss.

## Feel-Better Broth

Bone broth delivers extra-high levels of all those health-giving compounds, so it's not surprising that it can help prevent and heal many health problems, including...

- **Arthritis and joint pain.** By supplying collagen, glucosamine, chondroitin and other cartilage-nourishing factors, bone broth can repair and rebuild cartilage, preventing osteoarthritis or easing arthritis pain. In fact, bone broth might be the best food for osteoarthritis, which affects more than 30 million Americans.

***Compelling research:*** In a review of seven studies on osteoarthritis and melted collagen (collagen hydrolysate), researchers at University of Illinois College of Medicine in Chicago found that ingesting the compound helped create new cartilage, thus lessening pain and improving everyday functioning.

- **Digestive problems.** In the 19th century, broth and gelatin were widely prescribed—by Florence Nightingale and many others—for convalescents who lacked the strength to digest and assimilate food properly.

Sadly, nutritional therapy for digestive problems went out of fashion after World War II, replaced by pharmaceuticals.

***Example:*** A form of gelatin (gelatin tannate, or Tasectan) is being used as a digestive drug, with studies showing that it can help heal gastroenteritis (stomach and intestinal irritation). The new drug is being hailed as a "gut barrier protector"—but wouldn't it be better to prevent digestive diseases by strengthening your gut with bone broth?

- **Injuries and wounds.** The components in bone broth are crucial for healing broken bones, muscle injuries, burns and wounds—a key benefit for seniors, whose injuries can take longer to heal.

The use of cartilage (a main component of bone broth) for wound healing was championed by John F. Prudden, MD, whose published papers include "The Clinical Acceleration of Healing with a Cartilage Preparation," in the May 3, 1965, issue of *JAMA*. In his research, Dr. Prudden showed that cow cartilage could speed wound healing, produce stronger healing that was less likely to be reinjured and produce smoother, flatter and more natural-looking scars.

More recently, studies have shown that bone broth ingredients—particularly glycine and other amino acids—are uniquely effective at healing wounds, including hard-to-heal diabetic foot ulcers.

- **Infections.** Chicken soup—"Jewish penicillin"—is a classic home remedy for a cold, flu, pneumonia and other infectious diseases. Over the years, researchers studying broth and its components have noted their ability to strengthen immune cells, fight off viruses and calm down the overactive immune system caused by autoimmune diseases such as rheumatoid arthritis, Crohn's disease and psoriasis.

## How to Make Bone Broth (or Buy It)

Making a very healthful and delicious bone broth may seem daunting—but it's not. Here's a simple way to make a chicken bone broth. You can use the same method for any kind of animal bones. Beef bones (such as rib bones, short ribs and beef shanks) should be browned first in the oven for the best flavor.

***How to prepare bone broth:*** Whenever you eat chicken, save the bones. You can save skin and meat, too—the skin is rich in collagen, and there is some collagen in the meat. Just put all these leftovers in a zipper freezer bag, and store in the freezer until you have enough to fill a standard six-to-seven-quart slow cooker, about six to eight cups. Add a splash of vinegar and one sliced onion. Fill up the slow cooker with filtered water.

Slow-cook on low overnight. (If you don't have a slow cooker, you can make the broth by simmering it all day in a stock pot.)

In the morning, ladle the broth through a strainer and put the broth in the refrigerator. Fill up the slow cooker with water, and cook the bones again overnight, producing a second batch. As with the first batch, ladle the broth through a strainer. You now have about one gallon of chicken broth, which you can refrigerate or freeze.

***What to look for:*** A sign that your broth is rich in collagen is that it gels when chilled. To get a good gel, it is helpful to add chicken feet or a pig's foot to the bone mix.

You can use your broth as a basic ingredient in soups, stews, sauces and gravies. Or just add a little salt, heat it and drink it in a mug.

***Try this simple Thai soup:*** Two cups of chicken broth with one can of coconut milk, the juice of one lime and a pinch of red pepper flakes.

If you want to purchase healthful bone broth, good sources include Bare Bones Broth Company (BareBonesBroth.com), Osso Good (OssoGoodBones.com), Stock Options (StockOptionsOnline.com) and the Brothery (BoneBroth.com). These broths are available by mail order, but you may be able to find them in some gourmet and specialty shops.

# New Dangers for Supplement Users

Mark A. Moyad, MD, MPH, the Jenkins/Pokempner director of complementary and alternative medicine at the University of Michigan Medical Center, department of urology, in Ann Arbor. He is the primary author of more than 150 medical journal articles and author, with Janet Lee, of *The Supplement Handbook*.

By now, you know that the supplements you pop to stay healthy may turn harmful if you also take certain prescription and/or over-the-counter medications.

***What you may not realize:*** Scientists are still uncovering what the interactions are—and just how dangerous they can be. *What you need to know to stay safe...*

## The Latest Findings

When researchers at the University of Minnesota recently looked at data from more than 23 million scientific studies, they identified thousands of potential drug–supplement interactions—including some that have only recently been recognized.*

***The danger zone:*** Some supplements increase drug levels by slowing their breakdown in the body. Some accelerate drug metabolism/breakdown and reduce the desired effects.

***Other interactions are additive:*** Drugs and supplements can act on similar pathways in the body and increase the overall effects—and the risk for side effects.

## Particularly Risky

In the meta-analysis mentioned above, researchers discovered that echinacea, a popular herbal remedy for colds and other infections, reduced the activity of *exemestane* (Aromasin), a drug used for breast cancer. In fact, echinacea interferes with a number of chemotherapy drugs, including cyclophosphamide and fluorouracil. *Other drug–supplement interactions...*

- **Iodine.** Most Americans get enough iodine from salt, seafood, whole grains and other foods. But some people take supplements because they believe that extra iodine will improve thyroid health. The truth is, the supplement only helps if there's a true iodine deficiency.

***Serious interaction:*** *Levothyroxine* (Synthroid and Levoxyl), a synthetic form of thyroid hormone that treats low thyroid (hypothyroidism). High doses of supplemental iodine—300 micrograms (mcg) or more—can interfere with thyroid function. When this happens, a dose of levothyroxine that was previously effective can suddenly stop working.

***My advice:*** Do not take supplemental iodine unless you have been shown (via urine or blood tests) to be deficient, and your doctor approves it. Supplements often contain 500 mcg to 1,000 mcg of iodine—far more than the recommended daily allowance of 150 mcg.

***Helpful:*** Be cautious when taking any supplement that's dosed in micrograms. Anything that's measured in millionths of a gram requires careful minimal dosing.

- **Fish oil.** It has a number of proven benefits—lowering very high triglycerides (500 mg/dL and above)...improving pain from rheumatoid arthritis...slowing the progression of lupus...and even easing mild-to-moderate depression.

***Serious interactions:*** All blood thinners—including not only the popular prescription blood thinner *warfarin* and newer blood thinners, such as Eliquis and Xarelto, but also over-the-counter drugs with blood-thinning effects, including nonsteroidal anti-inflammatory drugs (NSAIDs) such as aspirin and *ibuprofen* (Motrin).

Fish oil has a blood-thinning effect because it inhibits the ability of platelets to stick together and form clots. This can be beneficial since blood clots in the arteries are the main cause of heart attacks. But combining

*To search for drug–supplement interactions, go to the National Library of Medicine's website NLM.nih.gov/medlineplus/druginfo...or the fee-based Natural Medicines Comprehensive Database, NaturalDatabase.com.

fish oil with other blood thinners can cause excess bleeding during surgery or dental procedures...or from wounds or internal injuries (such as ulcers).

***My advice:*** Ask your doctor if you can take fish oil along with your usual blood thinner. The blood-thinning effects of fish oil are dose-dependent—you're less likely to have problems at typical doses of, say, 2,000 mg or less daily.

***Don't make this mistake:*** If you're taking fish oil for high cholesterol, stop. A lot of my patients have been told that it lowers LDL "bad" cholesterol. Not true. At doses of 1,000 mg or more, it can actually raise LDL five to 10 points or more.

- **GABA (gamma-aminobutyric acid).** It's a neurotransmitter that's present in the brain and other parts of the body. In supplement form, it has a calming effect and is thought to lower cortisol, the body's main stress hormone.

***Serious interactions:*** Sedative drugs, including opioids (such as codeine) and antianxiety medications, such as *lorazepam* (Ativan) or *alprazolam* (Xanax). Taking these drugs with GABA can cause excessive sedation.

***My advice:*** Never combine sedatives—whether they're "natural" or pharmaceutical—without checking with your doctor.

- **St. John's wort.** This herbal supplement has been shown to be as effective as prescription antidepressants in treating mild-to-moderate depression—and with fewer side effects.

However, when combined with SSRI (selective serotonin reuptake inhibitor) antidepressants, such as *escitalopram* (Lexapro) or *paroxetine* (Paxil), or other types of antidepressants, the supplement can cause medication-induced serotonin syndrome. This dangerous "overdose" of serotonin, a neurotransmitter that affects mood, can cause swings in blood pressure and heart rate, along with such symptoms as heavy sweating, diarrhea and extreme agitation. But that's not all.

***Serious interactions:*** An increasing body of evidence shows that St. John's wort can interact with many other prescription drugs, including warfarin, *digoxin* and other heart medications, antiseizure drugs, certain cancer drugs and birth control pills. You must let your doctor know if you're taking St. John's wort.

- **L-arginine.** L-arginine increases blood levels of nitric oxide, a naturally occurring molecule that dilates blood vessels and can reduce blood pressure by 20 points or more. Some men take it for erectile dysfunction (ED).

***Serious interactions:*** L-arginine can interact with all prescription blood pressure medications, causing blood pressure to drop to dangerously low levels, resulting in dizziness, blurred vision or even a loss of consciousness. The supplement can also cause dangerous drops in blood pressure in men taking ED medication.

***My advice:*** Always check with your doctor before taking a blood pressure drug or ED medication with L-arginine.

## Heartburn Drug Danger

Long-term use (more than four consecutive weeks) of proton pump inhibitors (PPIs)—drugs such as *esomeprazole* (Nexium) and *omeprazole* (Prilosec), commonly taken for heartburn and gastroesophageal reflux disease (GERD)—speeds up the aging of blood vessels, which may increase risk for heart disease, kidney failure and dementia.

***Why:*** PPIs reduce the acidity needed to clear waste products from blood vessels, making them more susceptible to blockages.

John Cooke, MD, PhD, chair of cardiovascular sciences, Houston Methodist Research Institute.

## Are You Addicted to PPIs?

Jacob Teitelbaum, MD, board-certified internist and nationally known expert in the fields of chronic fatigue syndrome, fibromyalgia, sleep and pain. Based in Kailua-Kona, Hawaii, he is author of numerous books, including *The Fatigue and Fibromyalgia Solution, Pain-Free 1-2-3* and *Real Cause, Real Cure.* Vitality101.com

After reading about the downsides of proton pump inhibitors (PPIs), you may want to stop taking them—immediately. But you may not be able to!

Researchers in Denmark gave *esomeprazole* (Nexium) for two months to 120 people without heartburn. Within two weeks of stopping the drug, 44% of the study participants developed heartburn. In 22%, those symptoms continued for the next four weeks.

Why did healthy people stopping the drug develop heartburn? Because of the phenomenon that the researchers call rebound acid hyper-secretion. It's natural for the stomach to produce stomach acid. If you foil that function and then allow it to resume, it returns with a vengeance, generating huge amounts of stomach acid that cause heartburn.

***Best:*** Try the heartburn remedies below for two months, and then—under your doctor's guidance—start "tapering" your PPI, cutting the dose in half every week (or at the rate your doctor suggests). When you're at the lowest possible dose, switch to Tagamet, which decreases stomach acid without totally turning it off. The Tagamet can be stopped after one month.

### Safer Remedies

Your body produces stomach acid for a reason—to digest your food. Turning off that stomach acid with PPIs can decrease the pain from heartburn. But it doesn't treat the poor digestion that is causing your heartburn. To put it another way...your real problem isn't excess stomach acid—it's indigestion. Below are my recommendations to banish indigestion—you can try any of these remedies or even all of them at the same time if you wish. Continue to take a PPI drug at first while following these recommendations. You also may want to avoid foods that trigger heartburn, including citrus fruits, tomatoes, garlic, onions and chili.

***Important:*** If problems persist after two months, see your doctor.

- **For quick heartburn relief, try bicarbonate of soda (baking soda).** One-half teaspoon of alkaline bicarbonate of soda (baking soda) in four ounces of water can quickly neutralize stomach acid and relieve the pain. Over-the-counter antacids with alkalinizing minerals (calcium combined with magnesium, such as Rolaids) also work—as little as one-quarter tablet can squelch the pain of heartburn. But there is some evidence that long-term use of calcium is associated with increased risk for heart attacks in women.
- **Take digestive enzymes.** One of the primary reasons for indigestion in the US is lack of enzymes in food, which have been removed during processing. I recommend the enzyme-containing supplement Complete GEST from Enzymatic Therapy. Take two capsules with every meal to digest food properly.

***Caution:*** Some people find that digestive enzymes irritate the stomach. If this happens, start with GS-Similase—it's the gentler of the two products. If it causes irritation, don't use it. Instead, use the DGL licorice and mastic gum remedies (see below) until your stomach feels better, usually in a month or two—and then start taking digestive enzymes. The enzymes are used long-term to support healthy digestion.

- **While eating, sip warm liquid rather than cold.** Cold drinks slow and even can stop digestion. Drink warm liquids during meals to aid digestion.
- **Avoid coffee, carbonated beverages, alcohol and aspirin.** All of them can hurt your stomach. Once your stomach has healed, and indigestion and heartburn are a dim memory, you can use them again in limited amounts.

(You'll know you're using too much if indigestion and heartburn return.)

• **Take DGL licorice.** This herb helps resolve the symptoms of heartburn and underlying indigestion. In fact, research shows it's as effective as the H2 blocker *cimetidine* (Tagamet)—but unlike Tagamet, which has been linked to some of the problems caused by PPIs, DGL licorice is good for you. I recommend Advanced DGL by EuroPharm, which doesn't have the licorice taste. Take one capsule twice a day—after one to two months, it can be used as needed.

***Caution:*** You must use the DGL form of licorice. Other forms can cause high blood pressure.

• **Take mastic gum.** This gum (resin) from an evergreen tree is a wonderful remedy for heartburn and indigestion. Take mastic gum in supplement form. I recommend one or two 500-mg capsules twice a day for two months, then as needed.

## Dangerous Combo

Antacids with aspirin may cause bleeding. The side effect is rare—only eight cases have been reported since 2009. But people at risk for stomach or intestinal bleeding should be aware of it. Over-the-counter products such as Alka-Seltzer and Bromo Seltzer contain aspirin. People at bleeding risk include those age 60 or older...with a history of stomach or bleeding problems...who take blood-thinning drugs or medications such as *prednisone*...who take other medicines containing nonsteroidal anti-inflammatory drugs (NSAIDs)...and/or who drink three or more alcoholic drinks per day.

Karen Murry Mahoney, MD, deputy director, division of nonprescription drug products, US Food and Drug Administration, Silver Spring, Maryland.

### Sorry...There's No Room for Chocolate Candy in Weight Loss

Avoid chocolate candy when trying to lose weight. Stop eating it completely—trying to consume only a little typically leads to eating much more than you planned.

***Alternative if you want to consume healthful cocoa:*** Plain, low-fat yogurt mixed with two tablespoons of unsweetened cocoa powder...a drink made with skim milk and unsweetened cocoa powder.

Stephen Gullo, PhD, author of *The Thin Commandments Diet.*

## Go for Gelato

Gelato may be better for you than ice cream. Ice cream has more sugar, fat and calories per ounce than gelato. And because ice cream has a milder flavor and fluffier texture than gelato, it may feel less filling, causing you to eat more of it.

Lauren Slayton, RD, founder, Foodtrainers, New York City, quoted in *Self* magazine.

## Cool Exercise Treat

Having a slushy drink before a hot-weather workout may improve performance, recent research has found.

***Details:*** Runners were given about two cups of either a frozen or room-temperature drink 45 minutes before a 10K event in 82°F weather.

***Results:*** Those who drank the slushy ran an average of 15 seconds faster.

***Possible reason:*** The ice increased body heat storage capacity, which allowed runners to improve running time by avoiding overheating. Eating an ice pop may have a similar effect.

Jason Kai Wei Lee, PhD, head, human performance laboratory, DSO National Laboratories, Singapore.

## Paddleboarding for Fitness

Paddleboarding is great exercise and can be an enjoyable switch from a boring treadmill workout.

Also called stand-up paddling, paddleboarding requires you to stand and balance on a board while paddling on the open water, so the muscles of your core (abdominal) and those of your sides (external obliques) are constantly engaged in helping you to stay erect. Participating in the sport regularly will strengthen the muscles in that region, resulting in better balance and relief from any low-back pain. Cardiovascular benefits are more limited.

***Important:*** Though paddleboarding is a safe, low-impact sport suitable for those of any age, people with shoulder, back or balance issues should approach the sport cautiously to be sure they are not aggravating any existing issues. Wear a life vest and use a leash, which tethers you to the board and keeps it within reach should you fall. Slather on a waterproof sunscreen and wear a brimmed hat and sunglasses to guard against the sun.

Cedric X. Bryant, PhD, chief science officer, American Council on Exercise, San Diego.

## Two Minutes to Health

It's well known that sitting for several hours every day can lead to heart disease, diabetes and early death.

***Recent finding:*** Getting up for just two minutes during every hour of sitting and engaging in a light activity such as walking or housework can substantially lower these risks.

***Important:*** This strategy is not a substitute for the 150 minutes of moderate exercise that your body needs every week.

Srini Beddhu, MD, professor of medicine, University of Utah School of Medicine, Salt Lake City.

## Odd Weight-Gain Risk

Open living spaces may lead to overeating. In one study, students made 10% more trips to get food in an open setting, where there are no walls between the kitchen and dining room, and ate an average of 170 calories more than students in a closed floor plan, where the kitchen and dining room are two separate rooms.

Study led by researchers at School of Architecture, University of Notre Dame, Indiana, published in *Environment and Behavior.*

## A Better Way to Weight Train

Brad Schoenfeld, PhD, a certified strength and conditioning specialist and an assistant professor in exercise science at Lehman College in New York City, where he directs the Human Performance Lab.

To get the biggest bang from your exercise regimen, strength training is a must. It not only builds muscle and bone but also helps manage your weight and control chronic health problems such as diabetes and heart disease.

But not everyone relishes the idea of heaving heavy weights. And the practice can be risky for people with arthritis, osteoporosis and other conditions.

***Good news:*** Researchers have now discovered that people who repeatedly lift light weights get nearly the same benefits as those who do heavy-weight workouts.

***Why this matters:*** Whether you're using hand weights or exercise machines, the lighter-weight approach can make strength training safer and more enjoyable.

Men and women who lift light weights instead of heavy ones are also less likely to experience joint, tendon or ligament injury. Plus, the workouts are easier for older adults...those with arthritis or other health problems...and those who are new to weight lifting.

## The New Thinking

According to traditional thinking, you need to lift heavy weights to build your muscles. In practice, this meant identifying your one-repetition maximum—the heaviest weight that you could lift just one time. Then you'd design a workout that required lifting 65% or more of that weight eight to 12 times.

This approach is still favored by many elite athletes because lifting at the edge of your ability targets fast twitch muscle fibers, the ones that grow quickly and create an admirable physique. But studies now show that slow-twitch fibers, the ones that are stimulated to a greater extent by light lifting, can also develop and grow.

***Important finding:*** In a recent meta-analysis published in the journal *Sports Medicine*, people who lifted lighter weights for six weeks achieved the same muscle growth—although not quite as much strength—as those who lifted heavy weights.

Heavy lifting is still the preferred approach for people who need to develop their strength to the utmost—top athletes, construction workers, movers, etc. But those who simply want to look better and improve their functional capacity—the ability to carry groceries, work in the yard, play recreational sports, etc.—will do just as well with lighter loads.

***Bonus:*** Building muscle mass also helps control blood sugar.

## Less Weight, More Reps

Muscle growth occurs only when muscles are exhausted—when you simply can't move the weight one more time. So to get comparable benefits to a traditional heavy-weight workout requiring eight to 12 repetitions, you'll need to do 20 to 25 reps with lighter weights. Your weight workouts will take a little longer, but your muscles will be just as tired when you're done.

## A Light-Weight Plan

Lighter-weight workouts are easier on the joints than those done with heavy weights, and the results are still relatively fast—you'll likely notice an increase in strength/muscle size within a few weeks. *To start...*

- **Choose your weights wisely.** Instead of calculating percentages—a heavy-weight lifter, as described earlier, may aim to lift at least 65% of his/her one-repetition maximum—keep it simple. Forget the percentages, and let repetitions guide your starting weights. For example, do each exercise 20 to 25 times. If you can't complete that many, you're starting too heavy. Conversely, if you can easily do 20 to 25 reps, the weight's too light.*

***Important:*** You're not doing yourself any good if you can easily lift a weight 25 times. You need to strain. On a one-to-10 scale of effort, the last few reps should rate nine-and-a-half or 10.

- **Do multiple sets.** You'll progress more quickly when you do three sets of each exercise—for example, bicep curls. Complete 20 to 25 repetitions...rest for two minutes...do them again...rest...and repeat one more time. If you don't have the time—or the desire—to do three sets, opt for a single-set approach. You'll still notice increases in strength and muscle size, but your gains won't be as great as with a multi-set approach.

- **Work out at least twice a week.** You want to work each muscle group—arms, legs, chest, midsection, etc.—at least twice a week. Three or four times weekly will give even faster results.

***Important:*** Don't work the same muscles two days in a row. Growth occurs during the recovery phase...and injuries are more likely when you stress already-tired muscles.

***If you work out every day:*** Alternate muscle groups—for example, do leg and back exercises on Monday...arm and chest exercises on Tuesday...then more leg and back work on Wednesday, etc.

*Hand weights are available in neoprene, iron and vinyl at many retail stores and online. I recommend holding various weights in a store to choose the one that feels best.

## Exercises for Real Life

The strength-training exercises below will give you more confidence and power when doing your daily activities—follow the advice above for choosing your weights, repetitions, exercise frequency, etc.…

• **Bicep curls.** Exercising this upper-arm muscle will make carrying groceries a bit easier.

***What to do:*** Hold a hand weight in each hand. While keeping your elbows near your sides and your shoulders back, curl the weight toward your shoulder, then lower it back down.

• **One-arm triceps extensions.** This exercise will strengthen your triceps (muscles on the backs of the upper arms), which help balance the biceps—and give your arms a toned appearance. It will help when moving furniture or shoveling snow.

***What to do:*** While sitting, hold a hand weight over your head, with your arm straight up and your elbow close to your head. Bend your elbow and lower the weight just behind your neck, then raise it back up. Repeat with the other arm.

• **Lunges.** This versatile exercise targets the buttocks and thighs, along with the arms, making climbing stairs easier.

***What to do:*** With a weight in each hand, stand with your feet about shoulder-width apart. Take a long step forward with your right foot. As your foot lands, bend the knee until the thigh is nearly parallel to the floor. Pull your right leg back to the starting position, then lunge with the left foot.

# Blurry Vision After Exercise

Pamela Wartian Smith, MD, MPH, founder and director, Center for Personalized Medicine, Ann Arbor, Michigan. She is author of *Why You Can't Lose Weight*.

If you experience blurry vision after exercise, you could be having episodes of hypoglycemia (low blood sugar) because your body does not have enough calories for a strenuous workout. Low blood sugar can result in blurry vision, dizziness, weakness and headaches.

Exercise itself can lower blood sugar levels for up to 24 hours afterward, but there's no need to give up your workouts.

Keep your blood sugar stable by spacing out meals. Eat five or six small meals a day instead of three, and make sure to include high-fiber foods that help regulate blood sugar, such as most fresh fruits and nonstarchy vegetables, beans, legumes and many whole-grain breads and cereals.

This will help speed your metabolism and assist your weight-loss efforts, as well as provide you with enough fuel for your exercise program.

***Also important:*** Be sure to drink water before, during and after your workout so that you don't become dehydrated—this condition can lead to blurry vision and/or dizziness.

If these strategies don't help, you should see your doctor. Blurry vision can be a sign of many other health problems, including diabetes, cataracts and even multiple sclerosis.

# It's Your Butt!

Chris Kolba, PhD, PT, a sports medicine physical therapist and clinical instructor at The Ohio State University Wexner Medical Center in Columbus. He developed The Ohio State Tactical Rehab and Conditioning Program to meet the needs of firefighters, police officers and other tactical operators.

Want to get to the bottom of your persistent back, knee or hip pain? Look behind you, and you'll find the likely cause.

Dormant butt syndrome is the name that I've coined for a serious problem that affects millions of Americans, especially those who spend most of the day sitting. Did you pull a hamstring while playing with your grandkids? Suffer from an aching back after a few hours of TV watching? Weak gluteal (butt) muscles are often the common link. A lack of strength in this area forces other muscles to compensate and do jobs that they're not designed to do alone, resulting in pain in unexpected parts of the body.

## The Neglected Core

The big muscles in the buttocks do more than give it shape. They absorb shocks and control movements necessary for walking and other activities. When the gluteal muscles are weak, other muscles and joints definitely take the hit.

Dormant butt syndrome strikes people who are generally sedentary—whether they're sitting behind a desk, driving a car or watching their favorite sitcoms. When you're positioned on your derriere for hours on end, the glutes aren't "firing" and there's more tightness in the hip flexor muscles, which can lead to hamstring injuries or back, hip or knee pain. Runners and other athletes who do repetitive motion can also get tight hip flexors.

When I evaluate clients who have lower-body pain, I always check for adequate glute strength. To do this, I ask the patient to lie on his/her stomach and do a leg lift against resistance from my hand to determine how strong his glutes are.

I also put my fingertips lightly on the hamstring and gluteal muscles of the lifted leg to evaluate the "firing pattern" of muscles. Normally, the gluteal muscles will fire (or activate) first, followed by the hamstrings. If the pattern is reversed, I'll know that the gluteal muscles are weaker than they should be.

## More Bang for Your Butt

I advise clients to spend the majority of their waking hours standing, if possible. Since this isn't always practical, at least make an effort to increase your amount of upright time—staying on your feet when watching TV, for example, or standing (and pacing) when talking on the telephone. Six other movements that help—do each one twice a week (except for the hip flexor stretch, which should be done daily)...*

- **Glute bridge.** It is among the best exercises for targeting the glutes. It gives the abdominal core muscles a bit of a workout, too.

***What to do:*** Lie on your back with your knees bent and your feet flat on the floor. Contract your abdominal muscles slightly. Next, raise your hips up about six inches and hold for a few seconds...then slowly lower yourself back down. Repeat this movement 10 to 12 times.

- **Lunges.** They strengthen the gluteal muscles, along with muscles in the hips and thighs.

***What to do:*** Stand with your feet together and your hands on your hips. Take a step forward with your left leg, while simultaneously bending that leg until the thigh is parallel to the floor. Keep your front foot flat on the floor as you bend your knee (most of the weight should go onto your heel), and don't let the front knee extend farther forward than the toes. Return to the starting position, then repeat with the other leg. Work up to 12 to 15 reps on each leg.

***Note:*** If a deep knee bend is painful, don't go down as far.

- **Wall squats.** Squats are popular because they increase both gluteal and thigh strength. This exercise is easier than traditional squats because it requires only body weight and a wall for support.

***What to do:*** **Lean back against a wall with your feet shoulder-width apart and out a foot or two.** Keep your back and hips against the wall.

Slide down until your thighs are parallel to the floor. Hold the position until your thighs start to say "enough," then rise back up. In the beginning, your thighs might start shaking after just a few seconds. Over time, try to work up to holding the position for 30 to 60 seconds.

*Consult your doctor before beginning this regimen—or any other new exercise program, especially if you've had knee, hip or back surgery.

If you're out of shape or have weak knees, you can lower yourself about halfway to the parallel position. Don't let your knees collapse inward, and stop if you feel any pain. Work your way toward the full bend as you build strength.

• **Side planks.** For those with dormant butt syndrome, it's important to stretch/strengthen surrounding muscles as well as the glutes themselves. This exercise activates muscles in the midsection, including the hips.

***What to do:*** Lie on your right side, with your legs extended and "stacked" on top of each other. Prop up your upper body by supporting your weight on your forearm, keeping your shoulder aligned with your elbow. Contract the ab muscles and lift your hips and knees off the floor. Hold the position for 10 to 30 seconds, then lower back down. Repeat on the other side. Start with two to three sets, holding the position for 10 seconds, and gradually work up to one minute per set.

• **Single leg balance.** Most people lose some strength, balance and rotational motion (the ability of their joints to rotate) as they get older. This exercise is a good way to improve hip and core stability while challenging balance.

***What to do:*** Stand on one leg, with your arms held slightly away from your body for balance.

***Important:*** For safety, stand next to a counter to catch yourself if you start to topple over. Try to hold the position (without swaying) for 30 to 60 seconds. Then try it on the other leg. It's challenging at first! Once it gets too easy, lift the leg a bit higher and/or try to do it with your eyes closed. This is harder because vision helps the body orient itself.

• **Hip flexor stretch.** Tight hip flexors cause dormant butt syndrome. When these muscles are tight, there's compensatory movement throughout the lower back, which can lead to pain as well as disk damage in the lower back.

***What to do:*** Kneel on your left knee, with your left hand on your hip and your right foot flat on the floor in front of you—the right knee should be bent and the right thigh should be roughly parallel to the floor. Move your left hip forward until it extends beyond the left knee. Don't bend forward during the movement. Hold the position for 20 to 30 seconds, then repeat for three or four reps. Change position and repeat on the other side.

## "Barefoot Sneakers" for Muscle Gain

"Barefoot sneakers" strengthen legs and feet more effectively than regular sneakers. These minimalist shoes have stretchy-fabric uppers, zero heel-to-toe drop and a three-millimeter outer sole—with no midsole cushioning or arch support. Runners who used them for six months had 7% larger leg muscles and 9% larger foot muscles—while those who used regular sneakers had no muscle increase.

Study of 38 runners led by researchers at Hong Kong Polytechnic University, Hung Hom, Kowloon, published in *Clinical Biomechanics*.

## Help for Headaches While Working Out...

Alan M. Rapoport, MD, clinical professor of neurology, David Geffen School of Medicine at UCLA, and immediate past president of the International Headache Society. IHS-headache.org

About 10% of healthy adults develop mild-to-moderate headaches during or after a workout, a condition known as "primary exercise headache." The headache usually comes on suddenly and can be on one or both sides of the head. It is not caused by another disorder, and researchers believe that changes in blood flow to the brain can trigger the headache.

Fortunately, you can take steps to avoid this problem. Since sustained exertion can cause this type of head pain, ease into exercise by warming up for five minutes. Start with a slow pace and increase speed every minute until you are at your treadmill exercise pace. And don't skip the five-minute cool-down walk at the end of your session.

Also, stay hydrated by drinking water before, during and after exercising. *Naproxen* (Aleve) or a similar pain reliever, taken about an hour before your workout, may prevent an exercise-related headache.

Primary exercise headaches usually last from five minutes to two days. They typically go away within three to six months as the body adapts to a regular exercise program. To help your body adjust, take several weeks to increase your speed and incline on the treadmill.

If these tips don't seem to help, or if headaches are severe and/or are accompanied by other symptoms, such as weakness, numbness, and/or visual or memory problems, tell your doctor. You may need a neurological evaluation.

# You Can Work Out Like an Olympic Athlete

Timothy Miller, MD, director of the endurance medicine program, which specializes in treating endurance athletes, and associate professor of clinical orthopaedics at The Ohio State University Wexner Medical Center in Columbus. Dr. Miller is also a volunteer team physician for the US Olympic Track and Field Team.

Watching Olympic athletes perform their incredible feats can be awe-inspiring...and humbling. But don't despair.

Even if you're not an Olympic athlete, you can still perform at your highest potential by adding highly effective Olympic training routines to your own workout.

***Helpful:*** You can add all—or just a few—of the exercises below to your current fitness routine to increase your endurance, gain strength and boost bone density...*

## Fartlek Workout

***Which Olympic athletes do this?*** Cyclists and distance runners.

***Good for:*** Anyone who wants to add speed and endurance to a walking, running or cycling routine.

***What is it?*** Short bursts of high-intensity movement—a few seconds to a minute—that take place within a longer aerobic routine. Many people refer to this workout method as Fartlek (which means "speed play" in Swedish), but it is also known as interval training.

***How can I do this?*** Do a 30-minute walk or jog in your neighborhood. Begin with a 10-minute warm-up of a slower-paced run or walk (use a stopwatch to keep track of your time). Once you're warmed up, sprint (or walk fast) between two mailboxes (or telephone poles or any other regularly spaced marker)...then return to your regular pace for the distance of three mailboxes. Sprint or walk fast again, continuing the same interval pattern for 10 minutes. Afterward, return to your regular pace for 10 minutes. Then cool down for a few minutes with a slower run or walk.

For a 30-minute cycling routine, pedal slowly for a 10-minute warm-up. Then do 30-second sprints pedaling as fast as you can followed by one minute of slow pedaling for a total of 10 minutes. Then cycle for 10 minutes at a comfortable pace and end with a cooldown.

## Eccentric Exercises

***Which Olympic athletes do this?*** Power lifters and gymnasts.

***Good for:*** Anyone who wants to strengthen his/her calves, Achilles tendons and biceps.

***What is it?*** These exercises, which are the most efficient way to build strength, focus on working the muscle when it lengthens. In

*If you have a chronic medical condition or a recent injury, or are at increased risk of falling, consult your doctor before trying these exercises.

this phase, you consciously slow the descent of a weight (or gravity). This means that you use resistance twice—once while lifting the weight and once while lowering it.

***How can I do this?*** Biceps curls and heel drops.

***Biceps curl:*** To begin, choose a light hand weight (about three to five pounds)...or use small soup cans. Stand with your feet shoulder-width apart, elbows at your sides and forearms at 90-degree angles from your body, with your palms and weights facing up. Hold your left arm steady. Lift your right arm toward your shoulder for a count of two to three seconds, keeping your elbow at your side.

Lower the weight slowly and with control for a count of three to four seconds, keeping your muscles contracted. This is the eccentric phase of the exercise. Alternate arms for a total of 12 to 15 repetitions on each arm. Perform the whole set two to three times. When you can perform 10 reps easily, increase the weight.

***Heel drop:*** Stand with the balls of your feet on the edge of a stair. Drop your heels as low as you can in a slow, controlled motion, taking about three to four seconds to completely lower them. Then push your heels back up for a count of two to three seconds. Repeat 12 to 15 times. Do two to three sets.

### Plyometric Training

***Which Olympic athletes do this?*** High jumpers, gymnasts, sprinters and basketball players.

***Good for:*** Anyone who wants to build leg strength.

***What is it?*** Also known as "jump training," these exercises require your muscles to exert maximum force in short intervals.

***How can I do this?*** Box jumps. Most gyms have jump boxes of varying heights (six inches, 18 inches, etc.), or you can buy one at a sporting-goods store or online. Pick a height you can jump onto so that both feet land squarely on the box.

### Hate to Exercise?

Get a dog. Dog owners were 34% more likely to meet the recommended minimum of 150 minutes of moderate exercise a week—and 69% more likely to be physically active—than people who don't own dogs, recent research has found.

***Good idea:*** If you have a dog, work out with your pet. K9FitClub has lots of different classes in cities across the US. Go to K9FitClub.com.

Mathew J. Reeves, PhD, professor of epidemiology and biostatistics, Michigan State University, East Lansing.

Stand with feet slightly wider than shoulder-width apart, knees bent. Using your arms to help generate power, jump on the box landing softly on two feet, knees flexed. Keep your hands in front of you for balance. Then jump back down to the starting position. Repeat 10 times for a total of three sets.

## Why You Should Roll on a Ball on the Floor

Jill Miller, fitness therapy expert based in Los Angeles, author of *The Roll Model* and creator of the exercise program Yoga Tune Up.

Those bright, squishy balls little kids love to play with are for grown-ups, too! In fact, there's a way to "play" with these soft, tactile toys that can help you calm down...stand straighter...and breathe better.

It's inexpensive and easy to do, and it really works. You just have to get down on the floor, lie down with your ball under your abs...and roll around.

Here's how...

### A New Kind of Roll Play

Fitness-therapy expert Jill Miller, creator of Yoga Tune Up, author of *The Roll Model*, is so convinced that this exercise is effective that she's created an exercise program called Coregeous—rhymes with "gorgeous." The program uses soft balls to relieve stress and tension, improve posture and breathing, and even to break up deep internal abdominal scars from surgery.

***Here's the theory behind it:*** By lying on a soft ball pushed up against your abdomen, you stimulate the vagus nerve, which is deep inside and runs from your brain stem through your heart and lungs. In medical studies, stimulating the vagus nerve (through an electrical implant) has been shown to help relieve mood disorders such as depression and even help control epileptic seizures.

There's no research—and no such claims—for ball-rolling moves, but Miller has found that they can relieve stress. When you're anxious, she explains, and trying to breathe from deep in your belly—a good way to calm yourself—tense, tight abdominal muscles get in the way. They make it hard to inhale and exhale deeply and fully. But "when you lie face down on the floor with a ball positioned strategically under your abdominals, the pressure will make you aware of tension there that inhibits the full range of motion in your breathing muscles," she explains.

The muscle-and-tension-releasing effects of rolling on a ball also can improve posture. "The pressure of a ball under your belly puts you in touch with any unconscious tension you might be holding in your core," she says. Release that tension, and it's easier to reverse poor posture.

Belly rolling can also create an abdominal massage that mobilizes the fascia, the connective tissues of the body, letting them move the way that they they should. Tightness in these tissues can lead to aches and pains in almost everyone, says Miller.

She's also found that these moves can help break up adhesions—including deep, abdominal scar tissue from surgery, such as a C-section, gall bladder surgery or appendectomy. Since such internal scarring "creates compensation within muscles of the core that impact breathing, posture and stress," says Miller, "when you work on your scars, the muscles in your core are freer to get stronger—which in turn improves posture and breathing."

Ready to roll? Here are Miller's beginner tips—plus two moves to start you off. To better visualize the moves, visit one of Jill's videos on YouTube.com. Search Jill Miller Pin, Spin and Mobilize.

## Get on the (Right) Ball

Miller's Coregeous ball (available on her website) is specially designed for the exercises she has developed, but you also can use any very soft and squishy ball, such as a kids' Gertie (which costs about $8 at toy stores and online). "You even can use a small pillow or a rolled-up towel," Miller says. *Her tips...*

***Caution:*** Check with your doctor before doing these moves, especially if you've recently had surgery. It's best to wait until you're cleared for exercise.

- **Take a load off.** If rolling on a hard floor is too uncomfortable, try rolling on a bed or even against a wall. Both will reduce the pressure of your body weight on your stomach.
- **Go slow.** "At first, just the pressure of lying on a ball may be enough to unbind postural and emotional stress," says Miller. "Pay attention to your emotional reactions. Some people who have very negative feelings about their abs or feel ashamed of their bodies can feel vulnerable and even find the position unpleasant in the beginning."
- **Don't bounce back up too quickly.** When you finish with your rolling routine, stay on the floor for a few moments before standing, advises Miller. Jumping upright too quickly can make you dizzy.

Now here are the moves...

## Breath Reset

This helps you ease into the sensation of pressure on your abdominals, brings awareness of your diaphragm and breathing, and provides a gentle belly massage that will soothe your nervous system and help you relax.

- **Place the ball on the floor.** Lie face down on top of it, positioning it in the center of your abdomen. Extend your legs behind you with toes pointed. Bend your arms at the elbow, and let them rest on the floor on either side of your head.

• **Inhale...hold your breath...and then tighten your abs.** Hold for three to five seconds, and then exhale. Repeat five to eight times.

• **Keeping your weight on the ball, slowly shift your weight from side to side while breathing deeply.** Do this for two minutes.

## Pin, Spin, Mobilize

This exercise brings more movement to the fascia, which are tight and restricted in their movement in just about everyone. It's also a great exercise if you need to release scar tissue deep in the belly that can restrict breathing and throw off posture.

It will be most effective if you place the ball against your bare skin, so that your skin can grip the ball more tightly and provide traction. Do this only every other day in order to give your tissue time to remodel itself.

• **Position the ball under your abdominals in an area that feels especially tight and restricted.**

• **Use your hands and feet to slowly pivot your entire body in one direction until you feel a pinch.** Stop there, and breathe steadily for 30 to 90 seconds until the pinching feeling dissipates.

• **Then pivot a bit more in the same direction, just until you feel pinching again.** Stop and breathe until the sensation goes away.

• **Repeat the incremental pivoting for as long as the pinching is tolerable.**

***Note:*** You might have heard that the vagus nerve is involved in fainting—the kind that's triggered by things like the sight of blood, for example. Not to worry—this kind of mild exercise is very different from the body's reactions that can cause fainting.

Learn more about how the kind of abdominal massage provided by rolling on a ball might help manage autoimmune conditions, such as asthma, by reading a guest blog by yoga instructor Meredith Hutten Chamorro on the Yoga Tuneup site. Go to TuneUpFitness.com and search Roll Away Autoimmune Inflammation.

Meanwhile, if you want to keep your body and mind relaxed, be like old man river and just keep rollin'!

# Fitness Trackers Might Not Help You Lose Weight

Mitesh Patel, MD, assistant professor of medicine and health-care management at Perelman School of Medicine and The Wharton School at University of Pennsylvania, Philadelphia. HealthCareInnovation.upenn.edu

A study published in *JAMA* found that dieters who wore fitness trackers for 24 months lost significantly less weight than dieters who did not—7.7 pounds versus 13 pounds, on average. Fitness trackers are wearable digital devices that measure fitness data such as the number of steps taken each day and calories burned. Their makers often boast that these devices promote weight loss, something this study calls into question.

But other research suggests that while these devices alone often are not effective, they can be paired with "engagement strategies" to promote weight loss and fitness, such as using them in a social way.

***Example:*** The tracker's data could be shared with friends or family members for peer support...or a group of friends could wear fitness trackers and compete to see who can walk the farthest each week.

It also is worth noting that the recent study gave fitness trackers to people who already were participating in diet and exercise programs. In doing so, it might have accidentally undermined the healthy habits these people previously had established by asking them to change something that was already working.

***What to do:*** Before purchasing a fitness tracker, use a smartphone fitness tracker app—a popular one is Health Mate by Withings. These apps are not quite as accurate as full-fledged fitness trackers, but they are a good way for smartphone owners to confirm that they will use a tracker before investing money in one. One of the reasons that trackers sometimes are ineffective is that many people discontinue use within a few months.

As noted above, if you buy a tracker, share your tracker results with friends or, better yet, enlist those friends into a fitness-tracker competition.

Also, set reasonable fitness goals for yourself. Use your smartphone app or fitness tracker to determine your current daily activity level, and then set a personal daily target that is perhaps 1,000 to 2,000 steps above this. Increase this target slowly over time.

## If You Like to Hike… What to Do About Wild Animals

Bryan Bailey, an animal behaviorist in Memphis, Tennessee, and author of *Embracing the Wild in Your Dog.*

Hiking in the woods is great exercise, but how can you protect yourself from dogs, bears and other animals?

Remain vigilant at all times. Bears, mountain lions and wolves are predators with a very keen sense of smell and hearing (so are dogs), and they will detect you long before you are aware of their presence. In most cases, if these animals approach you, it is because they are curious and will likely flee once they realize you have detected them. Let them know you're on the trail by talking or singing and hike in a group, if possible.

***To stay safe:*** Carry bear mace (available at sporting-goods stores and online for about $25 and up), which can deter attackers at distances of up to 35 feet. If you do encounter an animal, remain quiet and slowly back away. Do not run.

## 15 Minutes to Better Health

People who worked out for only 15 minutes a day—half the widely recommended amount—had 22% lower risk for death (from heart disease, stroke, cancer and other causes) versus those who were sedentary, in an analysis of nearly 123,000 adults age 60 and older. Getting additional exercise lowered death risk even more—28% for those who worked out for 30 minutes…35%, for one hour or more.

***Note:*** Exercise needs to be moderate-to-vigorous intensity, such as brisk walking or fast biking.

David Hupin, MD, physician, department of clinical and exercise physiology, University Hospital of Saint-Étienne, France.

# APPENDIX 2: OPTIMUM AGING

## Look 10 Years Younger

Gail Sagel, CEO of FACES Beautiful cosmetics company, Westport, Connecticut. She is a makeup artist and creator of Brush-On Liquid Mineral Makeup. Sagel is author of *Making Faces Beautiful* and *FACE IT: Five Essential Elements for Living Beautifully—Tips for Beauties Over 50.* FacesBeautiful.com

If you are using the same makeup and skin-care regimen that worked for you 10 or 15 years ago, you may be looking older than you need to. As your skin texture and coloring change, your makeup and beauty routine should change, too. *Here, an expert's clever tips for looking fabulous...*

### Primer and Foundation

If you have never used primer, now is the time to try it. Primer is a base for foundation that gives a smoother finish and helps your makeup last all day. First apply moisturizer, then primer, then foundation. *Also...*

• **Don't use a heavy foundation**—heavy products settle into creases and pores, emphasizing them. Choose a lightweight, creamy foundation, or try a tinted moisturizer instead of foundation. Avoid powder foundations, which can be drying to the skin and emphasize fine lines.

• **Get the right color.** You may have heard that foundation color should be matched to the color of your neck, but that isn't a useful guideline for most women. Over time, many facial skin tones become progressively darker than the neck because the chin keeps sunlight from reaching the neck. A foundation color that is too pale looks artificial and aging.

Instead, find a foundation color that is midway between the color of your face and your upper chest. Also correct for ruddiness or sallowness by choosing a color that will help to neutralize these undertones.

***Example:*** If your skin has pink or red undertones, choose a color with a very slight yellowish cast. If you are naturally sallow with yellowish undertones, choose a color with just a touch of pink, which will make your overall color more radiant.

• **When you are testing a foundation color,** go outside to see if the color looks natural in bright, natural light.

• **Use a foundation brush rather than your fingers to apply foundation.** A foundation brush distributes makeup more sparingly and more evenly, creating an effect that is both polished and natural. To apply, either put a small amount of foundation on your hand and dip the brush into it...or put a few dots of foundation on your face and then spread with the brush. Try both methods to see which one works best for you.

### Concealer

Most women apply under-eye concealer before applying foundation. This can cause you to look older. Concealer, which typically is a heavier texture than foundation, will collect in the creases around the eye and call even more attention to wrinkles.

***What to do:*** Apply your other makeup first. Then step back and look at your face closely to see where you need concealer. You may need it in only a few small spots, or you may not need it at all.

Be careful when choosing your concealer color. Don't choose one that is too pale compared with your foundation—lighter colors highlight wrinkles. Use a color that is a similar color or just a touch lighter. A concealer that has a small amount of peach or rose in the color is very helpful in hiding dark circles.

### Liner and Eye Shadow

Eyes become angular with age. If you are using dark eye shadow to contour the orbital bone above the eye, you may be emphasizing those angles and adding years to your face. *Instead of classic contouring, I recommend the Side V eye shadow technique...*

**1. Apply eyeliner along the lash line above and below your eye.** Use a kohl pencil or a felt-tip liner—these glide much better than standard pencils, which pull at delicate eyelids. Or use eye shadow as a liner—put a drop of water on a fine brush, and dip the brush into an eye shadow that can be used either wet or dry.

**2. Sweep a light-colored shadow along your upper eyelid, from the lash line up to the crease.**

**3. Using a color darker than the lid shadow but lighter than the liner, brush a sideways "V" on the outside of the lid, with the open part of the "V" facing in toward the nose.** Then use a brush to blend the V from the outside corner of the eye inward. The sideways V gives eyes an uplifted appearance.

## Brows

Eyebrows thin out with age. Filling them in is recommended for a youthful, full brow. There are many brow-filling choices—brow balms, brow powders and brow pencils. Eyebrow pencils can make your brows look overdrawn and artificial. Brow balms and brow powders, which are applied with a small-angled brush, typically give the softest, most natural look.

## Lipstick

The lipstick that you have been wearing may not be the most flattering one for you anymore. Experiment with new lip colors. If you always thought a certain shade was off-limits for your coloring, try it anyway. If you are used to wearing subtle colors, try a bright color...if you typically wear deep colors, see what a nude color looks like on you.

Go to the cosmetics counter, and say to the consultant, "If I were to buy two new lipstick colors, what would make me look more beautiful?" Lipstick is relatively inexpensive—buy those two colors, and see what reaction you get when you wear them.

Using a gentle exfoliator (see below) on the lips when you cleanse is a great way to keep your lip area smooth from wrinkles. To prevent lipstick "bleeding," apply foundation on your lips as well as the rest of your face...then put a small amount of pressed powder on your lips...then apply lipstick. A good long-wearing lip liner can help prevent lipstick bleeding, too.

***Here's a trick:*** Apply lipstick first, then apply lip liner to the edges to define them. This also will make them appear more plump. This technique gives you younger- and fuller-looking lips, and it looks less harsh than outlining your lips first.

## Exfoliating Makes Skin Look Younger

How women (and men!) clean their facial skin affects how youthful they look. One secret to youthful, radiant skin is cleaning in a way that doesn't dry out your skin but actually forces exfoliation of the topical skin cells. Your body is constantly producing new skin cells and shedding old ones. Unfortunately, skin-cell turnover slows with age, leaving a buildup of dead skin cells that makes skin look dry and dull. Gentle daily exfoliation removes the older skin cells, revealing younger, more supple skin.

Men exfoliate by shaving, but to look their best, they need to exfoliate the rest of their face, as women do.

The simplest way to exfoliate is to clean with a gentle, hydrating, nonsoap, nondetergent facial cleanser using a clean, damp washcloth. A soap-based cleanser leaves buildup on your skin, contributing to the dull look.

At the end of each day, while applying a gentle facial cleanser, use the damp washcloth to gently massage cleanser into your skin. Rinse your face with lukewarm water.

Your skin should look slightly flushed after exfoliating but not bright red and inflamed. Too-rough treatment will damage the skin.

There are many types of exfoliators on the market. Not all of them are suggested for use on facial skin. Avoid using abrasive elements on your face such as loofahs and oatmeal scrubs, apricot scrubs or other cleansers containing abrasive elements. All of these have rough edges that can cause tiny lacerations on the face. But you can use these products on the rest of your body. Keep in mind that even pre-moistened towelettes, which seem mild, are made from paper, which can be harsh to older skin.

Facial cleansers and exfoliators containing fruit acids, such as mango, papaya and citrus extracts, are a very good choice for gentle exfoliation. Vitamin A topical serums and moisturizers stimulate more rapid turnover of skin cells, leading to a more youthful appearance. Start with a mild-strength product. Stronger ones may be too harsh for many skin types, especially older skin.

## Go Green, Live Long

Study titled "Exposure to Greenness and Mortality in a Nationwide Prospective Cohort Study of Women" by researchers at Harvard T.H. Chan School of Public Health, Brigham and Women's Hospital and Harvard Medical School, all in Boston, published in *Environmental Health Perspectives.*

The greenery that surrounds your home is more than eye candy. It also protects your lungs, helps ward off depression, protects you from cancer, improves your kidney health—and might even help you live longer.

So finds a study of more than 100,000 women living in nearly all US states. Researchers analyzed health records and compared them with geographic satellite data for "greenness"—a measure of chlorophyll, and a pretty good gauge of how much vegetation surrounded their homes.

Over an eight-year period, women who lived in the top fifth for greenery, compared with those in the bottom fifth, were 12% less likely to die. That was true regardless of age, race, socioeconomic status or whether the residents smoked. While this particular study was focused on women, similar health benefits for greenery have also been reported for men, the researchers note.

Why the green longevity bonus? Vegetation, the researchers note, helps protect against pollutants that can increase the risk for lung and kidney disease and cancer, improves mood and provides opportunities to be more active. Further analysis revealed that women surrounded by more greenery were less likely to have respiratory illness, kidney disease, cancer or depression. They also used fewer antidepressants. Living in green areas may allow for a healthier lifestyle—in fact, the researchers did find an increase in physical activity as well.

Nor was it just homes with big lawns that were healthier. While the relationship was strongest for the 250 meters surrounding the homes, it also held true (although to a slightly lesser degree) for an area of 1,250 meters—nearly a mile. So even if you don't have a big green property, if you live near parks and other green spaces, you're in the pink.

Forests, we're told, are the lungs of the earth. But the lawns and fields and trees that surround our homes also help our lungs—and our spirits. They may even help us hang around longer to enjoy the scenery.

If you live near clean grass, try walking on it barefoot to energize your body…and don't forget greenery inside your house. Even when you're in an office, you can stay mentally sharp by gazing at a green scene.

## "Super Ager" Secrets for Staying Sharp

Bradford Dickerson, MD, a behavioral neurologist, director of the Frontotemporal Disorders Unit at Massachusetts General Hospital and an associate professor of neurology at Harvard Medical School, all in Boston.

When it comes to research on memory loss, most studies have shown that it is very common in normal aging to have reduced memory, even in the absence of Alzheimer's disease or other late-life diseases.

But much of this research has been done on people who are in their 80s or older. What happens to memory in those who aren't quite that old? After all, by the time we've reached our 60s or 70s, most of us have memory lapses, whether it's misplaced eyeglasses or a forgotten name.

***Important recent discovery:*** By investigating somewhat younger adults, scientists are now uncovering a new breed of "super agers," who do as well on memory tests as those who are 40 or 50 years younger. This research is contributing to a growing body of evidence that could provide significant clues about new ways to prevent and treat memory loss.

Below, Bradford Dickerson, MD, a neurologist at Massachusetts General Hospital and a leading expert on brain changes and memory disorders, answers some key questions...

*How much does memory decline in the typical older adult?*

In clinical settings, memory can be tested in a variety of ways. One approach involves giving people a short list of words to memorize. When people in their 20s are presented with a list of 16 words—and given time to really study the list—they'll probably remember 13 or 14 of the words. Most people in their early or mid-70s might remember just eight or nine of the words. This would be considered "normal" memory loss.

***To test yourself:*** Study a list of 16 words for a few minutes and then see how many you can remember 20 minutes later.

*But some people do better on these tests?*

Actually, some do a lot better. Based on research conducted at Northwestern University, it is known that a small percentage of people who are age 80 or older—maybe about 10%—do as well or better on memory tests as people who are in their 50s and 60s.

Our study included adults closer to traditional retirement age. However, we found the same thing—some people simply don't experience the same degree of memory loss as their peers. This has huge implications.

If we can figure out why some people maintain robust memories, we might find ways to prevent or even reverse age-related memory loss—and possibly some forms of dementia, which can cause other cognitive problems such as impaired reasoning and behavior and personality changes.

*Do we know how the brains of super agers differ from those of other people?*

Even though the brain is roughly the same size in all adults (about the size of a cantaloupe and weighing approximately three pounds), we found in our studies of super agers that the size of specific brain areas correlated with memory: They were larger in those with exceptional memories and smaller in those with normal memories. This means that we now have a "biomarker" that may be used to study age-related memory changes.

*Is it possible to strengthen these brain regions and prevent memory loss?*

This is the million-dollar question. Some people, due to genetics, may simply be born with "young" brains. We know that exercise (see below) and following a Mediterranean-style diet with fruits and vegetables, fish, legumes and whole grains can stimulate brain growth. Good sleep and reducing stress can also make a difference.

*Do the brain changes that are associated with these or other activities lead to better memory?*

At the moment, we're not sure.

*How does exercise help?*

Aerobic exercise has been shown to reduce circulating cortisol, a stress hormone that can cause brain shrinkage. It also stimulates the release of growth factors (such as brain-derived neurotrophic factor) that prevent brain cells from shrinking and may even help new ones grow.

A recent study showed that sedentary older adults who take up moderate-intensity exercise—for example, a regular walking program for 30 minutes at least four days a week—for six months to a year show growth in the hippocampus (a part of the brain associated with memory) and also do better on memory tests. This reinforces the idea that exercise is protective.

***Important:*** Don't talk on your cell phone while walking or biking, since you may be more likely to fall. Head trauma raises risk for Alzheimer's disease.

*What about diet?*

Studies suggest that heart-healthy diets (such as the Mediterranean diet) can reduce the risk for Alzheimer's disease and other forms of dementia. We're just not sure whether the diet specifically improves brain functions.

However, in a recent study from Mayo Clinic, researchers found (based on MRI scans) that the brains of adults who consumed the most foods typical of a Mediterranean diet for a year—legumes, fish, whole grains and vegetables—had greater thickness in some parts of the cortex, which plays a role in memory, language and other cognitive functions. People who ate large amounts of carbohydrates, sugar and/or red meat had less cortical thickness.

*And stress reduction?*

In studies of older adults, those who participated in an eight-week meditation training program had improved connectivity between the frontal lobes and the hippocampus and other brain structures, which improves memory. It's possible that other relaxing practices, such as yoga, have similar effects. We're hoping to study this more.

*How important is sleep?*

Very! People who don't sleep well will obviously find it difficult to focus their attention and obtain and retain memories. Also, the brain consolidates memories during sleep (particularly during the deep, slow-wave stages of sleep)—the memories are shifted to brain regions where they become more stable.

It's important to remember, though, that we all require different amounts of sleep. Most adults seem to do best when they get seven to nine hours of sleep a day.

*Any other advice?*

Socialize. Studies show that adults who regularly connect with friends are less likely to develop dementia. Working past typical retirement age and/or volunteering after retirement also keeps older brains engaged.

# Take Years Off Your Face

Victoria J. Mogilner, CA, certified acupuncturist and acupressurist and owner of Total Rejuvenation Center, Scottsdale, Arizona. A specialist in facial rejuvenation, she is author of *Ancient Secrets of Facial Rejuvenation: A Holistic, Nonsurgical Approach to Youth & Well-Being.* VictoriaMogilner.com

Do you look older than you feel? You don't have to have cosmetic surgery to take years off your look. Facial acupressure, an ancient practice derived from Traditional Chinese medicine, involves lightly pressing certain points on the face. It can tighten the skin, create a youthful glow and promote the production of collagen, all without having to go under the knife.

## How Does It Work?

Traditional Chinese medicine focuses on restoring balance throughout the body and promoting the flow of energy, called qi (pronounced chee). Qi is circulated along a network of channels called meridians. There are 12 meridians in the body, each relating to a vital organ, such as the stomach, large intestine, gallbladder and bladder.

When the meridians become clogged because of poor diet, stress, dehydration or other factors, skin can age prematurely. When you put pressure on points on your face and open these pathways, circulation is improved, bringing blood and energy to the skin and other organs.

Digestion also is improved, ensuring the absorption of nutrients that are beneficial to the skin. And the lymphatic system, which drains damaging toxins and waste from the body, is stimulated. Improving the movement of qi and opening meridians result in a more youthful appearance. This may sound strange to you, but the techniques really do work, and they are very safe. If you do the exercises for 15 minutes a day, you will start to notice a difference within a week to 10 days.

## Getting Started

Acupressure face-lifts aren't difficult to do. *Just remember these guidelines…*

Set aside five minutes for the "pre-facial warm-up" and at least 10 minutes a day for the face-lift. To begin, choose one or two points (described below) to treat each day. As you become more experienced, you can spend more time and treat more points.

Don't worry about finding the exact point—as long as you are in the general area, you will affect each point along the pathway. As you continue, you will become more sensitive to the energy flow and your fingers will instinctively go to the correct points.

Touch and press each point with steady, gentle pressure on both sides of your face. Release after one minute.

***Important:*** Don't pull your skin, which is extremely delicate on the face. Just press with the pads of your fingers.

## The Acupressure Face-Lift

A successful acupressure face-lift isn't just "physical"—to reduce stress and help restore the flow of qi, there is a mental component, too…

***Pre-Facial Warm-Up:*** Sit away from distractions, where you feel safe, tranquil and nurtured. Begin to breathe steadily through your nose. Picture every part of your body, every pore, every cell receiving nourishment. Sit quietly, and relax your mind. As you breathe out, let go of stress. As you breathe in, repeat to yourself, *I let go of old thoughts. I work on myself to replenish myself at the cellular level.* Or you can make up your own affirmation. Do this for five minutes. Continue to be aware of your breath while doing the following exercises. While you focus on each affirmation, take a deep breath to the count of five, hold it for a count of five, breathe out to the count of five, and let your mind focus on your breath.

## Yang Brightness

The gallbladder meridian is a yang, or active, meridian and is the partner of the liver. The liver controls the eyes.

***Benefits:*** Stimulating the gallbladder meridian from the forehead improves circulation and stimulates collagen production, tightening skin and reducing forehead wrinkles. It also brightens eyes and improves mental clarity.

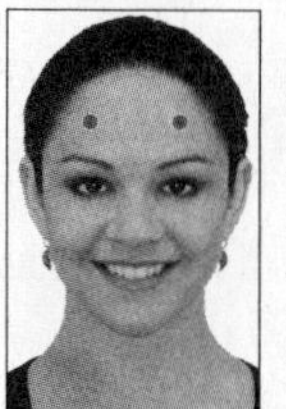

***How to do it:*** Place your middle three fingers right above the middle of the eyebrow at the highest point in the indentation of your forehead. Gently touch the skin as you say your affirmation.

***Suggested affirmation:*** *I release the negativity of the past and bring health and wellness into every pore of my being.*

## Pupil Bone

This point also works on the gallbladder meridian. The name refers to the acupressure point on the face—and the fact that it influences the eyes.

***Benefits:*** Increases blood flow to the eyes, restoring youthfulness to the skin around the eyes, particularly lessening crow's-feet—those stubborn wrinkles on the outer corner of the eye. This meridian also relates to decision-making, and by stimulating it, you can choose to create a more positive state of mind and physical health.

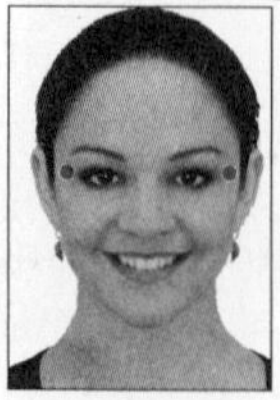

***How to do it:*** Place the middle three fingers in the hollows next to the eyes, and close your eyes. Do both eyes at once.

***Suggested affirmation:*** *As I move forward, I make the decision to release negative thought patterns and have a positive state of mind and inner well-being.*

## Receiving Cures

This point, on the stomach meridian, promotes digestion.

***Benefits:*** By stimulating the stomach pathway, nutrients are better absorbed, resulting in healthier-looking skin. This point also increases circulation and aids in the removal of toxins, which reduces the swelling and puffiness under the eyes.

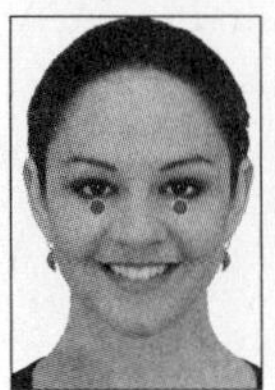

***How to do it:*** Place your middle three fingers in the indentations under the eyes. Close your eyes.

***Suggested affirmation:*** I receive all that life offers to nourish me. I connect with my inner self.

## Welcome Fragrance

On the large intestine meridian, this point is located next to the sinuses, aiding deep breathing.

***Benefits:*** Stimulates circulation and collagen production in the area under the nose, helping to eradicate fine lines and tighten skin in this area. Improves sense of smell and eases sinus congestion.

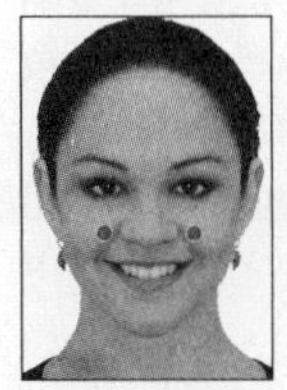

***How to do it:*** Place your middle three fingers next to your nose so that your ring fingers line up with the bottom of the nose. Gently touch the point.

***Suggested affirmation:*** I release my difficulties and problems regarding my spiritual essence, and I come home to my soul for guidance and protection.

## Lower Hinge

This point, along the stomach meridian, is located on the lower part of the jaw, acting like a hinge that helps the jaw relax.

***Benefits:*** Relaxes the cheek muscles and stimulates the production of collagen, smoothing the skin. Also relieves pain from teeth grinding and jaw tightness. Improves hearing and helps you to filter out negative self-talk.

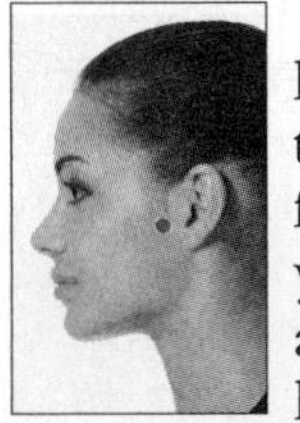

***How to do it:*** The jaw hinge is located about two inches from the tip of your earlobe. You can find it by opening and closing your mouth. Press gently upward as you breathe. Feel your jaw relax as you let go of stress.

***Suggested affirmation:*** I deserve to receive the best that life has to offer.

---

# What Your Hot Flashes Say About Your Health

Rebecca C. Thurston, PhD, director, Women's Biobehavioral Health Laboratory, professor of psychiatry, psychology, epidemiology, and clinical and translational science, University of Pittsburgh School of Medicine, Pennsylvania.

When is a hot flash not just a hot flash? When it's a window into future health—of your heart, your bones, your brain and your moods.

"We used to think that hot flashes were just an annoying quality-of-life issue, but now we are learning that they may signal something more about a woman's health," says psychiatry professor Rebecca Thurston, PhD, director of the Women's Biobehavioral Health Laboratory at the University of Pittsburgh in Pennsylvania.

To be sure, just having hot flashes is no cause for concern. After all, in the transition into and through menopause, almost 70% of women experience them. Most of the time, they are merely uncomfortable.

## The Variety of Hot Flash Experiences

The trouble is, in the run-up to menopause, when your hot flashes start, when they eventually stop, and how severe they are may be emerging clues to future risks for heart disease, diabetes, osteoporosis, dementia and depression.

Here's how to read those clues—and what to do about it.

As new research emerges, it's becoming clear that many of our assumptions about hot flashes have been way off base. Hot flashes can start many years before menopause and last for many years after your last period is a distant memory...arrive and depart in a year or two...or never happen at all. Now, thanks to a long-term research project called SWAN—it stands for "Study of Women's Health Across the Nation" and has followed about 3,300 women over 15 years—we're getting the real story. *While every woman experiences hot flashes differently, SWAN has identified four distinct trajectories...*

- **Early onset,** with the first hot flash about a decade before the last menstrual period and ending after the last period.
- **Later onset,** with the first hot flash appearing about the time of the final period, persisting several years and later declining.
- **The lucky few,** who have just a few hot flashes around the time of the final menstrual period that don't persist long afterward or never have hot flashes at all.
- **Super flashers,** who have frequent hot flashes from well before menopause and often well into the years afterward.

Women tend to fall fairly equally into these four groups, with the later-onset path being the most common (29%) followed by the lucky few (27%), super flashers (26%) and early onset (18%). SWAN and other studies are also uncovering key associations to health risks. *Here's what hot flashes tell us about...*

## The Heart

A SWAN study has reinforced the connection. Women were asked to track their hot flashes and underwent ultrasound to determine the thickness of the walls of the carotid arteries in their necks—a good measure of atherosclerosis, which increases the risk for heart disease and stroke.

***Result:*** Women who reported more frequent hot flashes (at least every other day) had evidence of atherosclerosis. Also, a different SWAN study found evidence of atherosclerosis in women who had early-onset hot flashes.

Bothersome hot flashes made little or no difference. "We have more often seen effects for frequency than severity," explains Dr. Thurston. But weight increased risk, she adds—if a woman was overweight or obese and had frequent or early-onset hot flashes, the heart risk connection was even stronger.

While the mechanisms aren't well-understood, it may be that women who have less-than-healthy blood vessels (but not yet actual cardiovascular disease) may be particularly susceptible to troublesome hot flashes. So the hot flashes serve as a kind of early warning signal for heart disease risk.

## Bones

Hot flashes may also be linked to bone density, osteoporosis and fracture risk. One Korean study found that women who had hot flashes, compared with those who never did, had lower bone density. That was true even after adjusting for other risk factors such as smoking, age, weight and exercise. (Lower bone density increases the risk that you'll develop osteoporosis.)

A separate American study analyzed data from nearly 30,000 women (ages 50 to 79) followed for more than eight years at 40 different medical centers. None were taking hormone therapy. Those with moderate-to-severe hot flashes, compared with those with no hot flashes, were 78% more likely to have a hip fracture.

## The Brain

This research is more preliminary, but there may be a hot flash link to brain changes that may increase a woman's risk for dementia. In a small study of 20 healthy midlife women who didn't have cardiovascular disease and weren't taking hormone therapy, hot flashes per se weren't linked with dementia risk, Dr. Thurston and her colleagues have found. But women who had more night sweats—hot flashes during the nighttime—were much more likely to have high levels of "white matter intensities" in their brains. "White matter intensities are a marker of small vessel disease," explains Dr. Thurston, "which is, in turn, a marker for increased risk for dementia." These associations were not accounted for by sleep quality or quantity or hormone levels.

## Diabetes

In a long-term Australian study, women who reported having severe, early-onset hot flashes were 55% more likely to develop type 2 diabetes during the 15-year follow-up period than women who had mild hot flashes. A separate SWAN study found that women who had hot flashes or night sweats tended to have more insulin resistance, a precursor to diabetes, than women without them.

## Depression and Anxiety

Women who have more hot flashes and night sweats are more likely to suffer from negative mood, such as increased depression and anxiety. These relationships are likely bidirectional—that is, the hot flashes and night sweats cause negative mood, and the negative mood also makes the hot flashes and night sweats less tolerable. In some studies—but not all—disrupted sleep accounts for the associations between night sweats and depressed mood.

## What to Do

The research on hot flashes' links to overall health is still new, so it's too early to draw firm conclusions about cause and effect. In some cases, early, frequent or severe hot flashes might be caused by underlying physiological problems—in other cases, especially with night sweats, bad hot flashes may just make it awfully hard to get a good night's sleep.

But if your hot flashes are frequent or severe, make it a wake-up call to take better care of yourself. "Women who are having a lot of hot flashes or who started having them early should stay on top of their health," says Dr. Thurston. "Watch your diet and remain physically active. Control cholesterol, triglycerides and blood pressure, and see your health-care provider at regular intervals for standard preventive health care." And if you smoke cigarettes, get help so you can quit. Controlling your risk for these factors may help level the playing field, she says.

If you're wondering whether treating your hot flashes will help minimize any or all of the above risks, well, unfortunately, there's no evidence for that.

***But one thing is clear:*** There's no reason to suffer. Hormone therapy, and nonhormonal medications and supplements, have been shown to reduce hot flashes, and mind-body disciplines such as hypnosis and cognitive behavioral therapy can be effective, too.

***The best approach:*** Redouble your efforts to improve your health habits to both curb hot flashes and improve your long-term health. Regular vigorous exercise, along with a largely plant-based diet, may also help reduce hot flashes—and reduce your risk for these chronic diseases. And if treating your night sweats helps you get restorative sleep again, you'll not only feel much better but will be doing your long-term health a world of good.

# A Pollen That Banishes Hot Flashes

Study titled "Nonhormonal Treatment of Perimenopausal and Menopausal Climacteric Symptoms" by James A. Simon, MD, CCD, NCMP, clinical professor of obstetrics and gynecology, The George Washington University School of Medicine, and René Druckman, MD, presented at the American College of Obstetricians and Gynecologists Annual Scientific and Clinical Meeting 2016. Dr. Simon is a Washington, DC–based physician who provides patient-focused care for women across the reproductive life cycle, from adolescence to childbirth, and through the menopausal transition.

For women going through the menopausal transition, there's no better discovery than a safe, natural, nonhormonal treatment for hot flashes that really works.

So a study just presented at the annual scientific meeting of the American College of Obstetricians and Gynecologists caught our eye. It focused on an over-the-counter botanical extract derived from pollen. Could such a simple remedy really improve symptoms and quality of life?

To learn more, we spoke with the study's author, James A. Simon, MD, an ob-gyn in private practice in Washington, DC, and professor at The George Washington University School of Medicine and former president of the North American Menopause Society.

## A Beekeeper's Discovery

Relizen, the brand name in the US of the botanical extract, was developed after an accidental discovery—a Swedish beekeeper noticed that when bees feasted on the pollen of a particular flower, they seemed more energetic. So he wondered if giving that pollen to men and women would make them more energetic, too.

"It didn't work," said Dr. Simon. "But menopausal women who took it said that their hot flashes were better." So the extract was developed using just the cytoplasm (material inside the cell) of the pollen—according to the manufacturer, that removes the pollen allergens. It's actually been available in Europe under different names for about 15 years, and it is backed up by peer-reviewed research. In a 2005 double-blind placebo-controlled study of 64 menopausal women, 65% of those who took it had fewer hot flashes—compared with 38% of those who took a placebo. It's been used by more than a million women in Europe.

In the recent study, 324 women going through the menopausal transition took Relizen daily for three months. To get into the study, the women had to be having hot flashes—and be bothered by them.

***Results:*** 86% had fewer hot flashes, and for 91%, their hot flashes were less severe. What the recent study adds is an emphasis on self-assessed quality of life—fatigue, irritability, sleep quality. These all got better, says Dr. Simon, who has no financial stake in the company that makes Relizen. "Their sense of well-being improved," he said. The mechanism—how this extract works—isn't well understood. Side effects, such as stomach upset, were rare and tended to go away after a week or two.

## An Additional Benefit for Breast Cancer Survivors

Because research has confirmed that it doesn't affect hormones, Relizen may have a particular role to play for women who have survived breast cancer and have been told that hormonal treatments aren't safe for them. Currently, the only nonhormonal FDA-approved prescription for relief of menopausal symptoms such as hot flashes is the antidepressant *paroxetine* (Brisdelle, which has the same active ingredient as the antidepressant Paxil). But this antidepressant not only has side effects such as headaches, nausea, weight changes, reduced sex drive and interference with the ability to have an orgasm—it may also interfere with the action of *tamoxifen*, the drug that is often prescribed after breast cancer treatment to prevent recurrence. Relizen, according to a recent study in *Menopause*, doesn't affect the action of tamoxifen.

## Should You Try It?

If you want relief from hot flashes and night sweats, Relizen is one of many options, said Dr. Simon. Hormone therapy, such as estrogen, is certainly the most effective for symptomatic relief, but many women want to avoid taking systemic hormones based on safety concerns.

Plant-based supplements that have estrogenic effects can help, and Dr. Simon occasionally recommends Remifemin, an over-the-counter product that contains the estrogenic herb black cohosh. "I double the dose on the package insert to achieve the best results," he said. Purified soy phytoestrogens also work for some patients, he notes. If you decide to pursue either option, he recommends that you work with a health-care professional, as there are safety questions for some women in taking estrogenic compounds, especially women with or at high risk of developing breast cancer.

Among nondrug approaches, he's seen success with hypnosis. Even acupuncture, which hasn't been shown in studies to be effective for hot flashes, appears to work for some people, said Dr. Simon.

What he likes about Relizen is that it's so safe—for any woman, including those with a history of hormone-sensitive breast cancer—that it's fine to try on your own. "A patient can acquire it by herself and see if it's beneficial—before seeing her practitioner," said Dr. Simon. "If it doesn't work after two or three months, she can see her health-care professional for other options." (*Note*: Relizen is currently available through the manufacturer's website.)

---

## Better Hot Flash Defense

Menopausal women who received up to 20 acupuncture treatments reported 36.7% fewer hot flashes after six months, according to a recent study. Hot flashes and night sweats increased by 6% in the women who did not get acupuncture.

### Exercise Can Reduce Hot Flashes

Researchers found that women who exercised reported 60% fewer hot flashes than women who did not work out. And women who exercised and who had hot flashes perspired less...had a much better ability to regulate their body heat...and had less intense hot flashes.

Study by researchers at Liverpool John Moores University, Liverpool, UK, published in *The Journal of Physiology*.

***Theory:*** Acupuncture may stimulate the production of endorphins, "feel-good" chemicals that help stabilize body temperature.

***To find an acupuncturist:*** Check the website of the National Certification Commission for Acupuncture and Oriental Medicine, NCCAOM.org.

Nancy Avis, PhD, professor of social sciences and health policy, Wake Forest School of Medicine, Winston-Salem, North Carolina.

---

## To Stop Hot Flashes, Keep This Diary

JoAnn E. Manson, MD, MPH, DrPH, chief, division of preventive medicine, interim executive director, Connors Center for Women's Health and Gender Biology, Brigham and Women's Hospital and professor of medicine and Michael and Lee Bell Professor of Women's Health, Harvard Medical School, Boston. She is author of *Hot Flashes, Hormones & Your Health*.

If you're experiencing hot flashes, the hallmark symptom of menopause, you're eager—OK, maybe desperate—to find ways to make them stop. Maybe you're wondering if you should consider supplements, a change in diet, breathing exercises, hypnosis or even hormone therapy.

But there is an effective approach you may have overlooked entirely.

You.

Understanding your own response to factors in your daily life that can bring hot flashes is the first step to minimizing them. It's also a good way to figure out whether anything you're doing is helping. All you have to do is live your life the way you already are—and jot down certain things that happen to you. Below are the exact steps to take—and we've even created a downloadable tracker to get you started.

### Hot Flash Triggers Are Personal ...so Get to Know Yours

Hot flashes seemingly come out of the blue, often at inopportune times—in a meeting at work, at a family event, in the middle of the night (waking you up). In reality, though, many hot flashes occur in response to a trigger.

Drinking a hot beverage or sleeping in a warm room are common triggers, but there are many others, according to JoAnn Manson, MD, an endocrinologist at Brigham and Women's Hospital and professor of medicine and women's health at Harvard Medical School. Other commonly reported triggers include spicy food, smoking, hot weather, alcohol, caffeine, exercising vigorously, becoming dehydrated and even using a hair dryer or curling iron.

***But here's the rub:*** Not every woman is affected by any particular trigger...and your set of triggers could be unique to you.

One woman may have hot flashes after drinking wine—while another is fine with wine but coffee sets her off. A nice warm bath? That's an invitation to an internal furnace for one woman, while for another it's a relaxing, soothing—even cooling—ritual.

Although there is little rigorous research on the role of "triggers," many are common sense and women are able to identify them quickly, explains Dr. Manson. If you can identify the foods, actions and scenarios that set off hot flashes for you, you can learn to avoid them. Presto—fewer flashes.

## The Tracking Edge

The best way to identify your triggers? Keep a hot flash diary. In addition to helping you notice physical triggers such as eating hot soup or sitting in an overheated room—which make immediate sense when you think about it—tracking can help uncover the less obvious triggers that you might not have imagined are setting you off, including other foods, activities and the powerful effect of emotional stress. Women can feel a hot flash coming on when they hear upsetting news or sometimes when they are preparing to speak in front of a group of people. Indeed, anything that stresses you, even the most mundane hassles, could be a trigger. And, once again, women don't all react to different stresses the same way—so learning how to deal with your stress triggers can be a "cool" thing.

Tracking your hot flashes is also a great way to monitor the effects of any actions that you take to minimize symptoms—to see if what you're trying is working. Maybe you'll try nutritional approaches such as soy and flax seeds or mind-body methods such as hypnosis, paced breathing or cognitive behavioral therapy. By tracking your flashes before you start and for a few weeks afterward, you'll know whether any new approach is helping.

Got an appointment with your health-care provider? Bring in your diary to inspire constructive discussion about what may help you, and continue using it if you start on a new medical treatment such as an antidepressant or hormone therapy.

How long should you track? It depends on how frequent your hot flashes are. If you get one or more every day, tracking for just a week or so should give you a good idea. If flashes come only a few times a week or even less, you may need to track for a month.

Women should feel empowered to play a role in managing their menopause symptoms, emphasizes Dr. Manson. She does offer a reality check, however. While many flashes occur because of triggers, others are simply physiological responses to fluctuating estrogen levels. So don't expect zero flashes. But if you're bothered by hot flashes, finding a safe and easy way to have fewer is always a good idea.

### Look Four Years Younger

Smile! In a recent study, 2,000 people were asked to estimate the age of women in photographs. A smile took two to four years off, while people with sad faces looked one year older.

DailyMail.com

## Menopause and Insomnia Speed Aging

Menopause—and the insomnia that goes with it—speeds aging. Women who start menopause at an earlier age are biologically older than those who begin menopause later in life. Researchers determined that menopause increases cellular aging by an average of 6%. Insomnia, which often accompanies menopause, also leads to faster biological aging, according to another study.

Two studies of more than 5,000 women led by researchers at David Geffen School of Medicine and Semel Institute for Neuroscience and Human Behavior, both at University of California, Los Angeles, published in *Proceedings of the National Academy of Sciences* and *Biological Psychiatry*, respectively.

## The One Sleep Habit That Most Helps Your Health

Study titled "Smoking, Screen-Based Sedentary Behavior, and Diet Associated with Habitual Sleep Duration and Chronotype: Data from the UK Biobank" by Freda Patterson, PhD, assistant professor of biobehavioral health and nutrition at University of Delaware, Newark, and colleagues published in *Annals of Behavioral Medicine.*

If you're trying to live a healthier life and resist the temptation to gobble down that extra piece of chocolate cake tonight and then blow off your workout tomorrow morning...here's a tip from the world of behavioral health science—go to sleep...earlier.

While lifestyle change is never easy, there's growing evidence that becoming less of a night owl and more of a morning lark is a good place to start. Hitting the sack earlier may not only help you get more sleep—a healthy thing in itself—but also make it easier to achieve other healthy lifestyle changes.

You've heard of gateway drugs. But an earlier bedtime may be the opposite...a gateway to healthier behavior.

Yes, you can change. Here's why you should —and how.

### Body Clocks, Watching TV and What You Ate Last Night

It's already well known that getting too little sleep, on a chronic basis, is strongly associated with an increased risk for heart disease, stroke, diabetes and other disorders. What the recent research found is that *when* you hit the hay is linked with three other behaviors that are major risk factors for disease.

The study, published in *Annals of Behavioral Medicine*, which analyzed data from 440,000 British adults, found that those who characterized themselves as "morning people" compared with "evening people" ate 25% more fruit and 13% more vegetables...and spent less time on sedentary activities such as watching TV (about 20 fewer minutes a day) and computer screens (about eight fewer minutes a day). "Morning people" also were 60% less likely to be smokers.

### Can Becoming a Lark Lead to Healthier Habits?

While the study does not show cause and effect, the study's lead author, Freda Patterson, PhD, assistant professor of health promotion in the department of behavioral health and nutrition at University of Delaware, believes there are good reasons to think that poor sleep habits lead to poor lifestyle habits—not the other way around.

One reason is a body of research about how people use time. People who go to bed later, Dr. Patterson noted, tend to have expanded evening recreation time, which might involve eating less healthy foods late at night and staying on the computer late at night. (Ask yourself—are you more likely to be eating fruits and veggies during the day...or late at night in front of the TV? Are those extra hours at the end of the day likely to be the ones in which you're exercising?)

Physiology plays a role, too. If you've had too little sleep, you may feel sluggish and need an energy boost in the evening...and eating sugary foods may feel like just the ticket. Smokers might get a similar lift from nicotine. Inadequate sleep is also related to stress and anxiety, added Dr. Patterson, which people might "treat" with these bad habits.

A good goal may be to shift your bedtime a half-hour earlier in five- to 10-minute increments, said Dr. Patterson. You'll likely spend less time watching screens and munching, and you may find you have more energy the next day to resist food temptations, eat healthier and be more physically active. "If we can get people to improve sleep, it may percolate to also improve these other risk behaviors," says Dr. Patterson. "Sleep may be the behavior that could facilitate improvements in cardiovascular and metabolic health."

---

# Is Your Body Clock Out of Whack? It Can Seriously Harm Your Health

Phyllis C. Zee, MD, PhD, professor of neurology, neurobiology and physiology in the department of neurology at Northwestern University Feinberg School of Medicine in Chicago and director of the school's Center for Circadian and Sleep Medicine.

---

The time you go to sleep at night and the time you wake up in the morning can be crucial to your health—and not only because you need enough sleep. It's also because you need to sleep at the right time of the night. For good health, you need to match your bedtime and wake-up times to your personal "clock genes"—genes that control your sleep/wake cycle along with many other biological fluctuations such as blood pressure and blood sugar. *If you don't, circadian disruption can result, putting your health in danger...*

## Circadian Disruption

Your biological rhythms are timed to Earth's 24-hour cycle of light and dark. B ut your body also runs on internally generated cycles that are a nearly perfect match for the 24-hour rhythm of day and night. Called circadian rhythms, these internal cycles are governed by the suprachiasmatic nucleus (SCN), a "body clock" located in the hypothalamus region of the brain.

Responding to light and dark, the SCN sends signals to every part of your body, regulating when you fall asleep and wake up, when you're hungry, when blood sugar levels rise and fall, when hormones are released—in fact, nearly every biological and behavioral process is regulated by the SCN.

In addition, there are clock genes that produce proteins that regulate rhythms within cells—scientists estimate that 20% of all genes are involved in the body's rhythms. Clock genes help determine whether you tend to go to bed early and wake up early ...or go to bed late and wake up late.

When the external rhythms of light and dark don't match your body's unique circadian rhythms—a condition called circadian disruption—your health suffers. Circadian disruption has been linked to many health problems (see list at end of article).

Fortunately, there are ways to prevent or reverse circadian disruption, including the following...

## Match Your Rhythm to Your Sleep Schedule

Some people have clock genes that run slightly faster than the 24-hour day-night cycle, making them tired earlier in the evening. Some people have clock genes that run slower, making them tired later in the evening. Which are you?

***How to tell:*** If you usually feel at your best—your most awake and alert—in the morning, you're what I call a "morning type." If you usually feel your best in the evening, you're an "evening type."

To be healthy, you must synchronize these genetic rhythms with your bedtime and wake-up time. In addition to timing, stability of sleep and wake times is important. When there's more than a two-hour difference between the time that is best for you to go to bed and when you actually go to bed, you're desynchronized—and your health is at risk.

***What to do:*** Establish a bedtime and wake-up time that reflect whether you're a morning type (*Example*: 10:30 pm bedtime and 6:30 am wake-up time) or an evening type (*Example*: Midnight and 8:00 am). Don't vary those times by more than one-half to one hour. If you work full-time during the week, don't vary those times by more than two hours during the weekend.

## Get More Light

One study compared people who worked near a window to windowless workers and found that those next to windows had better overall health and slept an average of 46 minutes more per night during the workweek over a one-month period—because daily exposure to light helped prevent desynchronization.

***What to do:*** Try to get natural light during the day. Even 15 or 20 minutes a day can help.

## Get Less Light in the Evening

While bright light in the morning and afternoon is synchronizing, bright light in the evening is desynchronizing—because it blocks the production of melatonin, a hormone that helps regulate the sleep-wake cycle.

***Recent research:*** Exposure to artificial light at night was linked to a 52% increased risk for breast cancer. But reducing artificial light at night—by using a bedtime reading lamp instead of overhead lights, for example—decreased risk by 81%. And a study published in *International Journal of Obesity* found that exposure to artificial light at night was linked to a 97% increased risk for obesity.

***What to do:*** Two to three hours before bedtime, turn off overhead lights to reduce brightness. Use table lamps instead.

At night, avoid the melatonin-suppressing "blue light" of electronic devices, such as computers, tablets and cell phones. LED TV screens give off blue light, too. If you must use blue-light devices at night, wear blue-blocking glasses or goggles, widely available online for less than $10. Or consider downloading an app such as f.lux or Twilight, both of which reduce blue light on your screens at night.

## Eat Regular Meals

A regular eating cycle is as important as a regular sleep-wake cycle in keeping you synchronized. Morning types tend to eat a big breakfast and smaller dinner. Evening types tend to favor dinner and skip breakfast.

***What to do:*** Whatever your type, try to eat your three meals at about the same time every day.

Finish dinner at least four hours before bedtime. That habit not only helps you stay synchronized but also helps prevent weight gain—studies show the closer to bedtime you eat, the more likely you are to be overweight.

## Structure Your Day

In addition to regular mealtimes, regular times for socializing, exercising and other daily activities help prevent desynchronization, improving sleep and memory—particularly in people age 55 and older.

***What to do:*** Exercise at the same time, several days a week. Get out of the house, and engage in regular, structured social activities such as going to the library or a place of worship. It's the day-to-day regularity of a structured schedule—doing one or more activities the same time every day, a minimum of three to four days a week—that helps create synchronization.

## Consider Taking Melatonin

Taking a melatonin supplement in the right dose at the right time can help restore synchronization and may benefit those evening types who can't fall asleep at bedtime.

***What to do:*** Take one-half to one milligram of melatonin five to six hours before your desired bedtime—that's the right amount and timing to maximize melatonin levels at bedtime.

## Dangers of Circadian Disruption

Circadian disruption has been linked to many health problems, including...

- **Insomnia**
- **High blood pressure, heart attack and stroke**
- **Obesity and diabetes**
- **Memory problems, dementia and Parkinson's disease**
- **Depression and bipolar disorder**
- **Heartburn, IBS and other digestive diseases**
- **Asthma, emphysema and chronic bronchitis**
- **Poor recovery from surgery**
- **Weakened immune system**
- **Cancer**

# Do You Ever Feel Dizzy? Here's What It Might Mean

Jack J. Wazen, MD, an otolaryngologist and otological/neurotological surgeon at the Silverstein Institute in Sarasota, Florida, where he is the director of research for the nonprofit Ear Research Foundation. He is one of the nation's leading experts on hearing and balance disorders and is coauthor of *Dizzy: What You Need to Know About Managing and Treating Balance Disorders.*

Have you ever felt dizzy and light-headed? Chances are the answer is yes. About 50% of adults experience dizziness at some time in their lives.

Feeling dizzy isn't just uncomfortable. It can be dangerous—for example, if you fall or lose control of your car while driving.

There are many different causes of dizziness or vertigo (the feeling that you or the world around you is spinning), so it can be tricky to figure out what's triggering your symptoms.

Here are the five most common causes—and important clues to determine which one is affecting you. Many causes of dizziness aren't serious, but some are, so it's always a good idea to get checked by your doctor.

- **Benign paroxysmal positional vertigo (BPPV).** Millions of tiny crystals, or otoliths, are attached to hair cells in the inner ear. They bend the hairs when you change position, which tells the brain that you've moved. When you have BPPV, the crystals break free and float into a part of the ear where they're not supposed to be.

***Result:*** A bout of vertigo that usually lasts 60 seconds or less.

***Important clues:*** Suspect BPPV when the attacks occur only after you've moved your head...there's a delay of three to five seconds between the head movement and the vertigo...and the severity decreases when you have multiple episodes over a period of minutes or hours.

***What to do:*** Ask your doctor to recommend a therapist who can show you how to do the Epley maneuver. Named after its originator, it consists of five steps that can eliminate symptoms in about 80% of patients. Other maneuvers practiced by therapists also can work.

The Epley maneuver includes reclining on a bed or table and then, in very particular ways, tipping your head to both sides, rolling over on your side and then sitting up, which causes the crystals to return to their usual location. Videos are available on YouTube.com.

- **Ménière's disease.** No one knows what causes Ménière's disease, although it's been linked to autoimmune diseases, viral infections, head injuries and other conditions. It causes intense dizziness, nausea and vertigo when a buildup of endolymph fluid in the inner ear causes pressure changes that interfere with balance.

The episodes come and go. Some people have attacks every few days. Others go weeks or months between attacks. Some people are lucky and have just a single attack—but this is rare.

***Important clue:*** Hearing loss in one ear that mainly affects lower frequencies (such as difficulty hearing a man's voice). This is the opposite of normal, age-related hearing loss, which usually affects high frequencies first.

***What to do:*** Reducing fluid in the inner ear is the cornerstone of treatment. Some patients can achieve this just by consuming less sodium. The FDA advises limiting sodium to no more than 2,300 milligrams (about one teaspoon daily of table salt). But most patients also will need to take a diuretic (sometimes referred to as a "water pill") that helps your body get rid of unneeded salt and water through urine. These include *acetazolamide* (such as the brand Diamox) or *hydrochlorothiazide* (such as the brand HydroDIURIL).

It's helpful to give up caffeine. Caffeine reduces blood circulation in the inner ear. Also, cut back on alcohol and sugar—these can increase dizziness in some people. Reducing stress can help, too. We don't know why, but stress can trigger attacks.

- **Acoustic neuroma.** This is a benign tumor that grows at the base of the brain and can affect a variety of nerves including the auditory nerve. About 3,000 Americans are diagnosed with one of these tumors every year. The symptoms include dizziness, a loss of balance and nausea.

The tumors aren't cancerous, but they can cause serious impairments and even death if they grow large enough. They typically grow about 2 mm (about one-eighth of an inch) a year.

***Important clue:*** Slight hearing loss (usually in one ear), along with the other symptoms mentioned above. Some patients also experience tinnitus, ringing or buzzing sounds in the affected ear.

***What to do:*** Because the tumors are slow-growing, your doctor might decide just to track your progress with periodic MRIs, especially if your symptoms are minor. But there's always a risk that a tumor will cause permanent hearing loss, along with damage to the facial nerve or other structures in the brain. If your doctor is concerned that an acoustic neuroma is dangerous, he/she will probably recommend either surgery or radiation to remove or shrink it.

- **Orthostatic hypotension.** Almost all of us have experienced the occasional dizziness that occurs when we stand up too quickly. For some people, these episodes happen often—this is particularly true for the elderly... those taking blood pressure medication... and people with certain conditions (including heart disease or Parkinson's disease).

***What happens:*** When you stand up, blood is pulled downward and away from your brain. It takes about a minute for your body to adjust to the change in position by increasing the strength of your heartbeat and tightening your blood vessels. In the meantime, a lack of circulation and oxygen to your brain can make you feel dizzy.

***Important clue:*** Suspect orthostatic hypotension when you experience dizziness or light-headedness only when you're changing position—usually when you go from a seated or lying position to standing.

***What to do:*** See your doctor. Orthostatic hypotension, while itself relatively harmless, can be caused by cardiovascular or nervous system disorders that are serious and require treatment. If you are on blood pressure medication, the dosage may need to be adjusted.

Whatever the cause of orthostatic hypotension, it helps if you change positions slowly to give your body time to adjust.

***Example:*** To get out of bed, swing your legs off the bed and sit up...but don't stand up yet. Wait a minute for your blood pressure to stabilize. Then stand up slowly.

- **Dehydration.** You might not think that skimping on fluids could cause your head to spin, but it's not uncommon.

***What happens:*** When you don't drink enough water, your blood volume falls. Reduced blood volume can reduce the amount of blood that circulates through the brain. The result can be dizziness or even fainting spells. Older adults are particularly at risk because the sense of thirst declines with age.

***Important clues:*** People who live in hot climates or take diuretics (the "water pills" often used to treat high blood pressure) are particularly prone to dehydration.

***What to do:*** Drink plenty of water throughout the day—and sip even when you aren't feeling particularly thirsty. Eight glasses a day is a good amount to shoot for. If you're taking a diuretic, ask your doctor whether switching drugs or changing doses might be helpful.

## Hot Flashes at 65...

Susan Davis, MBBS, PhD, chair of women's health, Monash University, Melbourne, Australia.

Many women experience hot flashes and/or night sweats (episodes of excessive sweating during sleep that can soak clothing and/or sheets) for 10 years or more after menopause.

When researchers at Monash University in Melbourne, Australia, studied 2,020 women ages 40 to 65, they found that 42% of women age 60 and older regularly experienced hot flashes and/or night sweats, and most also reported lack of sexual desire and vaginal dryness.

Women who smoke and those who are overweight were more likely to have long-lasting menopausal symptoms, so talk to your doctor about ways to lose weight if your body mass index (a ratio of weight to height) is more than 25. And if you smoke, you should quit!

Initiation of hormone replacement therapy is generally not recommended for women over age 65, but your doctor may prescribe a vaginal estrogen cream to relieve dryness and discomfort during sex.

A low-dose antidepressant, such as *paroxetine* (Paxil) or *venlafaxine* (Effexor), may also help relieve severe hot flash symptoms.

However, hot flashes and night sweats are not always due to menopause. For this reason, your doctor should check for underlying health conditions, such as high blood pressure, thyroid disease and diabetes.

Night sweats that occur without daytime hot flashes can also be an early symptom of some types of cancer, such as lymphoma or leukemia.

## Help for Brain Fog

"Brain fog" during menopause is normal and not a sign of cognitive decline. Women's handling of certain memory tasks declines as levels of estradiol (a form of estrogen) fall. This explains why up to 60% of women going through menopause complain of a kind of brain fog—forgetfulness, trouble concentrating and difficulty thinking clearly.

***Helpful:*** Exercise, and ask your doctor about short-term hormone therapy.

Emily Goard Jacobs, PhD, assistant professor, psychological and brain sciences, at Neuroscience Research Institute, University of California, Santa Barbara. She led a study of brain changes before and during menopause, published in *The Journal of Neuroscience.*

## The MIT Anti-Aging Pill

Michael Fossel, MD, PhD, a leading expert on the use of telomerase for age-related diseases. He is the founder and president of Telocyte, a company that is investigating telomerase therapy for Alzheimer's disease. He is author of *The Telomerase Revolution: The Enzyme That Holds the Key to Human Aging...and Will Soon Lead to Longer, Healthier Lives.* MichaelFossel.com

If there were a pill you could take to live longer, wouldn't you? Wouldn't we all?

Well, now there's a dietary supplement on the market that was developed by a famous scientist—from MIT, no less—that supposedly slows aging. It's called Basis. So we decided to take a hard look at it. Is it really a fountain of youth?

## The Basics About Basis

You may have seen some wild claims about the Basis pill. *So here's what you need to know to really understand it...*

• **It simulates the benefits of eating less.** When animals are underfed—given an adequate diet but one with about 20% or 30% fewer calories than normal—they live longer. We humans could try to eat less, too, but it's tough to sustain when food is widely available—so anti-aging scientists have homed in on compounds called sirtuins that are stimulated during underfeeding. The theory is that sirtuins—which are proteins that protect mitochondria, tiny energy factories in each of our cells—are responsible for the longevity effect.

• **It's based on science—mostly in animals.** Basis, marketed by a company called Elysium Health, contains two active ingredients that have been shown in animal studies to stimulate the body's production of sirtuins...

• Nicotinamide riboside (NR)—250 mg. Your body uses NR to make a coenzyme called nicotinamide adenine dinucleotide or NAD+. (Stay with us!) We have less NAD+ in our bodies as we grow older, and it's a hot area of research for scientists who study aging. In one recent mouse study, for example, published in *Cell Metabolism*, boosting NAD+ stimulated energy metabolism, prevented weight gain and improved insulin sensitivity, eye function and bone density. (The study didn't track whether the mice lived longer, however.) NR, also being studied to protect against hearing loss, is found in tiny amounts in many foods, including edamame (young green soy beans) and broccoli.

• Pterostilbene (PT+)—50 mg. Pterostilbene is similar to resveratrol, a compound found in grapes (and wine) that has been studied for its anti-aging and disease-prevention potential, including for Alzheimer's and osteoporosis—but PT+ is more bioavailable and in some ways more powerful. In animal studies, PT+ has had biological effects that may protect against cancer, neurological disease, inflammation, cardiovascular disease and diabetes. It may lower blood pressure and body weight, although some studies suggest that it may also raise cholesterol levels. It's found in tiny amounts in grapes and berries, especially blueberries.

• **Leading scientists developed it.** The scientist behind Elysium Health and Basis is the well-known and well-respected biologist Leonard Guarente, PhD, who has decades of research in aging under his belt. He runs a lab that studies the biology of aging at the Massachusetts Institute of Technology. Elysium Health's scientific board is packed with other big names in science and health, including six Nobel Prize winners.

• **It's probably safe.** As a dietary supplement, Basis isn't regulated by the US Food and Drug Administration, so it didn't need to undergo human safety studies before going on the market. But the safety research to date has been reassuring. According to anti-aging expert Michael Fossel, MD, PhD, who is not involved with Elysium Health or Basis, "I'm not aware of any safety concerns—and there may be none, but you never know."

• **It'll cost you a pretty penny.** Basis is available only online through the company's website. You can buy a single bottle—a one-month supply of the pills, which are taken twice a day—for $60. If you opt for an annual subscription, the monthly cost goes down to $40, or $480 per year.

## But...Will Basis Really Help You Live Longer?

We knew you'd ask that question. We suspect you know the answer, too—no one really knows. There's no scientific evidence that Basis works in humans. Elysium Health is studying the short-term effects of the pill in people—on body weight, blood pressure, blood sugar and more—and other human trials are planned on the active ingredients (in Japan, for example), but there are no published results yet. To be fair, it's challenging to study a longevity pill in humans, especially because we live pretty long anyway, so you can't expect actual longevity results for decades. But studies can find out whether Basis reduces risk factors for chronic disease, and we'll know that in the next few years.

Dr. Fossel, for one, isn't convinced that it will actually help us live longer. Yes, we lose NAD+ as we age, he explained, but he doesn't believe that simply pouring more of it into our cells is likely to keep us on this planet longer. "Sirtuins are just part of the longevity puzzle," Dr. Fossel said. He believes a better target to get at the root causes of aging is the telomere—the protective "cap" on our chromosomes that shorten with age.

***Here's why:*** "If I take a young cell, it's operating very nicely, but as it gets older, the pattern of gene expression changes, and that's modulated by the telomere," he said. Telomeres themselves don't cause aging, but they're the most "upstream" target that's currently within our grasp. Unfortunately, scientists still are many years away from safely and effectively being able to fiddle with telomere length and gene expression patterns in humans to extend life. "There is nothing on the market that is a miracle drug at this point," he said.

So go ahead and buy Basis if you want to—and can afford it. It's unlikely that it will hurt you, it may prime your mitochondria to work a little better, and it might reduce your risk for chronic disease. Whether it's a longevity pill is something we won't know—for ages.

If you are being treated for any health condition, let your health-care provider know that you're taking this supplement so you can be monitored for "the usual suspects," such as lipids (including cholesterol), liver function, complete blood count and blood pressure. According to Elysium, users report that they sleep better and have more energy and that their hair and nails grow faster—but that's purely anecdotal, of course. Concluded Dr. Fossel, "I think it probably has about as much efficacy as a good exercise program, a reasonable diet and a safe lifestyle." It is not, of course, a substitute for those things.

## To Live Longer, Cook This Way

Helen Vlassara, MD, professor emeritus and former director of the Diabetes and Aging Division at Icahn School of Medicine at Mount Sinai in New York City. She is coauthor, with Sandra Woodruff, MS, RD, and Gary E. Striker, MD, of *Dr. Vlassara's AGE-Less Diet: How Chemicals in the Foods We Eat Promote Disease, Obesity and Aging, and the Steps We Can Take to Stop It.* TheAge-LessWay.com

When it comes to our health, we often focus on what to eat and what not to eat. But just as important is how we prepare the foods we eat. Certain cooking methods can unleash chemical byproducts that have been linked to heart disease, diabetes, Alzheimer's and other chronic diseases.

### Glycotoxins

Sugar is a clingy molecule that attaches to amino acids and fats and changes their structures—a process known as glycation. This triggers a complex chemical reaction that culminates in the production of advanced glycation end products (AGEs). They're sometimes called "glycotoxins" because they trigger inflammation and can lead to cell injury and cell death.

Almost all foods contain AGEs. They're naturally produced by the body as well. But their number vastly increases during food preparation, particularly when you cook with dry, high heat.

Small amounts of AGEs aren't a problem—most are excreted through the kidneys. But the foods that many people prefer—particularly those that are high in sugar and fat and are cooked certain ways—are teeming with AGEs. The body can't cope with the excess, so the AGEs pile up over time. *This leads to...*

- **More heart disease.** AGE-modified proteins and fats can accumulate in blood vessel walls and stimulate clots—the cause of most heart attacks. AGEs also form chemical "cross-links" that stiffen blood vessels and cause high blood pressure.

• **Uncontrolled diabetes.** The high blood glucose (blood sugar) that is the hallmark of diabetes provides fuel for AGE formation. AGEs damage pancreatic cells (resulting in less insulin)...make insulin less effective... and increase diabetes complications, including nerve and blood vessel damage.

• **More cognitive decline.** AGEs damage the protective barrier that insulates the brain from the rest of the body. This allows AGEs to damage brain-specific proteins and produce amyloid plaques—the deposits that occur with Alzheimer's disease. In laboratory studies, animals given a high-AGE diet were much more likely to experience harmful brain changes than those given healthier foods.

• **More kidney disease.** AGEs can injure the blood vessels and other parts of the kidneys, causing them to become scarred and shriveled and greatly reducing their ability to excrete AGEs. As kidney function declines, AGE levels rise in the blood, flooding all tissues of the body and setting the stage for even greater damage to the kidneys and all other organs as well. Studies have shown that patients with chronic kidney disease who are treated with a low-AGE diet have a decrease in circulating AGEs, as well as in levels of markers of inflammation and oxidative stress.

The inflammation from excessive AGEs has been linked to many other conditions, including arthritis, obesity, vision problems and even skin wrinkles.

## Cut AGEs in Half

You can reduce your AGE levels by 50% in as little as one month. *Best steps*...

• **Add moisture, and reduce the heat.** Any form of high-heat cooking—mainly grilling, broiling, frying and roasting—greatly increases AGEs.

***Examples:*** The 500 kilounits (kU) in one serving of raw meat might increase to 5,000 kU after broiling. Moist-heat cooking methods—such as poaching, stewing and braising—are ideal. Consider one serving of chicken. It will contain 600 kU to 1,000 kU when it is stewed or braised, but up to 6,000 kU when it's roasted or grilled.

It is fine to have roasted or grilled food now and then. What's Thanksgiving without roast turkey! But try to limit how often you have these foods.

• **Marinate.** This is a good solution for meat lovers. The acidic ingredients in most marinades—such as lemon juice, wine, tomato juice and vinegar—greatly inhibit AGE formation even when meat is grilled. Depending on the meat's thickness, marinating it for one to two hours will reduce AGEs by up to 50%.

• **Choose lower-AGE foods.** In general, this means eating less meat, cheese and fat and more produce (see list at the end of this article). Beef, poultry and pork have the highest levels of AGEs.

***Important:*** Fatty meats tend to have more AGEs than leaner cuts, but even lean meats will readily produce AGEs when they're prepared with dry heat.

• **Eat minimally processed cheeses.** They aren't cooked, so why are some cheeses so high in AGEs? It is because they're heated during processing and because aging and the removal of liquids during cheese-making increase AGE formation.

***My advice:*** Eat lower-fat cheeses with shorter aging times that undergo the least processing. Cheddar cheese made with 2% milk, for example, has about half the AGEs of cheeses made with whole milk. Avoid Parmesan cheese (2,500 kU) and American cheese (2,600 kU).

• **Get more flavonoids.** These are naturally occurring compounds that appear to activate enzymes that deactivate AGEs, inhibit AGE-related oxidation and trap the molecules that can increase AGE formation.

***Good sources:*** Apples, chili peppers, berries, broccoli, kale and green or black tea. Spices and herbs that have similar effects include turmeric, cinnamon, parsley, rosemary and sage.

• **Go easy on the sweets.** Even though sugar and other sweeteners don't contain a lot of AGEs, levels increase when they're heated—when you're baking, for example, or during the factory production of breakfast cereals. High-sugar foods often contain fats and proteins, which increase the potential for harmful chemical reactions.

***Warning:*** The fructose in many soft drinks and processed foods causes a 10-fold greater rate of glycation than simple glucose. Dark-colored soft drinks (such as colas) are particularly bad because the color comes from caramelized (dry-heated) sugars. Diet colas contain nearly the same amount of AGEs as their sweetened counterparts.

## AGE Counts

• **Very Low (100 kU/serv or less)**—Bread • Eggs (poached, scrambled, boiled) • Fruits (fresh) • Grains (boiled, steamed) • Milk • Soy milk • Vegetables (fresh, steamed) • Yogurt

• **Low (101-500 kU/serv)**—Avocado • Fruits (dried, roasted, grilled) • Legumes (cooked, canned) • Olive oil • Olives • Pasta • Soy veggie burgers • Vegetables (roasted, grilled)

• **Medium (501-1,000 kU/serv)**—Cheese (reduced-fat) • Chicken (poached, steamed, stewed, braised) • Chocolate (dark) • Fish (poached, steamed) • Sunflower and pumpkin seeds (raw) • Tofu (raw) • Tuna or salmon (canned)

• **High (1,001-3,000 kU/serv)**—Beef or pork (stewed, braised) • Butter • Cheese (full-fat and processed varieties) • Fish (grilled, broiled, baked) • French fries • Nuts (raw) • Sweets (donuts, pies, cakes, pastries, etc.)

• **Very High (3,001-5,000 kU/serv)**—Chicken (skinless, broiled, grilled, roasted) • Fish (breaded and fried) • Pork chops (pan-fried) • Single cheeseburger (fast food) • Grilled cheese sandwich • Tofu (broiled, sautéed) • Turkey (roasted)

• **Highest (5,001 kU/serv or more)**—Bacon (fried) • Beef (roasted, grilled, broiled, well-done) • Chicken with skin (broiled, grilled, roasted) • Chicken (fried, fast-food nuggets) • Double cheeseburger (fast food) • Fish sandwich (fast food) • Hot dog • Sausage • Pizza

# Healthy Gums Tied to Longer Lives for Women

Rachel M. Bond, MD, associate director, Women's Heart Health, Lenox Hill Hospital, New York City.

Ronald Burakoff, DMD, chair, dental medicine, North Shore University Hospital, Manhasset, New York.

Michael LaMonte, PhD, MPH, research associate professor, epidemiology, University at Buffalo, New York.

*Journal of the American Heart Association*, news release.

Here's another reason to get flossing: Recent research suggests that gum disease is linked with earlier death in older women.

"Older women may be at higher risk for death because of their periodontal condition," said study author Michael LaMonte, PhD, MPH.

Dr. LaMonte is research associate professor in epidemiology at the University at Buffalo, in New York. His team published its findings in the *Journal of the American Heart Association.*

One cardiologist said the study raises an intriguing notion.

"Dental hygiene is an important part of our patients' overall health, and perhaps with this study it may prompt us to further investigate its direct impact on the heart," said Rachel Bond, MD, associate director for Women's Heart Health at Lenox Hill Hospital in New York City.

## Background

According to background information from the researchers, gum disease affects nearly two-thirds of US adults aged 60 and older. Complete tooth loss affects about one-third of US adults 60 and older, and often results from gum disease.

### The Study

But can poor gum health affect longevity? To find out, Dr. LaMonte's team tracked data on more than 57,000 women aged 55 and older.

Over nearly seven years, more than 3,800 of the women died, with 3,589 of those deaths due to heart disease.

According to the researchers, a history of gum disease was associated with a 12% higher risk of death from any cause.

Some women had particularly poor dental health, losing all of their teeth over the study period. These women also tended to have more heart disease risk factors, were less educated and had fewer dental appointments. They also had a 17% increased risk of death from any cause, the researchers said.

However, there did not appear to be an association between gum disease or tooth loss and increased risk of death from heart disease, the researchers added.

### Expert Commentary

Reviewing the findings, Dr. Bond stressed that a direct link between gum disease and heart disease is far from certain.

"Although this study highlights a valid point, it's not set up to prove any cause-and-effect relationship," she noted. So just because you're having more dental issues, that "doesn't mean you are setting yourself up for a heart attack," she said.

Ronald Burakoff, DMD, is chair of dental medicine at North Shore University Hospital in Manhasset, New York. He said the study's large sample size helps bolster its validity, but he concurred with Dr. Bond that the research can only point to an association.

"Additional studies are needed to see if treatment of periodontal conditions reduces the death rate for postmenopausal women, which would allow the researchers to establish a direct cause-and-effect," Dr. Burakoff said.

### Conclusion

Still, dental hygiene may have some role to play in overall health, he added.

"Perhaps the most important take-away message for postmenopausal women is that keeping your teeth has implications for avoiding [early] death," Dr. Burakoff said.

The U.S. National Institute of Dental and Craniofacial Research has more information on gum disease at NIDCR.nih.gov. Search "gum disease."

---

## Watch Pot Intake

Recreational marijuana use increased by 71% among adults over age 50 between 2006 and 2013.

***One concern:*** The concurrent use of marijuana and prescription drugs could increase physical/mental problems in older adults.

*Addiction.*

---

## Stand Tall and Live Longer!

Steven Weiniger, DC, managing partner and instructor at BodyZone.com, an organization devoted to improving posture as a way to promote health and longevity. Dr. Weiniger is also author of *Stand Taller–Live Longer: An Anti-Aging Strategy* and developer of the new app PostureZone.

---

Once you move out of your mother's house, probably no one reminds you to stand up straight. But good posture is not only important for looking your best, it's also essential for good health!

***Why:*** As human beings, our bodies are designed to stand upright, a position that helps us maintain balance. When your shoulders are hunched, you have an increased risk for falls. Plus, hunching causes other parts of your body to compensate to restore balance, which can result in upper and lower back pain, neck pain, headaches and other aches. Additionally, some research has linked bad posture to reduced lung function, poor circulation, digestive issues and much more.

## Why We Hunch

Let's face it—hunching is easier than standing up straight. Over the years, your body settles into its most comfortable position, and that becomes your "normal." The problem with this comfortable position is that it contributes to atrophy of the hip, shoulder, upper back and core muscles because they aren't being used to hold your body in alignment. Year by year, this muscle atrophy makes slumping more exaggerated and can lead to the health problems mentioned above.

Modern life also contributes to hunching. According to a 2016 Nielsen report, we spend an average of three hours each day hunched over a smartphone, computer or tablet...and another four hours slouched in front of a TV.

## Help for the Hunch

To develop good posture and lose the hunch, you need to strengthen the muscles mentioned earlier that help make standing up straight second nature. This simple routine takes no more than about four minutes to complete. If you do the exercises daily, you will start showing results in as little as two weeks.

### Exercise 1: Stabilize Shoulders Down

- **Lie flat on your back on a mat on the floor,** legs extended or knees bent (whatever is most comfortable), with your arms in a "T" position (elbows should be in line with your shoulders). Your face needs to be parallel to the ceiling.

- **Bend your elbows so that your fingers point toward the ceiling and your palms face your feet.**

- **Keeping your elbows on the floor,** pull your shoulders down toward your feet. Then bring your palms toward the floor as far as you comfortably can while keeping your shoulders down. Hold the position for three to five breaths (see below for the proper breathing technique).

### Exercise 2: Open Chest Up

- **Lie flat on your back and bend your elbows** so that your fingers point toward the ceiling and your palms face your feet as in Exercise 1.

- **Bring your hands backward toward the floor as far as you comfortably can.** Your arms will be in a "goalpost" position.

***Important:*** Keep your shoulders down as in Exercise 1. Do not shrug them.

Do this three to five times. Inhale as you point your fingers to the ceiling, and exhale as you bring your hands toward the floor.

### Exercise 3: Floor Angels

- **Lie flat on your back as above,** but with your arms flat on the floor in a goalpost position.

- **Keeping your forearms parallel,** and your shoulders on the floor, slide your arms up and down on the floor. Again, do not shrug your shoulders while performing this exercise.

Do this three to five times. Inhale as you slide your arms up, exhale as you slide your arms down.

Once you master this, make the exercise more challenging by holding and stretching an elastic exercise band between your hands as you move your arms up and down.

### Exercise 4: Pinkie Touch

- **Lie facedown on the floor,** with your forehead resting on the floor. Your arms should be straight at your sides with palms facing down.

- **Keeping shoulders down and elbows straight,** move your hands together beneath your torso so that your pinkie fingers are touching. (You'll have to raise your hips a bit to give your hands room to move.) Hold this position for three to five breaths.

## Better Breathing

As you perform these exercises, it's important to breathe from the belly, not the chest. *Why*: When you breathe from the chest, your shoulders naturally hunch...but when you breathe from the belly, your shoulders stay in place.

***To get the hang of belly breathing:*** Stretch an elastic exercise band across your lower back, with an end in each hand. Then crisscross the band in front of you, across your waist, about the level of your navel (you will need to exchange the band ends in your hands). Keeping your elbows bent at your sides, make the band snug but not tight. If you are breathing correctly, as you inhale, you will feel your belly pressing against the band, while your chest remains still. Exhale through pursed lips as your belly deflates.

### How to Monitor Your Posture

To track changes in your posture, ask a friend to take an annual photo of you from the front and side. Or use PostureZone, a free app.

### Self-Test for Hunching

Even people who don't think that they hunch their shoulders probably slump to some degree. *Try this simple exercise to find out if you're slumping (you can do this while standing or sitting)...*

- **First, bring your shoulders forward and in toward your chest,** and then bring them up toward your ears. This is an exaggerated hunch.
- **Next, pull your shoulders back and down toward your feet.** This is how your shoulders should be positioned for good posture. If this position feels uncomfortable or painful, you may have a hunching problem.

## Stave Off Cataracts

Jeffrey Anshel, OD, optometrist in private practice in Encinitas, California, and author of *Smart Medicine for Your Eyes.*

One of the leading causes of vision loss in older adults, cataracts can only be removed with surgery. But they tend to grow very gradually, and you may be able to slow their progression.

Vitamins C and E and the carotenoids lutein and zeaxanthin have, in some cases, delayed progression of cataracts for 10 years or more. If you are developing cataracts, your doctor can recommend an optimal supplement dosage, but you can reap the benefits of these nutrients by including them in your diet. Citrus fruits, strawberries and broccoli are high in vitamin C. Wheat germ, almonds and sunflower seeds are good sources of vitamin E. Get lutein and zeaxanthin in leafy greens.

Since ultraviolet light raises the risk for cataracts, also be sure to protect your eyes with sunglasses that block both UVA and UVB rays.

## Has Your Eye Color Changed?

Brett Levinson, MD, an ophthalmologist and cornea specialist in private practice in Baltimore. SpecializedEyeCare.com

Eye color (the color of the iris) does not normally change with time. However, as some people grow older, a change in the appearance of the cornea (the clear covering over the front of the eye) can cause the eyes to appear to have a bluish tint.

This condition, called arcus (or arcus senilis or arcus corneae), is harmless and often occurs with age.

Fat deposits in the cornea can cause a visible grayish-blue arc. This appears on the cornea where the white meets the iris. Arcus can start out as a partial arc and eventually become a complete circle, giving the appearance of a blue eye color when someone looks at his/her own eyes in the mirror. But on a comprehensive eye exam by an eye doctor, the iris color will appear the same and the arcus can be seen on the cornea.

Arcus does not affect vision and requires no treatment. In adults over age 60, arcus occurs for no known reason except for aging.

However, when arcus appears in younger people (under age 40), the condition can be a sign of high cholesterol levels that may require treatment.

***Also:*** People who have blue eyes can have a darkening of the iris color due to prostaglandin analog drops, such as *latanoprost* (Xalatan), used to treat glaucoma...or Latisse, a prescription product that lengthens and darkens eyelashes. In rare cases, the prostaglandin that is also an ingredient in Latisse may get into the eye and affect iris pigmentation. These changes can be permanent.

## Feeling Blue?

You may want to get your eyes checked.

***Recent finding:*** Older adults with cataracts were up to 50% more likely to suffer from depressive symptoms.

*Optometry and Vision Science.*

# Your Vision Is Great? Time for an Exam!

Study titled "Value of Routine Eye Examinations in Asymptomatic Patients" by researchers at University of Waterloo, Ontario, Canada, published in *Optometry and Vision Science.*

It's been a few years—OK, let's be honest, more than a few years—since you last had a comprehensive eye exam. But you can see fine with your current prescription. What are the odds that you really need a new exam?

Glad you asked—it's 58%!

That's the finding of a Canadian study of more than 2,500 people who went for a routine comprehensive eye exam. They were all "asymptomatic," meaning that they had no preexisting condition such as an eye disease or diabetes that would require more frequent eye exams.

The last time the 40- to 64-year-olds had been examined was nearly three (2.9) years earlier, on average. For those 65 and older, it was between one and one-and-a-half years earlier. *Findings...*

- **41% needed new spectacle prescriptions.**
- **16% had new "critical" diagnoses, such as glaucoma or cataracts.**
- **31% needed new "management,"** such as a referral to another doctor or a new treatment.

Put it all together and a full 58% of those who went in for a routine eye exam had some benefit from the visit. The older the patient, the more likely the exam turned up something, even if just a prescription change.

## How Often Should You Go for an Eye Exam?

The American Academy of Ophthalmology recommends that "asymptomatic" men and women get a comprehensive eye exam (which includes checking for glaucoma, age-related macular degeneration and cataracts)...

- **Age 40 through 54: Every two to four years.**
- **Age 55 through 64: Every one to three years.**
- **Over 65: Every one to two years.**

The recent research suggests that it may be prudent to follow the earlier side of those ranges. If your eye doctor recommends more frequent exams based on a specific condition or your health history, follow that advice instead, of course.

We're not talking about just getting your prescription tested by an optician—a full exam can pick up a long list of eye conditions, the earlier the better. The older you are, studies show, the more likely these exams will help not just adjust your prescription but reduce your risk for vision loss. In short, it's an appointment that could save your sight.

## Easier Glaucoma Treatment

A new contact lens is in development that slowly releases medication for up to one month. The lens works as well as eyedrops for treating glaucoma—and causes no changes in normal vision.

*Ophthalmology.*

## New Ways to Fight Dry Eyes and Protect Your Vision

Robert Latkany, MD, an ophthalmologist and founder and director of the Dry Eye Clinic at the New York Eye and Ear Infirmary of Mount Sinai and the Dry Eye Center of New York. He is actively involved in dry eye research and is author of *The Dry Eye Remedy, Revised Edition.* DryEyeDoctor.com

Once you're middle-aged or older, you may assume that it's normal to have dry, red, irritated eyes much of the time. But it's not.

Even though more than one-third of American adults endure this common eye complaint, it's a mistake to just put up with it.

Over time, dry eye can impair your ability to see clearly (usually temporarily but permanently in severe cases)...make it difficult to drive at night...and cause wrinkles on and around the eyelids that add years to your appearance.

***Latest developments:*** The FDA has recently approved new medication for treating dry eye—and another drug is being developed to increase levels of a protein that's needed for eye lubrication.

Sometimes you can control dry eye with lifestyle changes and the use of artificial tears. But whether you need medication or not, there are ways to largely eliminate these troubling symptoms and keep your eyes healthy.

### Tears: Not Just for Crying

Our eyes naturally produce about five to 10 ounces of moisture (tears) each day to help prevent the dry, scratchy and/or burning that results from dry eye. When we're exposed to dust, smoke, excessive sun, dry heat, air-conditioning and even hair dryers, most people produce even more tears.

Unfortunately, some people, for unknown reasons, simply don't produce enough tears. Tear production also tends to decline with age—particularly in women after menopause, when lower estrogen levels are to blame. Eye dryness is also on the rise among people who spend hours a day squinting at computers and smartphones. People who wear contact lenses while sleeping or use ill-fitting lenses are also subject to dry eye.

***Under-recognized causes:*** Literally dozens of prescription and over-the-counter drugs—including antihistamines...certain high blood pressure drugs such as diuretics...and antidepressants—can cause eye dryness as a side effect.

To find out if one of your medications may be causing dry eye, go to DailyMed.nlm.nih.gov. Enter the name of the medication and scroll down to see what adverse reactions, such as dry eye, have been reported. Dry eye can also be triggered by more serious underlying diseases, including diabetes and Sjögren's syndrome, an autoimmune disease.

### How Blinking Helps

To effectively control dry eye, you need to understand the blinking reflex. This is a natural process that stimulates the secretion of oil from approximately 50 tiny glands (the meibomian glands) in the lower and upper eyelids. The oil slows the evaporation of tears and improves their ability to cling to the surfaces of the eyes. At the same time, blinking spreads moisture across the eyes and removes dust and other contaminants.

***Important:*** The size of your eyes, along with their tear-producing capacity, can have a lot to do with dryness. Normally, the upper and lower eyelids come together at the conclusion of a blink. If your eyes are larger than normal—because of diseases such as overactive thyroid (hyperthyroidism), for example, or because they're just made that way—the lids don't completely close. This causes dryness in the lower half of the eyes.

What most people don't realize is that the frequency of blinking is highly individual—and it varies depending on what you're doing at any particular moment.

A study that looked at blink rates in healthy people found that the frequency was as low as 4.5 blinks a minute while reading or doing other engrossing tasks...or as high as 26 blinks per minute during lively conversations. One blink every four or five seconds is about average.

Even though blinking is among the most effective ways to prevent dryness, it isn't practical to spend your time willing yourself to blink.

***What works better:*** Break up your TV, computer or smartphone sessions by closing your eyes for 10 seconds or so a few times every hour.

## Artificial Tears

The first line of defense against dry eye is over-the-counter (OTC) artificial tears. There are many generic versions, including brands from major pharmacies, that work quickly.

***Popular brands:*** Refresh and Systane.

***My advice:*** Liquid drops are fine if you have only mild/intermittent dryness. Refrigerating the drops will make them feel more soothing. Preservative-free drops are more expensive, but they tend to be more soothing because the preservative can be irritating for some people. When eye dryness is persistent, use gel-containing drops—the gel keeps the eyes lubricated for longer periods.

***Popular gel brands:*** Refresh, Systane and GenTeal.

If you need a product that's even longer-lasting than liquid drops or gel, consider OTC lubricating ointments (such as Refresh PM). Many dry eye sufferers use an ointment every few hours instead of one or more times an hour for the liquid products. However, some people report blurry vision when using ointments. To avoid this, try the product at bedtime—especially if you wake up with dry eyes. Drinking lots of water and/or using a humidifier at night—or even near one's computer station during the day—helps, too.

***Also:*** Try omega-3 fatty acid supplements...or simply eat more fatty fish. A Harvard study that looked at more than 32,000 women found that those who ate fish more than five times a week were 68% less likely to develop dry eye than those who didn't. And patients who did have dry eye tended to have fewer symptoms.

The omega-3s in fish reduce inflammation and increase tear production. Fish-oil supplements probably have similar effects.

***Typical dose:*** 1,000 mg daily.

## Stronger Rx

If you follow these steps but your eye dryness doesn't improve within a month or two, it's wise to consult an ophthalmologist. He/she can offer additional advice and may prescribe medication. *For example...*

- ***Lifitegrast ophthalmic solution* (Xiidra), which was approved by the FDA in 2016, is an anti-inflammatory drop that's applied twice daily to each eye.** Reducing inflammation can increase tear production. Like other drops, it may cause irritation/blurred vision that typically lasts for minutes at a time.

- ***Cyclosporine ophthalmic emulsion* (Restasis) was approved by the FDA in 2002 for increasing tear production.** The downside is that it takes four to six months to reach its full effectiveness—and like Xiidra, it may cause irritation initially. The irritation usually fades after using it for about a month.

- **Lacripep is the newest eye drop for treating dry eye.** It's still in the early stages of testing. A large-scale clinical trial involving more than 200 patients will soon be under way. The drug contains a fragment of the protein lacritin, which is deficient in patients with dry eye. The protein is important for promoting healthy tears and maintaining the health of eye nerves involved in tear production. Unlike other drops, the drug isn't washed out by tears—it can still be detected 24 hours later. This means that it could potentially be used just once a day.

### When You Need More Help

If your dry eye is severe and does not improve with the approaches above, your doctor might recommend a simple office procedure that plugs the small openings (tear ducts) that drain tears away from the eyes. Blocking these openings with punctal plugs keeps tears in place longer.

Most people start with temporary plugs made from collagen or dissolvable suture material. The plugs break down on their own in about three months—long enough to see if this approach is helpful. If you're satisfied, the plugs can be replaced with permanent silicone plugs. Side effects, such as infection, are rare. Most health insurance covers the cost of this procedure.

## Delicious Dry-Eye Remedy

Pterostilbene (PS), a compound in blueberries, has been found to fight the oxidative damage linked to dry eye.

***Details:*** When PS was added to corneal epithelial cells in the lab, oxidative damage was significantly reduced, curbing the inflammation that leads to dry eye.

***Tip:*** Eat one-half cup of fresh or frozen blueberries daily.

De-Quan Li, MD, PhD, associate professor of ophthalmology, Baylor College of Medicine, Houston.

## More Muscle = Less Disease

Douglas Paddon-Jones, PhD, a professor in the department of nutrition at The University of Texas Medical Branch at Galveston, where he is the director of the physical activity and functional recovery translational research laboratory.

Have you ever stopped to think about what it is that makes people look old? Aside from superficial physical characteristics (such as gray hair and saggy jowls), the culprit that doesn't get nearly enough attention is the decade-by-decade loss of muscle mass.

Age-related muscle loss, known as sarcopenia, changes more than just your appearance. It is a slow, insidious process that can rob you of 1% of your muscle mass each year after age 40. It makes it harder to lift things...and more challenging to walk and maintain your balance.

Perhaps the biggest threat is that sarcopenia makes it harder to stay physically active, leaving one at increased risk for at least 35 chronic diseases ranging from heart disease, stroke, diabetes and arthritis to erectile dysfunction, cognitive dysfunction, depression and certain types of cancer.

### Diet Comes First

Many people assume that simply hitting the gym will help them preserve their muscles. That's simply not true. To maintain (or increase) muscle mass, you need both exercise and protein. In fact, dietary changes are the smartest place to start because they'll give your body the raw materials that it needs for muscle maintenance. *My advice...*

- **Increase protein.** The recommended dietary allowance calls for 0.8 g of protein per kilogram of body weight each day. (That's about 51 g for a 140-pound woman...or 65 g for a 180-pound man.) But that's not enough for people with sarcopenia. I recommend that adults with sarcopenia (or those at risk) get closer to 80 g to 90 g daily. Men and those who are physically active should check with their doctor about getting even more than this amount.

***Caution:*** People with kidney disease or other medical conditions may need to limit their protein intake. Ask your doctor for advice.

***To make it easier:*** Don't focus on total daily protein. Just make an effort to get 25 g to 30 g of protein with every meal—your body can only utilize about this amount of protein at a time to repair and build muscle tissue. If you need more, enjoy a protein-rich snack between meals.

***Good protein sources:*** A four-ounce serving of lean chicken or pork will provide about 30 g of protein. You'll get about 22 g from three ounces of salmon...11 g from one-half cup of pinto beans...and 12 g from one ounce of soy nuts.

- **Consider a supplement.** I mainly recommend food-based sources of protein, but people who have special needs—those who have trouble chewing, for example, or those who don't have the appetite for adequate meals—can take advantage of protein powders or bars. A scoop of plain whey protein powder (with added honey or fruit for flavor) contains 20 g to 30 g of protein.

***Important:*** Read the label, and avoid products that are high in sugar or fat. Choose one labeled "contains all essential amino acids." Amino acids serve as building blocks for protein used in the body.

- **Always eat breakfast—and make it hearty.** Many people skip it altogether...or make do with a bagel or a bowl of sweet cereal. Get in the habit of starting the day with a few eggs (two will provide about 12 g of protein), along with yogurt (11 g per cup of regular yogurt), almonds (6 g per ounce) or other protein-rich foods.

***Another good option:*** A breakfast burrito made with beef, beans, cheese and eggs.

- **Meat makes it easier.** Animal-based proteins are complete—they contain all of the essential amino acids. People who eat meat don't have to give protein a second thought as long as they meet the per-meal requirement of 25 g to 30 g.

But can you get enough protein if you're a vegetarian or vegan? Absolutely—but you'll have to be aware of the amino acids that are found in different foods, and you'll generally need to consume larger amounts because plant foods contain less protein than meats.

***Helpful hint:*** Eat complementary proteins—food combinations that provide all the essential amino acids needed to build protein in the body. For example, legumes combined with whole grains (such as lentil soup with whole-grain bread) will provide all the amino acids. So will combining dairy with grains or nuts (such as yogurt and granola).

## Muscle-Building Formula

Muscle loss occurs slowly, in part because people tend to reduce activity without realizing it. They start taking elevators instead of stairs...doing less yard work, etc.

Studies have shown that people who are physically active are less likely to develop sarcopenia—or they get it to a lesser degree—than those who are sedentary.

The best way to maintain and increase muscle mass is with protein—and resistance training.*

The American College of Sports Medicine recommends lifting weights two to three days a week—with eight to 15 repetitions of each exercise.

***My take:*** Resistance training doesn't need to be limited to lifting weights. Exercise that uses body weight, such as workouts with resistance bands, yoga, Pilates or even taking the stairs, is helpful.

## The Right Way to Exercise

Slow walks and easy gym workouts will help maintain muscle, but they won't build

*Check with your doctor before beginning any exercise program.

it. To boost your strength and gain significant amounts of muscle, you need to do progressive resistance training (PRT). "Progressive" means that you'll strive to lift heavier weights or increase the number of repetitions over time.

***Example:*** When you can easily complete an exercise, it's time to add additional sets. Rather than stopping at 15 repetitions, rest for two or three minutes, then do 15 more.

***Another choice:*** Increase the weight by 5% to 10% so that you can barely repeat the exercise eight times. Stay at that weight until you can easily do 15 repetitions. Then raise the weight again.

After about four or five months of PRT, people with sarcopenia will often add a few pounds of muscle, research has found. Once you've built muscle with PRT, talk to your doctor about a maintenance plan.

***To get a postworkout boost:*** Have a glass of low-fat chocolate milk after intense exercise. It has about 24 g of carbohydrates and 8 g of protein—the 3:1 ratio that's thought to be ideal for muscle growth. The carbs will quickly provide glycogen (to replenish postexercise energy), and the protein will jump-start muscle growth and repair.

# Stem Cells for Better Vision

Stem cells taken from the skin on a patient's arm and transplanted into the eye slightly improved vision—an important advance for treating macular degeneration, a leading cause of blindness.

The Association for Research in Vision and Ophthalmology.

# Is There a Ringing in Your Ears?

Murray Grossan, MD, an otolaryngologist at Tower Ear, Nose & Throat in Los Angeles. DrGrossanTinnitus.com

Tinnitus is the perception of ringing, clicking, buzzing or other noise in the ears when no sound is present. It's a fairly common condition that is usually caused by age-related hearing loss, ear damage or certain medications, such as nonsteroidal anti-inflammatory drugs (NSAIDs), including aspirin...loop diuretics...and some antibiotics. Tinnitus that comes and goes may be somatosensory tinnitus, a form of this condition that is caused by external stimulation of nerves in the ear. There is generally no hearing loss or vertigo involved.

Many things can trigger somatosensory tinnitus. Earwax can accumulate in the ear canal and press on the eardrum and auditory nerves. A drop or two of baby oil, eardrops or a warm saline solution applied with a syringe irrigator can soften earwax so that it will come out of the ear. Muscle tension in the face and back of the neck can irritate the auditory nerve. Briefly massaging these muscles when you feel tense may be all that you need to do to avoid tinnitus.

You may also have the jaw joint condition temporomandibular joint (TMJ) disorder, which has been linked to somatosensory tinnitus. While looking in a mirror, put a finger or two in front of each ear at the jawbone, then open and close your mouth. Do you hear the tinnitus sound? If so, the sound you hear may be the cracking of the jaw or another sensation caused by TMJ. Is the spot tender or painful? Is your jaw evenly centered when you open your mouth? If any noise, pain or misalignment causes concern, you may want to consult an otolaryngologist who can provide treatments, such as a mouth guard or exercises to help stretch and strengthen the jaw.

## Same-Day Hip Surgery

Matthew S. Austin, MD, an orthopedic surgeon and director of Joint Replacement Services at Thomas Jefferson University Hospital in Philadelphia. He is program director of the Joint Replacement Fellowship at the Rothman Institute and a professor in the department of orthopaedic surgery at Sidney Kimmel Medical College at Thomas Jefferson University.

Until recently, people who needed a hip replacement were operated on in a hospital, spent a few nights there and then went home or to a rehabilitation center to embark on a recovery period of up to three months or more.

***Now:*** An increasing number of people are receiving so-called "same-day" hip surgery—you arrive at a hospital or outpatient center in the morning, have the surgery (typically lasting about an hour or so), spend a few hours recovering from anesthesia and then go home at the end of the day.* Even though this approach may sound appealing, it is not necessarily for everyone.

To learn more about same-day hip surgery, we spoke with Matthew S. Austin, MD, a leading orthopedic surgeon who performs both traditional and same-day hip replacements and researches optimal recovery methods.

*First things first—who needs a hip replacement?*

It's mainly done in patients with arthritis- or injury-related hip damage that causes persistent pain. Surgery is recommended when people can no longer do the activities they enjoy and/or when they're suffering from chronic pain that isn't relieved by medications or the risks of taking painkillers outweigh the benefits.

*How is a hip replacement done?*

In a nutshell, the arthritic joint is cut and removed and then replaced with a synthetic "ball-and-socket" that works much like a natural joint...and much better than an arthritic/damaged joint.

Most hip replacements (including same-day surgeries) are done posteriorly. The surgeon enters the back of the hip to access the hip joint. The incision is typically about six to 10 inches long, although the same procedure can now be done with smaller incisions.

The operation can also be done anteriorly, with an incision on the front part of the hip...or anterolaterally (on the side). With these two techniques (both of which usually require an incision of about four inches or less), the surgeon moves muscles instead of cutting and reattaching them. A surgeon who's experienced in any of these three surgeries can complete the operation in about an hour.

*Is there a preferred technique for same-day surgery?*

It makes no difference. The different surgeries have similar success rates—roughly 20 years after surgery, about 85% will still have their implant. Same-day surgery is a different process, not a different surgery.

*What do you mean by "process"?*

It has to do with the care that's given during the time before and after surgery. The same-day approach involves more of a team effort than conventional surgery...and the process begins well before the actual operation.

Patients have to be medically optimized to reduce the risk for complications and allow them to recover at home instead of in the hospital. A diabetic patient, for example, will be encouraged to stabilize his/her blood sugar before having the surgery. Someone who's obese might be advised to lose weight. Even though these recommendations also apply to people having a conventional hip surgery, they are crucial if a patient wants to go home the same day as the surgery.

The same-day approach also requires an extensive support system. Patients having same-day surgery might meet with team members, such as nurses and physical therapists, to learn such things as how to get around on crutches (usually needed for a couple of

*If you go to an outpatient center, look for one that's affiliated with a major medical center and/or has accreditation from the Accreditation Association for Ambulatory Healthcare.

weeks)...how to safely climb stairs...how to bathe and use the toilet...and how to manage postsurgical nausea. A discharge planner will ensure that they have adequate support at home—for example, a spouse or a friend who can help them with meals, etc.

In addition, you're encouraged to stay in close contact with doctors, nurses and other support staff. A nurse or doctor should be available 24/7 to answer questions.

*Isn't this riskier than staying in the hospital?*

Not necessarily. As long as patients are ready for the procedure—in terms of overall health, at-home support, etc.—they'll do about the same as hospitalized patients. The overall complication rate—from blood clots, joint dislocation, poor wound healing or infection—is less than 5% in both same-day and conventional hip replacements.

*Who should—or shouldn't—have same-day surgery?*

A patient who's 85 years old, lives alone, can barely get around the house and has a variety of health problems would probably be advised not to go home the same day.

On the other hand, a 50-year-old who's in great shape will probably be physiologically able to go home the same day—but you have to consider motivation, as well. It may be easier for some in a hospital, where help is a button-push away.

*What about recovery?*

The evidence suggests that it's about the same regardless of the type of hip replacement. You can expect to walk a bit soon after surgery, while full recovery might take three months or more. Patients may do physical therapy exercises to strengthen the thighs and hips for six weeks or more.

*Do all medical centers offer same-day surgery?*

It's not available everywhere, so you'll have to ask your primary care doctor or surgeon or call around. Insurance coverage will probably be similar for inpatient and outpatient procedures.

***Important:*** Whether or not you're considering same-day surgery, choose a board-certified surgeon who does at least 50 hip replacements a year. Studies have found that that's the number at which complication rates start to level off.

Also make sure that the surgeon is experienced in the same type of surgery (anterior, anterolateral or posterior) that you are getting.

***To find an experienced surgeon:*** Check the website of the American Academy of Orthopaedic Surgeons, AAOS.org...or the American Association of Hip and Knee Surgeons, AAHKS.org.

## Better Joint-Replacement Recovery

Peripheral nerve blocks (PNBs)—the injection of an anesthetic near nerves to block pain in a specific area during surgery—improve pain control after joint replacement.

***Now:*** An analysis of more than one million knee- and hip-replacement surgeries found that PNBs also improve complication rates, resulting in fewer infections and shorter hospital stays than reported in patients who did not receive a PNB.

***Possible reason:*** Patients with PNBs have less need for opioids to control pain and fewer side effects than when general anesthesia is used and are able to participate in rehabilitation sooner after surgery.

Stavros G. Memtsoudis, MD, PhD, attending anesthesiologist and senior scientist, Hospital for Special Surgery, New York City.

## Feeling Old?

You could be at greater risk for health problems, according to recent research involving more than 10,000 adults. People who think of themselves as old (no matter their real age) are more likely to be depressed and in poorer health...have more cognitive decline...and are up to 25% more likely to be hospitalized.

***To feel young at any age:*** Get regular exercise...don't believe negative stereotypes about aging...and stay connected with family and friends.

Yannick Stephan, PhD, associate professor, University of Montpellier, France.

## Don't Call Me Nana

Pamela Redmond Satran, author of *How Not to Act Old* and cofounder of the baby-name website Nameberry.com.

A grandparent nickname might seem like a silly thing to fret about, but these names are more than what our children's children call us. They define how we see ourselves.

It turns out that unconventional grandparent names are popular. Former President George W. Bush is Jefe. Actress Goldie Hawn is GoGo. Singer Naomi Judd is Mawmaw. These names are more fun than conventional names, which in comparison seem old-fashioned and, well, old.

But if you want to have a say in your grandparent nickname, say so early on. If you fail to push a particular name by the time your oldest grandchild starts speaking, he/she might choose one for you.

Some grandparents have names such as Bubbles, G-Dawg, Muddy, Muffer, MaxiMa, Jeepers, Punky, Paddles and Peppers. If a young grandchild tries to hang one of those on you and you don't like it, find a private moment and tell him that he's looking at years of itchy sweaters for his birthday if he doesn't do a quick rethink. That ought to set things straight.

# APPENDIX 3: VERY PERSONAL

## Sexy and Safe: Are You Wearing the Wrong Underwear?

Richard Bennett, MD, an associate professor of urology at Michigan State University in East Lansing and Oakland University William Beaumont School of Medicine in Rochester.

Unless you're the type of person who shares lots of personal information, you probably don't discuss your underwear with your doctor. Perhaps you should. There are certain types of underwear that may be better for you than others. *What you need to know about underwear—but may have been too shy to ask...*

### Panties vs. Thongs

Once favored mainly by the young and daring, the G-string has become the go-to underwear for women of all ages who want to avoid panty lines.

Unlike panties, thongs press tightly against the genitals/anal area. Some experts speculate that this could cause irritation and skin damage—and that the back-and-forth movement of the "string" could spread the bacteria that cause vaginal or urinary tract infections and/or irritate hemorrhoids.

Over the years, I've heard anecdotes about a few thong-wearing patients who got infections. It makes intuitive sense that anything that transfers bacteria from one area to another could cause infection. But I'm not aware of any studies that have proved it.

***My take:*** Wear a thong if it feels comfortable and you like the look. Women have been wearing thongs for a long time. If they were causing an increase in infections, we would have seen it by now.

### Breathable or Not?

"Pretty" panties and thongs are often made from rayon, nylon or other nonbreathable fabrics. These fabrics trap heat and moisture and can lead to maceration (skin damage) as well as infection.

***Scientific evidence:*** Research published in the *European Journal of Obstetrics & Gynecology and Reproductive Biology* found that synthetic underwear was one of the factors associated with yeast infections. Synthetic "shapewear" such as Spanx, which limits air circulation, could cause similar problems.

***My take:*** For all-day wear, cotton or other breathable fabrics are healthier than synthetics. It's fine to wear lacy/sexy underwear under a cocktail dress or when you're planning a romantic evening, but consider these fabrics "for recreational purposes only." After a few hours, change into cotton.

***Another choice:*** Synthetic thongs/panties with cotton liners. You'll get the look you want without sacrificing breathability.

### Antibacterial Underwear

Undies impregnated with bacteria-killing triclosan or nanosilver (small silver particles with antimicrobial properties) are relatively new to the men's and women's underwear market. Manufacturers claim that killing bacteria reduces odors.

Does antibacterial underwear work? Maybe. The same products are often made with moisture-wicking fabrics, which might have more to do with reducing odors than the chemicals.

***My take:*** You'll do just as well by wearing breathable underwear and changing it regularly. I worry that the chemicals could migrate and increase yeast infections by changing the vagina's bacterial balance.

### Going Commando

Do you need to wear underwear? Not for health reasons. In fact, going bare gives the genital and anal areas a chance to air out. If you live in a hot, humid climate, it can be good for the skin. It can also help those who are overweight or obese—that's because yeast can proliferate in thigh creases, under the belly or in other sweaty areas.

Forgoing underwear could cause chafing when delicate skin rubs against pant seams, but this isn't a problem for everyone. For women, going underwear-free could allow traces of natural discharge to end up on clothing, but this is an issue only if it bothers you.

***My take:*** If you enjoy the airy feeling, go for it!

## Change Them Daily—or Not?

It makes sense to change out of damp or dirty underwear. But, in general, how often should underwear be changed?

***My take:*** There's no health reason to change clean underwear more often than once a day.

However, if your underwear gets damp from urine—even a few drops—swap them as soon as possible for a fresh pair. Odor is an obvious problem, but dampness increases the risk for yeast infections on the skin.

## Extra Protection...

If you "leak" now and then, you may benefit from disposable or washable incontinence briefs (available in several styles and all sizes) that look like regular underwear and aren't visible under clothing.

***Alternative:*** Both women and men can wear thin disposable pads (such as Butterfly Men's Body Liners or Depend Shields for Men...or, for women, Poise Liners or Equate Thin Liners) that slip inside regular underwear and wick moisture away from the skin.

# For Some Women, Sex Gets Better at Midlife

Holly Thomas, MD, assistant professor, medicine, University of Pittsburgh.

Jan Shifren, MD, director, Massachusetts General Hospital Midlife Women's Health Center, and associate professor, obstetrics, gynecology and reproductive biology, Harvard Medical School, Boston.

North American Menopause Society, annual meeting, Orlando, Florida.

Here's good news for middle-aged women who fear their sexual satisfaction is destined to decline: Aging can provide benefits that might make lovemaking even more enjoyable, a small study suggests.

Interviews with more than three dozen women ages 45 to 60 revealed that some were more satisfied with sex at midlife even though they had it less often.

These women "felt more confident and more comfortable in their own skin as they got older, and this allowed them to feel more free in the bedroom," said study lead author Holly Thomas, MD.

"They had a better knowledge and understanding of their own bodies as they got older. And they felt more comfortable and empowered to communicate their sexual needs to their partner than when they were younger," said Dr. Thomas, an assistant professor of medicine at the University of Pittsburgh.

Other research has examined the rates of problems for older women, such as low libido and vaginal dryness.

These studies "typically show that sex gets worse as women move through middle age," said Dr. Thomas. "We used a different technique, speaking to women face-to-face using interviews and focus groups, to try to see if there was more to the picture."

## Study Details

The researchers interviewed 20 women and also conducted three focus groups with a total of 19 participants. Their average age was

58, and roughly half were white. All but two said they were heterosexual.

Jan Shifren, MD, director of the Massachusetts General Hospital Midlife Women's Health Center, said, "It's important for people to realize that everything that happens with aging is not doom and gloom, and there can even be some positive things in terms of sexuality." She wasn't involved in the study.

Some women in the study talked about "negative" changes in their sex lives as they aged, such as less frequent sex, vaginal dryness and difficulty reaching orgasm. But they were more likely to blame family and work stressors than biological factors like menopause, the researchers said.

Dr. Shifren said women are often urged to turn to hormone treatments when their sex lives decline. But, she added, the women in the recent study are "telling us they're experiencing these changes because they're experiencing a lot of midlife stressors. We should not automatically say that sexual changes are just biologic. We have to remember this is a complex time in women's lives."

The women who reported negative changes were more likely to say that they adapted to them. A smaller group of women said the changes distressed them, Dr. Thomas said, and a few reported indifference.

The study, partly funded by the U.S. National Institutes of Health, was presented at the North American Menopause Society's annual meeting in Orlando, Florida.

## Recommendations

What are the lessons from these findings for midlife women?

"Focus on what you can change," Dr. Shifren said. "Think about what's bothering you and what can you do to make it better, and focus on reducing other midlife stressors."

Problems such as vaginal dryness, for example, can be treated with low-dose vaginal estrogen and lubricants, she said. And it can be helpful to urge male partners to seek treatment for erectile dysfunction if that's an issue, she added.

What else can partners do to help?

"If there are changes due to aging and your female partner seems to be getting less pleasure from sex, think about what you can do to make it more pleasurable, such as other ways you can increase intimacy," Dr. Shifren said. "Some couples adapt by being more creative, by adopting new positions and activities."

For more information about sexuality in later life, visit the U.S. National Institute on Aging website, nia.nih.gov, and search "sexuality in later life."

---

# Good Sex Good for Older Women's Heart... Not So Great for Men?

Hui Liu, PhD, associate professor, sociology, Michigan State University.

Gregg Fonarow, MD, professor, cardiology, University of California, Los Angeles.

*Journal of Health and Social Behavior.*

---

An active sex life appears to have no bearing on older women's risk for heart attack. And older women who described their sex life as enjoyable, pleasurable or satisfying emotionally and/or physically saw some health benefit, a recent study found.

On the other hand, sexually active older men may be more likely to have a heart attack, heart failure or stroke compared with their less lusty peers, the research suggests.

What's more, older men who say they enjoy frequent sex also appear to face a higher risk for such serious cardiovascular events, the study authors said.

But at least one cardiologist said he was reluctant to accept the study findings until more research is carried out.

## The Study

The study researchers evaluated survey responses from more than 2,200 seniors who participated in the U.S. National Social Life, Health and Aging Project. Participants answered sexual behavior questionnaires in 2005-2006 and again five years later. All were 57 to 85 years old at the time of the first survey.

***Among the findings:*** Older men were more likely than older women to say they were sexually active. In the two surveys, about 70% and 50% of men, respectively, said they had had sex in the past year, compared with roughly 40% and 23% of women.

Men were also more likely to say they had more frequent sex. In the two polls, between 20% and 25% of men said they had sex once a week or more in the prior year, compared with 11% of women.

Finally, men were more likely than women to say their sex was "extremely physically pleasurable"—36% versus 23% in the first survey. And 37% of men said their sex was "extremely emotionally satisfying," compared with 25% of women.

Survey responses were then compared with key cardiovascular measures, including blood pressure readings, rapid heart rate, elevated C-reactive protein levels, and incidence of heart attack, heart failure and/or stroke.

Compared with older men who said they weren't sexually active, those who had sex once a week or more were almost twice as likely to experience a heart attack, heart failure or stroke by the second survey.

And men who found sex enjoyable also faced a higher risk for such heart illnesses, the study authors said.

Neither risk was seen among women. Women who said their sex lives were extremely pleasurable or satisfying had a lower risk for high blood pressure than women who didn't, the study found.

The study findings appear in the *Journal of Health and Social Behavior*.

## Possible Explanations

"The result for men is indeed surprising for us, given our general assumption that sex is always good for health," said study lead author Hui Liu, PhD, an associate professor of sociology at Michigan State University.

Dr. Liu pointed to several potential explanations.

"When men get older, they may have more difficulties reaching an orgasm for medical or emotional reasons," she noted, perhaps leading to overexertion, exhaustion and cardiovascular stress.

Also, medication and supplements to improve sexual function "may have negative effects on their cardiovascular health," Dr. Liu added.

"Moreover, having quite a high frequency of sex may indicate problems of sexual addiction, sexual compulsivity or sexual impulsivity," she said. These may be related to the onset of anxiety and/or depression, which can negatively affect the heart, Dr. Liu said.

## Expert Reaction

Gregg Fonarow, MD, professor of cardiology at the University of California, Los Angeles, voiced caution about the findings, however.

"Most studies suggest that maintaining an active sexual life seems to be associated with men's cardiovascular and overall health," he said.

Prior studies, Dr. Fonarow added, "have suggested that high frequency of sexual intercourse is associated with lower risk of cardiovascular events and great longevity for men."

Contrary to the recent research, "studies have shown that a reduced frequency of sexual activity was an independent risk factor for cardiovascular events in men," he said. "In addition, studies have documented the risk of cardiovascular events during sexual activity to be very low in absolute terms."

With that in mind, Dr. Fonarow stressed that "the findings of the present study require replication before further consideration."

## Advice

Dr. Fonarow encouraged seniors to broach the subject with their doctors.

"Seniors with or at risk for heart disease should not be shy about talking to their physician about their sex life, implications for heart health, and any concerns," he said.

For more on heart disease and sex, visit the American Heart Association website, heart.org, and search "sex and heart disease."

# Better Sleep Could Mean Better Sex for Older Women

JoAnn V. Pinkerton, MD, executive director, The North American Menopause Society, and professor, obstetrics and gynecology, University of Virginia Health System.

Steven Feinsilver, MD, director, sleep medicine, Lenox Hill Hospital, New York City.

Jill Rabin, MD, co-chief, division of ambulatory care, Women's Health Programs-PCAP Services, Northwell Health, New Hyde Park, New York.

*Menopause*, news release.

A more satisfying sex life may be only a good night's sleep away for women over 50, recent research finds.

## The Study

Researchers led by Juliana Kling, MD, MPH, of the Mayo Clinic in Scottsdale, Arizona, tracked data from nearly 94,000 women aged 50 to 79.

The investigators found that 31% had insomnia, and a little more than half (56%) said they were somewhat or very satisfied with their sex life.

But too little sleep—fewer than seven to eight hours a night—was linked with a lower likelihood of sexual satisfaction, the findings showed.

"This is a very important study since it examines a question which has tremendous potential impact on women's lives," said Jill Rabin, MD, who reviewed the findings. She's co-chief of the Women's Health Program at Northwell Health in New Hyde Park, New York.

Age played a key role in outcomes. For example, the study found that older women were less likely than younger women to be sexually active if they slept fewer than seven to eight hours per night.

Among women older than 70, those who slept fewer than five hours a night were 30% less likely to be sexually active than women sleeping seven to eight hours, Dr. Kling's team found.

The study was published in the journal *Menopause*.

## Implications

The findings highlight how crucial sleep is to many aspects of women's health, medical experts said.

"Seven hours of sleep per night will improve sexual satisfaction and has been shown to increase sexual responsiveness," said JoAnn Pinkerton, MD, executive director of The North American Menopause Society.

Besides putting a damper on sex lives, she said, poor sleep is also tied to an array of health issues, such as "sleep apnea, restless legs syndrome, stress and anxiety." Other health problems linked to insomnia include "heart disease, hypertension [high blood pressure], arthritis, fibromyalgia, diabetes, depression and neurological disorders," Dr. Pinkerton added.

Steven Feinsilver, MD, directs sleep medicine at Lenox Hill Hospital in New York City. He reviewed the recent findings and stressed that they can't prove cause and effect. "It certainly could be possible that many underlying problems—for example, illness, depression—could be causing both worsened sleep and worsened sex," he noted.

Dr. Rabin agreed, but said there's been "a paucity of studies" looking into links between sleep and sexual health, especially during menopause.

"We know that obstructive sleep apnea and sexual dysfunction are positively correlated," she said. "Other factors which may lead to a decreased sleep quality include a woman's general health; various life events, which may contribute to her stress; chronic disease; medication; and degree and presence of social supports, just to name a few," Dr. Rabin explained.

And, "in menopause, and due to the hormonal transition, women may experience various symptoms which may impact the duration and quality of their sleep patterns," Dr. Rabin added.

"We and our patients need to know that quality sleep is necessary for overall optimum functioning and health, including sexual satisfaction, and that there are effective treatment options—including hormone therapy—which are available for symptomatic women," she said.

The U.S. National Institute on Aging website has more information about sexuality later in life at nia.nih.org. Search "sexuality in later life."

# The Mystery of the Female Orgasm Solved?

Gunter Wagner, PhD, professor of ecology and evolutionary biology, Yale University, New Haven, Connecticut.

Mihaela Pavlicev, PhD, assistant professor, Cincinnati Children's Hospital Medical Center.

Yale University, news release.

The female orgasm—famously faked by Meg Ryan in "When Harry Met Sally"—may have its true roots in evolution as an aid to conception, recent research suggests.

## New Research

In their study, researchers at Yale University noted that while the male orgasm's role in getting the sperm to meet the egg has long been clear, the female orgasm's role has been a mystery.

It has no obvious role in the success of reproduction or in the number of children, so scientists have long tried to determine why women have orgasms, said a team led by Yale professor of ecology and evolutionary biology Gunter Wagner, PhD.

He and coresearcher Mihaela Pavlicev, PhD, assistant professor, Cincinnati Children's Hospital Medical Center, studied other mammals for clues into how the female orgasm evolved. They looked at non-human mammals and focused on a specific reflex that goes along with orgasms in women—release of the hormones prolactin and oxytocin.

In many mammals, this orgasm-linked reflex plays a role in ovulation—specifically, helping to stimulate the release of eggs from the ovaries.

## Conclusions

Despite the fact that mammals vary widely today, this trait may have been necessary to ovulation in species that were ancestral to humans. "This [orgasm-linked] reflex became superfluous for reproduction later in evolution, freeing [human] female orgasm for secondary roles," according to a Yale news release.

The study authors also noted that the clitoris appears to have shifted in anatomical position throughout evolution—so that it now is less likely to be directly stimulated during intercourse.

The study was published in the journal *JEZ-Molecular and Developmental Evolution.*

The Society of Obstetricians and Gynecologists of Canada has more information on female orgasm at SOGC.org. Click on "Resources and Publications" and scroll down to "Female Orgasms: Myths and Facts."

# For Women, a Zesty Path to Better Orgasms

Elena Ratner, MD, assistant professor, department of obstetrics, gynecology and reproductive sciences, Yale University School of Medicine, New Haven, Connecticut, and a board-certified gynecologist oncologist. Dr. Ratner has no financial connection to the manufacturer of Zestra.

The advice for menopausal women who want to continue to enjoy sex starts with the well-known, but often neglected, basics—use a vaginal moisturizer once or twice a week and a lubricant before sex...and practice Kegel exercises daily.

But there is also some unexpected wisdom for these women. An over-the-counter botanical formula called "zester oil" (brand name Zestra) that a woman applies to the area around her clitoris and labia a few minutes before sex.

Why? It enhances sexual response and improves orgasm. Interested? Here's what you need to know.

## A Warming Sensation

Zester oil is a blend of botanical ingredients and nutrients...

- **Borage seed oil,** a source of the polyunsaturated fatty acid gamma-linolenic acid (GLA), which has been shown to reduce inflammation.
- **Evening primrose oil,** another source of GLA.
- **Angelica root (aka the Chinese herb dong quai),** which has estrogen-like effects and improves blood flow.
- **Coleus forskohlii,** a botanical in the mint family, which relaxes muscles.
- **Theobromine,** a stimulant found in chocolate.
- **Vitamins C and E,** antioxidants that sustain the formula's shelf life.

According to the manufacturer, the ingredients are safe to ingest—they are "derived from natural botanical ingredients that are often used in dietary supplements and have well-established safety profiles."

How Zestra works, and what role each of the botanicals plays in that process, isn't known, but there is some evidence that it does work. In two randomized, controlled, peer-reviewed clinical studies—albeit sponsored by the manufacturer—it was compared with a placebo (tinted, flavored soybean oil). The larger study involved 256 women over four months.

***Results:*** Zester oil improved measures of desire, arousal and sexual satisfaction...both in women with and without sexual issues. It was effective for women taking SSRI antidepressants, which often have libido-dampening side effects, as well. And, Zestra can improve sensation and arousal in many different groups of women, including cancer survivors and postmenopausal women.

The manufacturer recommends applying zester oil first and then using a lubricant (coconut oil is a good one). Within two or three minutes of applying it, a woman should feel a warming sensation, which lasts about 45 minutes, although it peaks after the first 10 minutes or so. The only known side effect—about 15% of women report a mild-to-moderate burning sensation in the genitals. The product is widely available online.

Zestra is generally safe for most women, and no serious side effects have been reported in the five years it has been on the market, according to the manufacturer.

***But there are some cautions:*** A woman should not use Zestra if she has an active vaginal infection, genital lesions or genital irritation...has a hypersensitivity or allergy to any of the ingredients...or is pregnant, breast-feeding or trying to conceive. And while there are no known drug interactions, women taking medications should check with their doctors before using it.

## Paths to Sexual Satisfaction

When it comes to enjoying a satisfying sex life before, during and after menopause, zester oil is just one tool. Other tools include hormones such as estrogen or testosterone, botanicals, prescription drugs and integrative practices such as Reiki and acupuncture. Women should expect to continue to have normal sex lives after menopause. Sex changes, but those changes should not be negative. If they are, talk to your doctor.

# When Sex Hurts: Intrarosa Is a New Way to Short-Circuit Pain

Andrew L. Rubman, ND, medical director, Southbury Clinic for Traditional Medicines, Southbury, Connecticut. SouthburyClinic.com

If you're a woman approaching menopause or you're already there, you may have discovered a not-so-great fact about the facts of life—during this particular stage of life, sex can hurt.

***Here's why:*** As you transition into and through menopause, you'll have lower levels of estrogen, the hormone that keeps the tissue of the vagina and vulva healthy and lubricated. Vaginal tissue becomes drier and thinner, which can lead to uncomfortable sex, including pain. The medical name for painful sex is *dyspareunia*.

Women who have it might label it with another name—killjoy.

Vaginal moisturizers, used every few days, as well as lubricants right before sex, can help. But for many women these are not enough to offset thinner, drier vaginal tissue, so there is still some discomfort or pain. In that case, the primary options that women have had from their health-care providers have been prescription vaginal inserts, including rings, or creams that contain estrogen. These are generally safe, since little of this estrogen is absorbed into the bloodstream, and there is no evidence that it increases the risk for uterine or breast cancer. But many women, especially those with a history of breast cancer, are uncomfortable with any circulating estrogen and prefer an approach that doesn't introduce estrogen into the body.

Now they have one. It's a new prescription product that helps you build your own estrogen back in the one place in your body where you need it most for pain-free sex.

## What's a Dietary Supplement Doing in a Vaginal Suppository?

The U.S. Food and Drug Administration (FDA) has approved Intrarosa, a novel treatment for dyspareunia due to menopause. It comes in the form of a vaginal suppository that's inserted once a day.

The clinical trials submitted to the FDA for approval were conducted by the manufacturer, but many other trials have also found that it's beneficial. In one year-long study, for example, Intrarosa significantly reduced pain—and increased lubrication, orgasms and sexual satisfaction—in postmenopausal women.

What's novel about Intrarosa, and what sets it apart from current treatments for vaginal dryness and dyspareunia, is that its active ingredient is prasterone, which most people know as a dietary supplement called dehydroepiandrosterone (DHEA).

As a vaginal insert, rather than as a dietary supplement, however, DHEA works in a novel way. It's the raw material that vaginal cells use to produce their own estrogen. Don't be confused by the idea that a woman in menopause is able to make her own estrogen. While it's true that the ovaries stop producing estrogen once you've reached menopause, many cells in your body can still produce small amounts of the hormone used within the cells themselves. In this case, the estrogen is actually manufactured, in tiny amounts, by the vaginal tissues.

Even in menopause, the cells that line the vagina and are responsible for its health, including the ability to stay lubricated, remain richly supplied with receptor cells for estrogen (and progesterone). When small amounts of DHEA are applied topically, it stimulates these tissues to convert the DHEA and produce estrogen locally. Voila, natural lubrication, reducing friction—and pain—during sex.

Is this brand new? Not entirely. DHEA creams, both over-the-counter and prescription-only, have been available for many years. Naturopathic physicians regularly prescribe vaginal DHEA creams, for example. But FDA approval makes this approach available to women from any MD, including their primary care doctors. (*Note*: Intrarosa, manufactured by a Canadian company, doesn't yet have a US distributor but is expected to have one within a few months.) In truth, it's a validation from conventional medicine of an approach that naturopaths have used for years, and that's a good thing.

While Intrarosa is approved for women in menopause, it may be beneficial in perimenopause, when levels of estrogen fluctuate but are still declining. Your health-care provider can let you know with a test called a "maturation index evaluation," done with a Pap smear, what your vaginal estrogen level is. If it is low, you may want to discuss whether Intrarosa is a good idea for you.

## Is It Safe?

I believe that prasterone is safe, primarily because it does not affect levels of circulating estrogen at all. So there are none of the concerns, for example about increased risk for breast cancer, that come into play with increased levels of circulating estrogen.

Side effects are minor. In clinical trials, about 6% of the women who used it experienced vaginal discharge—primarily from the product itself, since it melts at body temperature. It may affect the results of a Pap smear, and while it's not a safety concern, it's a good idea to remind your doctor before a Pap smear that you're using this product. For a more accurate Pap smear, stop using it three days before your test. There's no need to monitor your hormone levels if you're using Intrarosa.

## How Quickly Does It Work?

Vaginal cells turn over rapidly, so a woman who starts using Intrarosa can expect to experience its feel-good effects fairly rapidly—in three to 10 days. After that, with daily use, there may be no need at all to apply an external lubricant to have the enjoyable, pain-free sex you want. It's even OK to skip using Intrarosa for a day or two if you're having a romantic long weekend and don't want to…be disturbed.

# What Happens During Sex Therapy?

Barry McCarthy, PhD, a professor of psychology at American University in Washington, DC, and a certified sex and couples therapist who has practiced for 42 years. In 2016, he received the Masters and Johnson award for lifetime contributions to the field of sex therapy. He is author of 14 books, including *Sex Made Simple* and *Rekindling Desire*.

*Admit it*: You're curious. When you hear the phrase "sex therapy," you wonder who actually goes and why. What do people do in sex therapy? And could it help me?

It's not as mysterious as it sounds. The point of sex therapy is to help partners or spouses—and sometimes singles not in committed relationships—regain an active and satisfying sex life. Sex therapy can be done individually, but it is more successful when done as a couple.

***An under-recognized problem:*** More people could benefit from this specialized therapy than actually seek it—sexual problems, including low libido, premature ejaculation and erectile dysfunction, are more prevalent in the US than the incidence of anxiety and depression combined.

When a couple's sex life is going kaput, forgoing this valuable tool may endanger one's relationship. That's because couples—both heterosexual and homosexual—often underestimate the importance of a mutually pleasing sex life to their overall bond.

***Important finding:*** A study cited in the *Journal of Marital & Family Therapy* reports that contented partners attribute only between 15% and 20% of their happiness to a pleasing sex life, while unhappy mates ascribe 50% to 70% of their distress to sexual problems.

In addition, one of the major causes of divorce in the first five years of marriage (whether it's a first marriage or a second marriage) is sexual problems or dysfunction.

Here's what sex therapy is all about and how it may help you…

## The Biggest Bedroom Problem

Back in the 1970s, the biggest issues centered on arousal and orgasm. Now the major problem is desire—or lack thereof.

Perhaps surprisingly, healthy long-marrieds tend to be more sexually satisfied than others, even though they might not have sex as often as they used to. The most vulnerable time for couples to stop being sexual—defined as having sex fewer than 10 times a year—is within the first few years of marriage, after heady romance fades and day-to-day drudgery sets in. Many spouses have trouble transitioning to a more humdrum existence where they view each other as life partners and intimate friends but begin to de-eroticize the other person.

***Danger points:*** It's during stress points such as childbirth or long-term infertility treatment when major sex problems, such as lack of desire, tend to spike. Other reasons people go to sex therapy include unwanted sexual fetishes, painful sex (resulting from a chronic medical condition, for example, such as arthritis) and/or poor body image (due to being overweight, for example, or a disfiguring operation). Sex therapy can also facilitate recovery for victims of sexual abuse and assault.

## No Nudity Required!

Nudity or sexual touching isn't part of office-based therapy sessions. In the office, talk therapy is front and center, helping couples identify the anxiety, inhibitions and/or unrealistic expectations that interfere with their sexual pleasure.

A sex therapist will assure patients that they won't be pressured, and explain that he/she needs to understand each partner's psychological, relational and sexual strengths and vulnerabilities.

***Homework:*** After each weekly or biweekly session—which, for most couples, continues for three months to a year—sex therapists assign partners homework. These exercises typically include talking, touching and setting up erotic scenarios.

***Examples:*** A woman might practice her ability to veto touch she doesn't like and express her pleasure in touch she enjoys. A man might be given an exercise that involves the wax and wane of his erection.

About half of sex therapy takes place in the couple's home. If a couple has difficulty with an exercise at home, they can take a break and reestablish comfort and trust by holding each other and remaining calm before trying the exercise again.

## Overcoming Barriers

Some people avoid seeking sex therapy because they're afraid of exposing themselves, whether physically or emotionally. Others, unfortunately, fall victim to a common public misconception that sex therapists don't work with mainstream, traditional couples. But most couples are traditional in the sense that they value their couplehood and maintain a traditional agreement about not having sexual relationships with others.

***Shaking off shame:*** Many partners silently worry that their mate wouldn't love or respect them if they knew their deepest sexual secrets—unusual turn-ons, colorful histories, long-ago rape or abuse or a sexually transmitted disease. But confronting these issues in sex therapy typically reveals acceptance, not intolerance. Partners learn that their secrets no longer control them.

## The Best Sex Therapists

Finding a qualified sex therapist isn't always an easy task. Most marital therapists are not trained to deal with sexual issues directly. In traditional couples therapy, sex problems are almost always considered to be a symptom of relationship problems, so sexual attitudes, behaviors and feelings are not directly addressed. Also, most states don't have licensing requirements for sex therapists.

The nonprofit American Association of Sexuality Educators, Counselors and Therapists (AASECT), AASECT.org/referral-directory, offers an easy-to-use online tool to help locate certified sex therapists in most parts of the US. Unfortunately, most health insurers don't reimburse for sex therapy.

To find the right therapist, look for a practitioner who...

- **Has a degree in mental health, such as a doctorate of psychology (PhD) or a master's in social work (MSW).**
- **Is certified by the AASECT to practice sex therapy.**
- **Has at least three years of experience working with couples—including signifi-**

**cant experience dealing directly with sexual issues.**

It's worth the effort to find a therapist whom both partners like and respect. Talk to several therapists on the phone or e-mail a few to get a feel for who might be a good fit.

---

# Sex Tips to Stay Safe from STDs

Melanie Davis, PhD, a certified sexuality educator and copresident of the Sexuality and Aging Consortium at Widener University in Chester, Pennsylvania, and founder of the website SaferSex4Seniors.org. Through Honest Exchange, LLC, she trains health-care providers, medical students and educators about sexuality and communication.

---

For older men and women, the fun game is no longer shuffleboard. It's sex. And that's a great thing—except that sexually transmitted diseases (STDs) are on a meteoric rise in this age group. *The latest stats...*

- **Between 2007 and 2011,** chlamydia infections among Americans age 65 and over increased by 31%.
- **Syphilis infections in this age group rose by 52% in the same period.**
- **17% of new cases of HIV infection are in people age 50 and older.**

## The New Sexual Revolution

One big reason for the rise of STDs—also called "sexually transmitted infections" or STIs—is that more people continue to be sexually active well into their golden years. "The generation of people now hitting this stage of life came of age during the sexual revolution—they're healthier and fitter and expect to keep having sex," explains Melanie Davis, PhD, copresident of the Sexuality and Aging Consortium at Widener University in Chester, Pennsylvania, and founder of the website Safer Sex for Seniors.

Viagra and related erectile dysfunction (ED) drugs play a role, too. One study found that men (average age 61) who used these drugs were twice as likely to have STDs compared with men who didn't. As women become more savvy about managing sexual health after menopause, they also find sex easier to enjoy. It's also liberating for many women to be able to have sex without worrying about getting pregnant.

Being able to enjoy sex later in life, with more comfort and no worries about pregnancy, is all good. But it also opened the door to the new epidemic of STDS.

It has even become an issue in long-term-care facilities. Many STDs are asymptomatic, but most nursing homes and assisted-care facilities don't screen for them. And even if they did, all it would take is one conjugal visit with an infected nonresident for an infection to spread, according to Dr. Davis. Plus, people with chronic conditions may be more susceptible to infection, including STDs.

If you're sexually active, especially if you have recently had multiple sexual partners (or your partner has), being tested for STDs should be a regular part of your preventive medical care. It's so important for the health of seniors that Medicare now covers STD testing as a free preventive service. But as with everything related to health, prevention is always better than treatment. Here's how to stay safe—and still enjoy yourself.

## How to Have More Fun in Bed...Safely

The single best way to prevent the spread of infection during sex—heterosexual or homosexual—is to use a barrier form of protection such as an external or internal condom or dam, says Dr. Davis.

As bodies change, though, it can take new skills to use barrier protection right. For older men, for example, "the use of an external condom can be tough if he has challenges achieving a firm erection or if his erection waxes and wanes during sex," she explains.

This doesn't mean, however, that it can't be done. Nor does it mean people struggling with this issue must either consign themselves to a having a risky sex life or going back to shuffleboard. *Some tips...*

• **Hold on.** If you change position while wearing a condom during sex, either partner can reach down and keep the condom in place by holding the bottom of it (the part closest to the man's body). One slip and the protective quality of a condom goes down the drain.

• **Try an "innie."** An internal condom (aka a female condom) can be the perfect alternative to a conventional external (aka "male") one. Basically an elongated tube of pliable plastic, this disposable device has soft rings at either end. One ring is inserted into the vagina to hold that end of the condom in place. The other end stays outside the body. "It can look a little weird," says Dr. Davis, "and it takes a little practice, but it has some real advantages. The material it is made of transfers heat well, and that can feel better and more natural for both partners than an external condom," says Dr. Davis. It's fine to use an extra lubricant, but it's often not necessary. "The lubrication inside and outside of the internal condom helps with comfort," she explains. "It's pretty slippery." The female condom is more protective as well. "A conventional condom doesn't cover the base of the penis, which is where the herpes virus likes to hang out," explains Dr. Davis. "Not only does an internal condom solve that problem, it covers the entire labia, essentially providing a barrier against any other organisms as well."

• **Practice safe oral sex, too.** Pretty much any STD you can get on your genitals you also can get in your mouth, according to Dr. Davis. "Use an external condom if you're performing fellatio or an internal condom if you're performing cunnilingus," she advises.

***Another option:*** A "dam," which uses a square of material (similar to a female condom) designed for just this purpose. Says Dr. Davis, "They make flavored condoms and dams for a reason—to be used during oral sex."

• **Lube it or leave it.** With age, vulvar and vaginal tissue gets thinner and dryer so that, even during gentle sex, it can be more easily torn—basically opening the door for a sexually transmitted organism. A woman can increase her pleasure and decrease her risk for infection by using a lubricant. Dr. Davis advises using a silicone-based lube. "It stays viscous longer than water-based lube," she explains. If dryness is a significant problem, talk to your doctor. You may benefit from a topical estrogen cream or another product that moisturizes the tissues. (A condom is still essential for protection, of course.)

• **Tinker with toys.** Safety is only one part of the satisfying senior sex equation. Men and women of a certain age also just want to have fun. "In terms of pleasure," says Dr. Davis, "adult toys are a great idea." For both genders, the older the body the more time and direct stimulation is needed for both arousal and orgasm, she explains. So don't just play it safe—it's fine to just play, too. "Small bullet-style vibrators are great for targeted stimulation of the clitoris," she explains. "Palm-sized vibrators, about the size of a computer mouse, are easy to hold against the vulva, while longer vibrators or dildos (elongated, without vibrations) are good for internal play and keeping the vaginal muscles flexible. For penises, masturbation sleeves, vibrating or not, can be pleasurable—lubricant increases comfort and sensation."

• **Try a little tenderness.** "Consider other types of 'toys' as well," says Dr. Davis. "Brushing a partner's hair is very sensual—with zero STD risk." So is a partner massage. "Massage oil can also enhance sexual experiences," she added.

---

## Get Your Hair Back

Ivan S. Cohen, MD, associate clinical professor of dermatology at Yale University School of Medicine and director of the Center for Hair Transplantation in Fairfield, Connecticut. He is board-certified by the American Board of Dermatology and the American Board of Hair Restoration Surgery. DrICohen.com
Harvard Health Publications, Health.Harvard.edu

Men who lose their hair can still look great. But some are really bothered by it. And women, who are nearly as likely as men to experience some degree of age- and hormone-related hair loss, are more likely to suffer from feelings of unattractiveness.

If you're losing your hair and it bothers you, here's what you need to know about the latest treatments...

## Medications

• ***Minoxidil* topical (Rogaine).** This treatment is effective for men and women. Studies have shown that it is about 60% to 70% effective at stopping hair loss, stimulating growth and making hair thicker and longer. It works best when started soon after hair loss begins—it will not cause hair growth in areas that already are bald. It causes no serious side effects, although some people may have a little scalp irritation.

***How to use it:*** Minoxidil is sold over the counter as a liquid or foam. The newer foam version is less irritating and may be more effective. Men apply it twice a day and women once a day when hair and scalp are dry.

***What to expect:*** Most people notice improvement after about two months, with peak improvement after four to six months. You'll need to keep using it—if you stop, hair loss will resume.

***Cost:*** About $20 a month.

• ***Finasteride* (Propecia, Proscar).** Finasteride, an oral drug sold by prescription, works by blocking *dihydrotestosterone* (DHT), the androgen hormone that causes hair loss in men. It is not FDA-approved for women, and there is little reliable evidence it's effective, although some studies suggest that women who don't respond to minoxidil may benefit from the addition of the androgen receptor-blocking drug *spironolactone.* Rare side effects include diminished sex drive and weight gain. Women of reproductive age should not take these drugs. Men usually take 1-mg. tablet daily; women per their clinician's directions.

***What to expect:*** Growth may improve within a few months, but it can take up to a year to show the full benefit. You will need to continue the treatment—if you don't, hair loss will resume.

***Cost:*** $20 to $50 a month.

## Transplants

Today's hair transplants are much more sophisticated than the unsightly plugs from the past because hairs are transplanted exactly as they grow naturally, in follicular units (groupings of one to four hairs).

The outpatient procedures are minimally invasive and often can restore a full head of hair (unless you lose more hair in the future).

***How it works:*** The scalp is numbed. Follicular units are extracted from areas where there's still hair and then implanted where they're needed using one of three techniques (below). Because the "donor" hairs are impervious to androgens, they'll continue to grow indefinitely. It takes six to nine months before there's full improvement. Most patients with limited hair loss require only one procedure. Patients with more extensive baldness may need a second procedure. Most patients can return to work after a few days, using existing hair or a hat to cover up the surgical area.

Three types of surgical transplants...

• **Follicular unit transplantation (FUT).** This is an older method that's still commonly used. A narrow strip of hair is removed from the back of the scalp. Technicians separate the hair units, and the surgeon implants the units in an equivalent number of tiny slits in thinning areas. It might take 1,000 to 1,500 grafts to "fill" a bald area.

***Cost:*** About $5,000.

• **Follicular unit extraction (FUE).** Rather than taking a strip of donor hair, the surgeon uses a punchlike device to remove individual hair units, which are then implanted.

***Advantage:*** There is less postoperative discomfort and less chance of visible scarring in the donor area than with the FUT procedure described earlier. However, the results with FUE are less predictable, and the cost is 20% to 30% more.

• **Robotic follicular unit extraction.** This technique is the same as follicular unit extraction except that hairs are extracted robotically. A device using cameras and a computer precisely calculates cutting angles and can remove hairs without damaging the roots. It's more accurate than manual FUE, and the operating time is shorter. The downside is that it costs more.

***Cost:*** About $8,000.

### Platelet-Rich Plasma

This new treatment isn't yet FDA-approved for hair loss. But it is effective in more than half of patients and is a good choice for those who don't want to take a drug or submit to surgery.

***How it works:*** A tube of blood is drawn from the patient. Platelets are separated out, processed and then injected into the scalp. The concentrated platelets contain growth factors that stimulate hair follicles and thicken hair.

Patients are treated again at three months...six months...and once a year thereafter. When the procedure works, improvement becomes visible within a few months. It can be a stand-alone treatment or used in conjunction with other treatments. The only side effect may be some mild swelling of the forehead lasting one to two days.

***Cost:*** About $1,000 to $1,200 per treatment.

### Laser Therapy

This is a safe, nondrug and nonsurgical treatment that has been cleared by the FDA. In my experience, it's less effective than minoxidil, finasteride or platelet-rich plasma, but it helps in some cases. Studies reported a 37% increase in hair count in women after four months of treatment (and a 35% increase in men).

***How it works:*** The scalp is exposed to low-level laser light. This can be done in a doctor's office or by wearing a cap (or using a comb) with light-emitting diodes. The light increases blood flow and the release of nutrients and other stimulating factors. There is no discomfort or skin damage. People typically use the devices for 10 to 15 minutes, three times a week.

---

## Hair Products Linked to Hair Loss

Tina Sigurdson, assistant general counsel for the Environmental Working Group (EWG), a nonprofit environmental health research and advocacy organization. EWG maintains a database called Skin Deep, which offers health and safety ratings for thousands of personal-care products. EWG.org/skindeep

---

More than 21,000 consumers have lodged complaints about WEN Cleansing Conditioners, a line of hair-care products heavily advertised on television. Many of the complaints cite significant problems such as hair loss and serious skin irritation. But despite this flood of complaints...an alert issued by the Food and Drug Administration (FDA)...and at least one class-action lawsuit, the products remain on the market. It's not clear which ingredients in the WEN conditioners may be causing the problems—which contributes to the FDA's inability to address the issue more strongly.

Hair-care and other personal-care products including cosmetics, toothpaste, mouthwash, baby wipes, baby powder, shaving cream and body wash are virtually unregulated by the government. The FDA has no authority to recall these items, and manufacturers are not required to confirm that the products are safe to use. Legislation that would increase FDA oversight of personal-care products is being considered by the Senate. But any changes are unlikely to take effect for many months.

***What to do:*** Never assume that a product is safe because its packaging or advertising features words such as "Natural," "Healthy" or "Gentle." The use of these words is unregulated when it comes to personal-care products, so they often mean little or nothing.

***Example:*** The makers of WEN Cleansing Conditioners have used the word "Natural" in their marketing materials even though these products contain synthetic chemicals—including at least one known to cause allergic reactions.

# Beware Tight Hairstyles

Tight hairstyles that pull on the scalp, such as braids and knots, can lead to traction alopecia, the most common form of hair loss among African-American women.

*Journal of the American Academy of Dermatology.*

# Hair Dye and Psoriasis

Melissa Kanchanapoomi Levin, MD, dermatologist and director of clinical research, Marmur Medical, New York City.

If you've developed psoriasis on your scalp, you can still dye your hair. *But you need to take some precautions...*

- **Avoid hair dyes during a flare-up,** when scaly patches are painful and inflamed. Since chemicals in the dying process can make it worse, it is advised to wait until the inflammation has subsided to color your hair.

- **Carefully choose your hair dye.** The most common chemical that can cause irritation or allergic reactions is paraphenylenediamine (PPD). Other chemicals that can irritate the scalp are peroxide and bleaches. And dyes labeled "natural" or "organic" do not always mean that they are safe. Some of these products can be high in alcohol and should be avoided, since alcohol can dry the skin and worsen scalp psoriasis.

***What to do:*** Put a small amount of dye on your scalp first and check for a reaction within two days. Minimize skin contact with the dye by applying a protective coat of petroleum jelly to your forehead, neck and ears before dying your hair.

# Why Acne Can Strike Women After the Teen Years

Debra Jaliman, MD, assistant professor, dermatology, Icahn School of Medicine at Mount Sinai, New York City.

Bethanee Schlosser, MD, PhD, associate professor, dermatology, Northwestern University Feinberg School of Medicine, Chicago.

*Journal of the American Academy of Dermatology.*

Why does acne still plague some women into adulthood? A recent study offers some hints.

Researchers from Italy who looked at 500 women uncovered some factors related to the risk of acne after the age of 25—including a low intake of fruits and vegetables, high stress levels and a family history of adult acne.

The findings do not prove that those things cause acne in some women, but it's plausible that they are involved, dermatologists said.

"We see that people who have a diet of junk food tend to break out more," said Debra Jaliman, MD, an assistant professor of dermatology at the Icahn School of Medicine at Mount Sinai in New York City.

Specifically, Dr. Jaliman said, research has implicated foods with a high "glycemic index"—which cause blood sugar to surge. Some high-GI foods include white bread and rice, chips and crackers, and sugary baked goods.

Similarly, Dr. Jaliman said, chronic stress takes a toll on overall health, and that could show up on the skin.

## Background

Over 80% of teenagers have bouts of acne. The good news is, most see their skin clear up after age 20, according to a team led by Luigi Naldi, MD, of the Study Center of the Italian Group for Epidemiologic Research in Dermatology in Bergamo, Italy.

Still, anywhere from 20% to 40% of adults continue to have breakouts, the researchers added.

"Women tend to get adult acne more often than men," Dr. Jaliman said. "It's often due to changes in hormone levels and or hormonal imbalances."

Women may get acne before their menstrual period, for example, or when they start or stop birth control pills, Dr. Jaliman said.

But it's not completely clear why some women continue to have acne, while others don't.

## Study Details

To look into the question, Dr. Naldi's team surveyed women seen at dermatology clinics in 12 Italian cities. Overall, 248 were diagnosed with acne and 270 were diagnosed with other conditions to serve as the control group.

The researchers found that certain lifestyle factors were tied to the risk of an acne diagnosis.

Women who ate fruits and vegetables, or fresh fish, on fewer than four days out of the week were more than twice as likely to have acne, compared with women who ate those foods more often.

The findings were published in the *Journal of the American Academy of Dermatology*.

## Expert Commentary

It's not clear, though, whether fruits and veggies specifically ward off acne, according to another dermatologist who reviewed the study.

Women with diets low in those healthful foods may eat a lot of high-GI fare—which could be the culprit, explained Bethanee Schlosser, MD, PhD, an associate professor of dermatology at Northwestern University Feinberg School of Medicine in Chicago.

She also noted that the study found no connection between dairy intake and acne, which conflicts with the researchers' own previous work.

It's possible, Dr. Schlosser said, that the diet factors tied to acne might be different for different age groups.

### Natural Relief for Constipation

Eating three dried figs a day can relieve chronic constipation, according to a recent eight-week clinical trial.

*Asian Journal of Clinical Nutrition.*

## Stress, Hair, Heredity and Hormones

Along with diet, women's stress levels were linked to acne risk. Those who reported "high" or "very high" stress levels had a threefold greater risk of acne, compared with women who were less stressed.

Acne risk was also higher among women whose parents or siblings had adult acne. The same was true of women who'd never been pregnant or had hirsutism—male-pattern hair growth on the face or body.

According to Dr. Jaliman, those latter findings may reflect the effects of polycystic ovary syndrome (PCOS)—a hormonal disorder that causes fertility problems, hirsutism and acne.

In fact, Dr. Schlosser pointed out, the study included women with a diagnosis of PCOS or other disorders that boost testosterone levels. And that limits the potential to extend the findings to the "general population of women" without hormonal disorders, she said.

## Recommendations

But even though this study does not prove fish, fruit or stress reduction will clear a woman's acne, it's always wise to be mindful of diet and lifestyle, Dr. Jaliman noted.

"I recommend doing something that you find relaxing for yourself daily," she said, pointing to meditation as an example.

Dr. Jaliman also advised eating plenty of fruits, vegetables and fish—which are clearly good for overall health.

The American Academy of Dermatology website has more information on adult acne at AAD.org. Search "adult acne."

## A Natural New Treatment for Polycystic Ovary Syndrome (PCOS)

Andrew L. Rubman, ND, founder and medical director, Southbury Clinic for Traditional Medicines, Southbury, Connecticut. SouthburyClinic.com

Study titled "Effects of resveratrol on polycystic ovary syndrome: a double-blind, randomized, placebo-controlled trial" by Antoni Duleba, MD, and colleagues at University of California-San Diego and Poznan University of Medical Sciences, Poland, published in *Journal of Clinical Endocrinology and Metabolism.*

Women with polycystic ovary syndrome (PCOS) may now have a new and better therapy for their condition. Resveratrol, an anti-inflammatory compound found in grapes (and wine), berries and nuts, is the first natural compound that has been shown in a clinical study of PCOS to reduce the higher-than-normal levels of testosterone that are the hallmark characteristic of this very common but hard-to-treat endocrine disorder that affects one out of 10 American women of childbearing age. (Although we think of testosterone as a man's hormone, women also need it but in much smaller quantities.)

If you have PCOS or know someone who does, you'll want to keep reading...

### Current Treatments Increase the Risk for Clots

Symptoms of PCOS, such as irregular and painful periods, excess facial and body hair and weight gain, are distressing enough on their own. For women who want to have children in the future, the effects are particularly disturbing—the increased testosterone levels may interfere with normal ovulation and thus reduce the ability to become pregnant. There are serious long-term health concerns, too. Women with PCOS are at higher risk for diabetes, stroke and heart disease.

While PCOS is a chronic condition that is not well-understood and can't be cured, symptoms can be somewhat managed with birth control pills, which can help reduce testosterone levels, and the drug *metformin*, which can improve insulin sensitivity (reducing associated diabetes risk).

Oral contraceptives, though, come with an increased risk for blood clots—exactly what women with PCOS don't need because they already face a 50% higher risk for blood clots than women without PCOS. Indeed, women with PCOS who take oral contraceptives are twice as likely to develop blood clots compared with women who don't take the pills.

It's clear that there is a pressing need for a safer treatment method. Resveratrol could be it.

### Resveratrol: From Bench to Bedside

First, a little background: Researchers at Poznan University of Medical Sciences in Poland and University of California-San Diego had already determined that exposing certain ovarian cells that produce testosterone to resveratrol reduces the cells' ability to produce the hormone—without affecting production of progesterone, an important hormone needed to keep the uterine lining healthy. But that was a test-tube study using cells from rats.

For the recent study, the first ever clinical trial of its kind, the researchers randomly assigned 34 women with PCOS to receive either resveratrol or placebo pills for three months. At the start and end of the study, all of the women had tests to measure body mass index, insulin resistance, levels of various hormones and cholesterol. Because some of these values change naturally throughout the month, testing was done at the same time for each woman's cycle.

***Results:*** After three months, the resveratrol group showed a 23% reduction in testosterone levels...a 22% reduction in a marker for DHEA, the precursor compound for both testosterone and estrogen...and a 66% increase in insulin sensitivity (a good thing) from their baseline levels. The women in the placebo group did not see any improvements in these measurements. Cholesterol levels stayed level in the test group but rose for those taking placebos.

***Even better:*** The drop in testosterone was greater than the decline seen after three months of treatment with birth control or with metformin.

## A Promising Approach

To better understand the research, we spoke with Andrew L. Rubman, ND, a naturopathic physician and medical director of Southbury Clinic for Traditional Medicines, in Southbury, Connecticut. He found the study promising—with caveats. "For women with PCOS whose symptoms are being treated conventionally with hormones and/or metformin, resveratrol may be a better alternative—in the short term," said Dr. Rubman. Why the caveat? It's a small study, for one, and the first of its kind to study resveratrol's effects on PCOS. It's also a short-term study, so it doesn't address whether taking resveratrol long-term might affect estrogen production, which could happen from the decrease in DHEA. Nor do we know whether there are long-term effects on adrenal steroids, such as cortisol, which are closely linked to sexual steroids, adds Dr. Rubman.

With those caveats, he certainly thinks resveratrol is a supplement women with PCOS should discuss with their health-care providers, who can monitor hormonal and metabolic responses over time. It can be part of a complementary medicine approach to PCOS, which involves diet, exercise and weight loss as well as other supplements—including cinnamon, flaxseed, spearmint tea, B multivitamins and glucomannan, a fiber supplement that helps with appetite and blood sugar control. (While these are each beneficial in different ways for women with PCOS, none of them directly affects testosterone levels, as resveratrol does.) Stress control makes a difference, and acupuncture may also help.

Dr. Rubman pointed out that although PCOS is a chronic condition, symptoms may not always be bothersome, so women may be able to wean themselves off treatment. "Women with PCOS may not need treatment all the time, and the dose of resveratrol can potentially be reduced over time," he explained. "The most important time to take resveratrol is a few days before, and during, ovulation, when follicle-stimulating hormone (FSH) surges," says Dr. Rubman. "It is regarded as beneficial throughout the cycle as well."

## If You Decide to Try Resveratrol

The dosage of resveratrol used in the study was 1,500 milligrams (mg) per day, about three times the normal dose in an over-the-counter preparation. Although 1,500 mg is a potent dose, most women should be just fine taking it, said Dr. Rubman, although some may notice bowel irritability, which should go away in a few days.

For women who want to give resveratrol a try, Dr. Rubman recommends Nutrigenomic Super Berry POWder manufactured by Eclectic Institute. Its resveratrol is derived directly from berries rather than synthesized, and the supplement contains other healthful compounds as well. (*Note*: While berries are very healthful, you can't eat enough to get anywhere near the dose of resveratrol studied.)

***Bonus:*** Resveratrol may also help protect against osteoporosis.

---

# Limit Caffeine Before Conception

Caffeine consumption before conception can increase risk for miscarriage. Miscarriage risk rises when either the woman or the man consumes more than two caffeinated drinks a day (one drink of coffee is eight ounces) in the weeks leading up to conception. To be on the safe side, both people may want to limit caffeine when the woman is trying to become pregnant. And women should talk with their doctors about taking a daily multivitamin before conception and through early pregnancy—this also reduces miscarriage risk.

Analysis of data on 344 pregnancies, 28% of which ended in miscarriage, by researchers at US National Institute of Child Health and Human Development, Bethesda, Maryland, published in *Fertility and Sterility.*

# Less-Invasive Fibroid Treatment May Be "Under-Used"

Prasoon Mohan, MD, assistant professor, interventional radiology, University of Miami Miller School of Medicine.

Anne Hardart, MD, assistant professor, obstetrics, gynecology and reproductive science, Icahn School of Medicine at Mount Sinai, New York City.

Society of Interventional Radiology, annual meeting, Washington, DC.

A minimally invasive procedure for uterine fibroids may be "under-used" in US hospitals, compared with surgery, a recent study suggests.

The study looked at a national sample of hospitals and found that fewer fibroid patients are undergoing hysterectomy—surgical removal of the uterus.

But hysterectomy remains much more common compared with a less-invasive procedure called embolization.

## About Fibroids

Fibroids are non-cancerous growths in the wall of the uterus that are usually harmless. But when they cause problems—such as persistent pain and heavy menstrual bleeding—treatment may be necessary.

According to the US National Institutes of Health, up to 80% of women develop fibroids—most often in their 40s and early 50s. Usually, fibroids cause no symptoms. But some women develop pelvic or low back pain, heavy menstrual bleeding or frequent urination.

Short of surgery, women can use pain relievers or hormonal drugs to help shrink the fibroids.

For women with severe symptoms, the go-to has traditionally been hysterectomy, or sometimes surgery to remove the fibroids only. Another less-extensive procedure is endometrial ablation—where the lining of the uterus is removed.

## About Embolization

There are other options, though. One is embolization, which involves injecting tiny particles into the small uterine arteries supplying the fibroids. The particles block the fibroids' supply of nutrients and cause them to shrink.

Embolization has been a widely accepted treatment for 10 to 15 years, said Prasoon Mohan, MD, lead researcher on the recent study.

Yet, his team found, it still lags far behind hysterectomy. From 2012 through 2013, hysterectomies were performed 65 times more often than embolization at US hospitals.

When embolization was done, it was usually at a large medical center. Few women treated at smaller or rural hospitals had the procedure, the study found.

That points to a discrepancy in women's access to the treatment, said Dr. Mohan, an assistant professor of interventional radiology at the University of Miami.

How often "should" embolization be done? There's no way to define that, but Dr. Mohan said it seems clear that it's not offered often enough.

"I think it's definitely under-used, considering it's minimally invasive, has a shorter hospital stay and is less expensive," he said.

## The Study

On average, Dr. Mohan's team found, total hospital charges for embolization were about $21,600, versus $33,100 for hysterectomy.

"Every patient should be told about all of her options, so she can make an informed decision," he suggested.

For the study, Dr. Mohan's team used a national database on US hospital stays. Between 2007 and 2013, the annual number of women undergoing a hysterectomy for fibroids dropped by more than half: from more than 168,000, to just under 78,200.

Still, the surgery remained far more common than embolization. For the years 2012 and 2013, there were fewer than 2,500 embolization procedures for fibroids, the researchers found.

Dr. Mohan presented the findings at the Society of Interventional Radiology's annual meeting, in Washington, DC.

## Expert Reaction

Anne Hardart, MD, is an assistant professor of obstetrics, gynecology and reproductive science at Mount Sinai's Icahn School of Medicine, in New York City.

Dr. Hardart agreed that embolization is an "important minimally invasive option for some women with symptomatic fibroids."

But not all women are good candidates for embolization, said Dr. Hardart, who wasn't involved in the study.

"The size, number and location of fibroids can all affect how well (embolization) works," she explained.

Plus, Dr. Hardart said, the findings from smaller and rural hospitals highlight another issue. Those centers may simply lack the resources for the procedure.

Overall, Dr. Mohan's team found, only 0.4% of all embolization procedures were done at rural hospitals, while 8% were performed at "small hospital systems."

"Embolization requires specialized equipment and interventional radiologists to perform it," Dr. Hardart said. "And most of these specialists are located in more-populated areas where their services can be accessed by a larger number of patients."

## Conclusions

Dr. Mohan agreed that embolization is not for everyone. For example, if a woman wants to become pregnant after treatment, surgical removal of the fibroids is a better choice, he noted.

What's important, Dr. Mohan said, is that women know the benefits and risks of all their options.

He added that one longer-term risk from embolization is "ovarian failure" and earlier menopause, because the procedure may also disrupt the ovaries' blood supply.

The best choice for any one woman depends on her personal situation and preferences, Dr. Mohan said.

The U.S. Office on Women's Health has more on uterine fibroids at womenshealth.gov. Search "uterine fibroids."

# Lyrica Linked to Birth Defects

The drug Lyrica is prescribed for epilepsy, fibromyalgia, anxiety and other health problems.

***Recent finding:*** Women taking Lyrica (*pregabalin*) were as much as six times more likely to have a baby with a major defect in the central nervous system than women not taking the drug.

Study of 164 women who took Lyrica during their first trimester, compared with 656 pregnant women who did not take the drug, by researchers at Lausanne University Hospital, Switzerland, published in *Neurology*.

# Pregnancy Complication Linked to Eye Problems

Women who have preeclampsia during pregnancy have 1.6 times higher risk for retinal detachment and nearly twice the risk for other retinal diseases versus women who do not develop preeclampsia.

Study of more than one million women by researchers at University of Montreal Hospital Research Center, Quebec, Canada, published in *Obstetrics & Gynecology*.

## Question Ovary Removal

Removal of normal ovaries does more harm than good in women who are not at high risk for ovarian or breast cancer. The procedure, called prophylactic oophorectomy, is commonly done during hysterectomy to reduce the risk for cancer.

***But:*** Ovary removal raises the risk for colorectal cancer by 30%, possibly because oophorectomy decreases a woman's levels of estrogen and androgens. Oophorectomy also raises the risk for cardiovascular disease and osteoporosis and can result in impaired sexual health.

Josefin Segelman, MD, PhD, senior consultant colorectal surgeon, department of molecular medicine and surgery, Karolinska Institute, Stockholm, Sweden.

## Help for Itchy Breast Rash

Intertrigo is a common skin condition called intertrigo, an inflammation that develops in skin folds and can turn into a fungal or bacterial infection. Women are susceptible to intertrigo if their breasts sag and the lower part of the breast rests on the skin just below.

Intertrigo often becomes a fungal yeast infection, especially in large-breasted women who sweat a lot. This rash is caused by the yeast Candida, the same yeast that is responsible for vaginal infections. Prescription nystatin cream applied very lightly (so lightly that you can't see the cream after applying it) four times a day will often clear this up in less than a week.

Use over-the-counter Zeasorb powder to keep the area dry, and wear a bra that wicks moisture away, such as an all-cotton bra or a quick-drying sports bra.

Neal Schultz, MD, a dermatologist in New York City. NealSchultzMD.com

## Fix for Smelly Feet

Holistic treatment for smelly feet: Black tea. Soak bad-smelling feet in strongly brewed, cooled black tea for 30 minutes daily for seven to 10 days...then once a week for maintenance. The tannic acid in the tea dries out the sweat glands responsible for foot odor in many people.

Jane E. Andersen, DPM, doctor of podiatric medicine, Chapel Hill, North Carolina, and spokesperson for the American Podiatric Medical Association, quoted in *The Wall Street Journal*.

## Stop Toenail Fungus Spread

Toenail fungus (onychomycosis) is not highly contagious, but spores can live in warm, moist areas such as shower stalls. Help protect your family by spraying this area with a cleaning product that contains bleach every day. Also, wear flip-flops around public pools or showers. Wear socks to bed to help protect your spouse or yourself, and the family should not share towels, nail clippers or other items with the family member who is infected.

Fungal infection on toenails is difficult to eradicate. Two laser treatments (they may not be covered by insurance) given three months apart plus a topical medication, such as Formula 3, produce the best results for my patients.

I also recommend the SteriShoe, a product that uses ultraviolet light to eliminate fungi and germs from shoes ($150 at SteriShoe.com)...or antimicrobial shoe sprays such as Clean Sweep or Gehwol Foot & Shoe Deodorant (about $30 each).

Johanna Youner, DPM, podiatric surgeon, New York City. HealthyFeetNY.net

# INDEX

## D

## E



## F



## G

## N



## O



## P



## Q

## R



## S



## T